Chiropractic Peripheral Joint Technique

Chiropractic Peripheral Joint Technique

Raymond T. Broome DC FCC

Former Clinic Director and Lecturer
Anglo-European College of Chiropractic
Bournemouth, England

Post-graduate Lecturer
Institut Français de Chiropractie
Paris, France

Post-graduate Lecturer, Nordisk Institut for Kiropraktik og Biomekanik
Odense, Denmark

Private Practitioner, Oxford, England

With contributions from

Christopher J. Good DC MA(Ed)
Daniel J. Proctor BSc, DC(Hons) FCCS(C)
Peter McCarthy PhD
Susan C. Hill DC, DACNB
Daniel P. Lane BSc(Chiro) DC

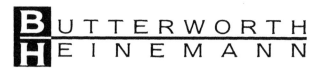

EDINBURGH LONDON NEW YORK OXFORD PHILADELPHIA ST LOUIS SYDNEY TORONTO 2000

BUTTERWORTH-HEINEMANN
An imprint of Elsevier Limited

First published 2000
   Reprinted 2003, 2004

ISBN 0 7506 3289 5

British Library Cataloguing in Publication Data
A catalogue record for this book is available from the British Library

Library of Congress Cataloging in Publication Data
A catalog record for this book is available from the Library of Congress

Notice
Medical knowledge is constantly changing. Standard safety precautions
must be followed, but as new research and clinical experience broaden
our knowledge, changes in treatment and drug therapy may become
necessary or appropriate. Readers are advised to check the most current
product information provided by the manufacturer of each drug to be
administered to verify the recommended dose, the method and duration
of administration, and contraindications. It is the responsibility of the
practitioner, relying on experience and knowledge of the patient, to
determine dosages and the best treatment for each individual patient.
Neither the Publisher nor the editors/contributor assumes any liability
for any injury and/or damage to persons or property arising from this
publication.

The Publisher

 your source for books,
journals and multimedia
in the health sciences
www.elsevierhealth.com

Composition by Scribe Design, Gillingham, Kent
Transferred to digital printing 2006
Printed and bound by CPI Antony Rowe, Eastbourne

To Anne, Ute, Alex and Chris

Contents

Contributing authors

Christopher J. Good DC MA(Ed) CCSP
Associate Professor, New York Chiropractic College; Private practitioner, Romulus, New York, USA

Daniel J. Proctor BSc DC(Hons) FCCS(C)
Assistant Professor, Canadian Memorial Chiropractic College, Toronto; Post-graduate faculty member, Canadian Memorial Chiropractic College, Toronto; Private practitioner, Toronto, Canada

Peter McCarthy PhD
Senior Lecturer, School of Applied Sciences, University of Glamorgan, Pontypridd, Wales

Susan C. Hill DC DACNB
External Lecturer, Anglo-European College of Chiropractic, Bournemouth, England; Co-ordinator, Wessex Faculty, British College of Chiropractors; Private practitioner, Dorchester, England

Daniel P. Lane BSc(Chiro) DC
Chairman, Oxfordshire Faculty of the British College of Chiropractors; Co-ordinator, BCA Vocational Training Scheme, UK

Foreword

The manipulation of the extremity joints is a skill which every undergraduate chiropractor learns, but one which can easily fade thereafter, given the dominance of spinal complaints in practice. This can put practitioners at risk of a gradual loss of expertise in peripheral joint techniques throughout their practising lives.

Raymond Broome is a master chiropractic technician of international standing who has for years been in constant receipt of requests to give courses on peripheral joint techniques. In this volume, however, his students will find much more. Here is a comprehensive range of procedures, in numbers which could never be absorbed in an instructional course. These are carefully catalogued, systematically explained and well illustrated so that readers with a basic chiropractic background will find themselves able to transpose each explanation into a skill. However, this book contains many more techniques than would normally be covered in an undergraduate curriculum; each of them built on the concept of direction of motion restriction in individual joints. Part Two of the work is, in effect, a manual of techniques, many of which relate to the 'joint play' and 'fixation' schools of Mennell and Gillet. The foundations of these and other basic premises upon which the techniques are built are set out and reinforced throughout the work. A number of the procedures, notably the 'short lever' ones, are of the author's own invention, but even the more traditional technique 'setups' carry his unmistakable stamp.

This book is timely in a further respect. As Broome's co-authors reveal in Part One, the integrated function of the neuromusculoskeletal system is becoming much better understood, widening the options in chiropractic rehabilitation. However, many rehabilitation strategies require a comprehensive repertoire of manual techniques to accompany them. The book therefore makes an important contribution to the rehabilitation of the spine, especially through its chapters on the shoulder and lower limb complexes.

I would also commend this work to non-chiropractic students, that is, to those who wish to understand some of the 'nuts and bolts' of chiropractic, but approach from a different background. The information they will find here, while definitely not superficial, will provide a feel for the technical discipline of chiropractic which does not deny any of the other aspects of patient care in which a practitioner must be proficient. They will find the index and glossary especially helpful.

In *Chiropractic Peripheral Joint Technique*, students of chiropractic, whatever their current experience of the topic, will find a reference work of enduring value. Although future developments in the understanding of management and underlying mechanisms may eventually merit revisions, the procedures themselves are timeless. In the following pages, the reader will find a unique mixture of flair and rigour which reflects the personality and expertise of the author himself. This book combines scholarship and skill in a volume which will sit proudly in any chiropractic library.

Alan Breen DC PhD
Research Director
Anglo-European College of Chiropractic

Preface

This book has been written with the intent to meet a longstanding need in the chiropractic profession. The primary purpose is to provide a comprehensive volume of practical, clinically well-tried adjustive methods for the peripheral joints, reflecting the rich diversity of mainstream peripheral joint techniques available to the modern chiropractor, together with methods of evaluating accessory joint motion for the application of those techniques, the neurological implications of peripheral joint problems and the role of exercises as a supportive therapy.

It was not the intention to produce an exhaustive manual of every known peripheral joint technique. Indeed, many more techniques were considered only to be discarded later on the grounds of poor mechanical efficiency, impracticality, or when they were found to be merely minor variants of major methods already included. Bryner (1989) in a survey of indications for manipulation of the knee alone, in which 247 techniques were researched from 27 sources, also found considerable duplication.

Wherever possible, however, several alternative manoeuvres for the more common joint problems are included, for several reasons. It is essential to provide alternative techniques to cater for the variation of anatomical structures and sizes of patients. The diminutive practitioner faced with treating large patients or vice versa produces very different technique demands. Patients with degenerative joint disease or who have other special requirements due to frailty also require a versatility of technique approach. Apart from this, it is necessary to cater for practitioner preference and also variable skill levels.

The book is divided into two parts. In Part One, the first chapter gives an overview of the relevance of peripheral joint technique in everyday practice. The second chapter discusses the major technique types utilized in the technique section of the book, their clinical advantages, disadvantages and methods of delivery. The third chapter describes the peripheral joint kinematics, followed by a chapter on passive osteokinematic motion palpation of the peripheral joints which outlines the necessity for the practitioner to have the fullest understanding of joint mechanics. The fifth chapter discusses the neurological significance of biomechanical problems of the peripheral joints and the effects of chiropractic treatment when applied to them. The final chapter in Part One gives an outline for the rationale, the role of exercises and the types of exercises used in therapy and rehabilitation in clinical practice to enhance the chiropractic treatment of the peripheral joints.

Part Two of the book contains two chapters. The first section deals with the evaluation of the five major biomechanical problems and methods of correction of the temporomandibular joint (TMJ). Although the TMJ is a joint of the axial skeleton, this chapter has been included because of the neurological significance of the joint.

The second chapter has two major sections dealing with the mobility evaluation and adjustments for the joints of the appendicular skeleton. For each joint, there is a description of how to evaluate the joint play (Mennell, 1964) motion status, followed by techniques to apply to those findings. The author concurs with the statement made by DuBarry (1996) that 'There is no standardization for describing technique in the chiropractic literature'. An attempt has been made to keep as close as possible to the DuBarry codification proposal and each technique description follows the same outline – of the direction of joint play loss, the patient's position, the chiropractor's stance, the contact and the procedure for carrying out the adjustment.

It was not intended that this manual should be all-inclusive for the differential diagnosis and case management of peripheral joint problems, which would include the taking of a case history, physical examination, laboratory testing and imaging, each of which would fill a book themselves. The use of soft tissue diagnosis and therapy are also omitted, and for these the reader is referred to other excellent available texts.

It is hoped that the text will do what it is intended to do, which is to provide the student and practitioner alike with a clear, easy to use guide and manual for the manipulative methods of peripheral joint technique.

BIBLIOGRAPHY

Bryner, P. (1989) *A Survey of Indications: Knee Manipulation. Chiropractic Technique.* Baltimore, MD, Williams & Wilkins.

DuBarry, E. (1996) Classifications for adjusting procedures. DC, vol. 14, no. 2.

Hammer, W. (1991) *Functional Soft Tissue Examination and Treatment by Manual Methods.* Gaithersburg, MD, Aspen Publishers.

Hoppenfeld, S. (1976) *Physical Examination of the Spine and Extremities.* New York, Appleton–Century–Crofts.

Mennell, J. McM. (1964) *Joint Pain.* Boston, MA, Little Brown & Company.

Plaugher, G. (1993) *Textbook of Clinical Chiropractic. A Specific Biomechanical Approach.* Baltimore, MD, Williams & Wilkins.

Acknowledgements

In a book entitled *Truth to Tell*, David Pawson wrote 'No book is the work of one person'. No statement could be more accurate than when applied to a text such as this. Quite apart from the chapters by the contributing authors, its very nature is composite. It has been drawn from decades of published and unpublished works, from personal contacts and communications with colleagues and from various lectures attended. Personal innovations are also included, gleaned from and honed by the varied demands of clinical practice derived from more than 30 years in the field.

Wherever possible, credit has been duly given to all known authors and developers of techniques. However, many techniques have been in common chiropractic usage for a very long time, appearing in a number of different texts, often with only slight variations. This gives rise to the thought that, where chiropractic techniques are concerned, there may well be something to the saying that 'There is nothing new under the sun'. All sources used have been acknowledged and I am indebted to those colleagues who first pioneered and then disseminated their knowledge to the profession through the years, enabling others to learn and use their techniques to benefit suffering patients.

I have been most fortunate in enlisting the help of my contributing authors in the preparation of this book, each one being an acknowledged expert in their field. All have willingly and unstintingly given of their time and skills for the benefit both of this text and ultimately for their profession. These chapters are included to help increase the knowledge of the relevance of peripheral and extra-vertebral joint problems and the role they play in neuro-musculoskeletal diagnosis. In addition, they are also included to help increase the practical expertise of students and practitioners alike, in the correction of peripheral joints in both everyday practice and in the more specialized applications such as the treatment of sports injuries.

I wish to record my thanks to a host of people, colleagues, patients, family and friends, for their encouragement to write this book.

My thanks go to David O'Neill, Librarian at the Anglo-European College of Chiropractic, and his staff for the retrieval of records.

Special thanks go to David Antrobus of Atlas Clinical Ltd. for more than one reason. First for his generosity in lending me the excellent, versatile variable height treatment table used in the photographs of the techniques, and also for devoting his time to giving invaluable advice on camera angles.

For the photographs of the techniques, Paul Godfrey's renowned camera expertise has enhanced the book, providing it with the essential visual impact. My grateful thanks go to him, and also to Jeanette Pihl for acting as the model for the techniques.

My thanks go also to the audio-visual department of the New York Chiropractic College for the excellent photographs for the chapters written by Christopher Good.

My grateful thanks go especially to my wife, Anne, for many reasons, amongst which are her unfailing patience and good humour during the many hours of preparation, for encouraging me not only to write this book, but also to take time out of a busy practice in order to do so! My thanks also for the countless hours she has spent typing and correcting the manuscripts. It is a certainty that without her assistance this book would not have been written.

Last but not least, I thank my editors, Mary Seager, Hannah Tudge, Claire Hutchins and all the team at Butterworth–Heinemann, for their guidance and thoughtful comments. Without them, none of this would have been possible.

Part
1

Biomechanics

The relevance of peripheral joints in clinical practice: an overview

Raymond T. Broome

Since the early days of chiropractic its practitioners have treated the extraspinal joints. D.D. Palmer (1910) recorded his treatment of toes not long after his discovery. Since then, a multiplicity of different adjustive procedures to treat the peripheral joints have been advanced and developed by the practitioners of its art.

What is the rationale for treating peripheral joints? Amongst the reasons advanced by Laedermann (1984) which may encompass the major grounds, are the treatment of local biomechanical problems, reflex triggered functional syndromes, a time prescription, psychological reasons and a placebo effect. The first three reasons imply an active participation by the chiropractor but the last three could signify an active or passive role by the chiropractor. Let us consider each of these reasons in turn.

THE PSYCHOLOGICAL REALM

The caring attitude of the practitioner, the placebo effect of examination by a therapist, followed by the application of skilful treatment are inextricably woven together. The actual amount of psychological benefit to the patient, however, remains difficult to quantify, but it is accepted as extremely important in the patient's recovery. Laedermann (1984) relates the widely held importance of looking at, and of course touching, not just what may be a vertebral level of cause but also the extremity where the symptom may be felt. He rightly poses the rhetorical question 'How often is a patient heard complaining that their former practitioner focused their examination only on the spine for the cause of their problem or for that matter, remained at their desk reaching for the prescription pad and did not even look at the area in the extremity where the patient's symptoms were experienced?'

LOCAL BIOMECHANICAL PROBLEMS

These are the easiest to identify since it is mostly pain, swelling, paraesthesia and sometimes a combination of pain and fear which prompts patients to seek our assistance. These local biomechanical problems include plantar fasciitis (Ambrosius and Kondracki, 1992), sprains, strains, joint insufficiency as in foot pronation, and athletic injuries.

TIME PRESCRIPTION

What Laedermann meant by a 'time prescription' is the increased quality of life afforded to a patient when they are treated palliatively or more especially for self-limiting conditions such as a shoulder capsulitis, to ease them through a trying time.

REFLEX TRIGGERED FUNCTIONAL SYNDROMES

As a result of local dysfunction, a series of structural and/or neurological events may follow. Janse (1976) noted that faulty body mechanics are usually a consequence of a serial distortion rather than a single lesion. Both Hoppenfeld (1976) and Bergmann, Peterson and Lawrence (1993) give similar illustrations showing that disturbance in one part of the kinetic chain can affect another part in either direction, proximally or distally. This can be due to a variety of causes: mechanical deficiency such as a leg discrepancy (Jones, 1953; Beech, 1965) and mechanical or muscular insufficiency leading to foot pronation or valgus knee (Kenel, 1965).

Gillet (1964) ventured his hypothesis that fixations in the lowest part of the kinetic chain, the foot, can cause reflex fixations in the spine and its appendages. Phenomena also commonly observed during examination of patients are the hypotonic states of various muscles attached to the trunk which respond with a significant positive effect when manual treatment to the foot is applied (Greenwalt, 1981) (Blennerhasset, 1997; Walther, 1981). There are very few scientific studies to determine the efficacy of these phenomena but sufficient important features are there to the observer/clinician to maintain the value of their identification.

It is significant that Curchod (1971) traced an incidence as high as 4–5% where the foot was the direct cause of sciatic pain. No wonder then that Gillet (1964) recorded that, as a matter of routine when treating a typical 'chronic spine' (with or without radiating pain) after several visits and successfully clearing the vertebral fixations, he examined the foot and corrected any fixations there.

Gillet (1964) also recorded a case of chronic sacro-iliac 'slip' of 2 years' duration which recurred repeatedly in spite of frequent local treatment. After correction of the tarsal fixations, the sacro-iliac joint was found to be spontaneously corrected.

Although these latter examples are subjective and anecdotal, there are many chiropractic clinicians who have observed similar evidence-based phenomena and would corroborate them as being commonplace (Lening, 1991). The examination and treatment of the peripheral joints should be considered as an integral part of the diagnostic procedure and case management of the musculoskeletal system, and to ignore them must be to the detriment of the patient and cause frustration for the chiropractor.

Initial examination of the peripheral joints begins as a patient first enters the room. Always working from the general to the specific, the chiropractor observes critically as the patient approaches, and when invited to sit for the interview. Alteration of gait, obvious foot pronation or abnormal wear and tear to the footwear, toeing in or out during ambulation, hesitation in bending knees or ankles when sitting, are all noted. Absence of normal elbow flexion when walking and difficulty in reaching out to shake hands, local swelling in hands or fingers are also clues to be observed. The initial clues may be numerous, but this may not always be the case. Where there is no obvious sign of peripheral joint dysfunction, the routine case history may reveal more clues. The value of a carefully taken case history can never be over-estimated. MacBryde (1970) states, 'It is widely recognized by experienced clinicians that a skilfully taken history with a careful analysis of the chief complaints and of the course of the illness will more frequently than not indicate the probable diagnosis even before a physical examination is made or any laboratory tests are performed.'

According to Major and Delp (1962), 'the history of the patient is absolutely essential to the physician who is attempting to make a diagnosis. In some diseases, a physical examination is of little value; in other diseases, the reverse obtains; but in all diseases the history is of great importance'.

In the case of reflex-triggered functional syndromes, the patient will most likely be totally unaware that their persistent upper thoracic spinal pains have anything to do with a metatarsal or tarsal dysfunction or that their relatively asymptomatic metatarso-tarsal joint, upsetting normal proprioceptive function, is the reason for a recurrent sacro-iliac problem. Only a painstaking and skilful local examination can reveal this factor in the equation.

As a general principle, the method of approach to the examination of structural integrity, whether or not the patient is experiencing peripheral joint pain, remains essentially the same.

Examination approach to skeletal integrity of peripheral joints has the following components:

- *General observation, as discussed above.*
- *Case history, as discussed above.*
- *Detailed observation:*
  (a) *Static comparison of one side to the other for asymmetry, malformations, atrophy, swelling, limb length discrepancy, vascular changes and skin conditions, evidence of trauma or self abuse.*
  (b) *Gross limb and trunk movements for gait changes and evidence of painful disability on weight-bearing compared to non-weight bearing.*
- *Muscle testing for local peripheral joint integrity and for testing the strength of the muscle stabilizers of the hip, knee and ankle, etc. Bilateral grip strength should be tested by dynamometer.*
- *Orthopaedic tests – for the extremities as well as those for the spine should be performed (Schultz Villnave, 1983).*
- *Neurological assessment includes sensory function and motor function tests and the deep tendon reflexes and tests for tremors, vibratory sense and clonus, together with observation for muscle atrophy.*
- *Static palpation is invaluable for detecting comparative details of one limb to the other, when swelling and subtle differences of joint alignment, temperature differences and taut and tender fibres will be observed.*
- *Double weighing scales in conjunction with a plumb line and grid will indicate distortions, stresses and inequality of weight-bearing. These tests are simple to perform and give easily accessed information on the strains with which the axial and peripheral structures must contend.*
- *Motion palpation of normal joint ranges and the detection of hypermobility as well as the presence of hypomobility. Motion palpation into joint play is necessary to fully detect joint integrity and the methodology is described in detail in Chapter 8.*
- *Imaging in the form of MRI scans or by radiography, especially in post-trauma cases, may be necessary.*

Following this detailed examination procedure, the clinician can then assess whether manual treatment would be to the patient's benefit and should be applied to the problems presented.

In addition to chiropractic treatment, the clinician should bear in mind that rehabilitation in its various forms, including strapping, cryotherapy, non-weight-bearing stretching exercises and orthotics, may also be necessary in some cases to support the manipulative procedures applied.

The examination for, and the application of manipulation to the extravertebral and peripheral joints presents a rewarding field of practice and one to which all chiropractors should aspire. The student and practitioner must be mindful, however, that the examination and adjustive procedures for the extremities require no less dexterity, skill and practice than those for application to the spine and pelvis. Accuracy of the application of psychomotor skills remains paramount.

REFERENCES

Ambrobius, H. and Kondracki, M. (1992) *Plantar Fasciitis. European Journal of Chiropractic* **40**(2).

Bergmann, T., Peterson, D. and Lawrence, D. (eds) (1993) *Chiropractic Technique.* New York, Churchill Livingstone.

Beech, R.A. (1965) The fundamentals of the short leg syndrome. *Ann. Swiss Chiro. Assoc.* **III.**

Blennerhasset, G. (1997) Personal communication.

Curchod, G.A. (1971) Sciatic pain and the foot. *Ann. Swiss Chiro. Assoc.* **V.**

Gillet, H. (1964) *Belgian Chiropractic Research Notes*, 5th edn. Brussels, Belgian Chiropractic Association.

Greenwalt, M.H. (1981) *Spinal Pelvic Stabilization*, 2nd edn. Dubuque, IA, Publishing Division, Foot Levelers Inc.

Hoppenfeld, S. (1976) *Physical examination of the Spine and Extremities.* New York, Appleton–Century–Crofts.

Janse, J. (1976) In *Principles and Practice of Chiropractic. An Anthology.* (R.W. Hildebrandt, ed.) Lombard, IL, National College of Chiropractic, pp. 8, 116, 117.

Jones, S.L. (1953) *The Postural Complex.* Springfield, IL, Charles C. Thomas.

Kenel, F. (1965) Purpose of sole and heel lifts and their effects on spine and pelvis. *Ann. Swiss Chiro. Assoc.* **III.**

Laedermann, J.P. (1984) The rationale of extra-vertebral joint manipulation. Lecture given at the European Chiropractors Union Convention, Zurich, May.

Lening, P.C. (1991) Foot dysfunction and low back pain – are they related? *ACA J. Chiro.* **May**, 71–74.

MacBryde, C.M. and Blacklow, R.S. (1970) *Signs and Symptoms. Applied Pathology, Physiology and Clinical Interpretation*, 5th edn. Philadelphia, J.B. Lippincott Company.

Major, R.H. and Delp, M.H. (1962) *Physical Diagnosis*, 6th edn. London, W.B. Saunders Company.

Palmer, D.D. (1910) *The Chiropractor's Adjustor.* Davenport, IA, Palmer School of Chiropractic.

Walther, D.S. (1981) *Applied Kinesiology*, Vol. I. Abriendo, CA, Systems, DC.

2

Techniques employed in the biomechanical correction of peripheral joints

Raymond T. Broome

Adjustive techniques are nothing more and nothing less than tools designed to achieve a desired neuro-biomechanical effect. The efficacy and validity of techniques lack firm documentation but it is a common assumption that manipulation increases the quality and quantity of joint motion. The comparative manual assessment of joint function by skilled practitioners before and after the use of adjustive techniques remains the present benchmark for identification of their value.

As Droz (1971) points out, 'the manipulative act is a passive manoeuvre (for the patient) applied to vertebral or extra-vertebral articulations; it consists of a quick, sharp, deft thrust whose line of forces passes along the articular plane'.

Much has been written about techniques, and in the past they have evoked an emotive response and partisanship within the chiropractic profession. Fundamentally, however, they must each be judged on their mechanical efficiency and practicality to do the job required with the least possible force in order to minimize trauma to the holding elements of the joint.

There are four basic criteria that form the essential requirements for all techniques when treating the peripheral joints:

1 *They must use minimal force commensurate with the therapeutic aim.*
2 *As far as possible, the force must be confined solely to the joint being treated.*
3 *They must always be performed within the patient's tolerance.*
4 *The line of force has to pass along the articular plane.*

to acquire an efficient working knowledge of the widest selection of techniques. Paucity of knowledge denies the practitioner the opportunity of using a rational approach to the patient's case demands, and possible symptomatic changes, and encourages the imposition of an inappropriate method or force resulting, at best, in an indifferent clinical response.

On the one hand, the chiropractor must be prepared to alter technique choice, which is dependent on numerous factors presented by the patient such as case type, severity, chronicity, pain thresholds, age, anatomical variables and sometimes just from sheer size of the patient or even their frailty. On the other hand, the practitioner's limitations must be considered. The technique changes or modifications needed are determined by personal variable skill levels, inherent dexterity and aptitude, the availability, or lack of availability, of suitable equipment, the level of personal body fitness and physique and the lack of confidence in attempting and performing some types of available manipulative procedures. Lastly, there is a possibility of insufficient time being set aside to develop new skills.

All these foregoing factors have a bearing in technique selection. There are no hard and fast rules for choice of technique, since adjusting is practised as an art and chosen by utilizing the aggregate of sound knowledge of joint mechanics, practical observation, thorough examination and constant close experiential acquaintance with the multitude of case types presented before the practitioner. There is no substitute for clinical experience because, apart from general rules, there cannot be any rigid or set way to perform any joint manipulation.

TECHNIQUE CHOICE

All too often the chiropractor is faced with treating peripheral joints exhibiting variable states of degenerative joint disease. These cases require the clinical decision to modify a favourite technique or to select an alternative one to assist in maximizing the function of an irreversible condition. This emphasizes the necessity for the chiropractor

TECHNIQUE SKILLS

No one would be advised to attempt to use the psychomotor skills described in this book without the long years of chiropractic training, in order that they may be applied with skill and safety. 'Manipulation is an art that requires much practice to acquire the necessary skill and competence. Few ... have the time or inclination to master it' (Cassidy et al.,

1983). In addition, it is also equally important to have the knowledge and expertise to know when to halt therapy or when not to apply it, as it is to know how and when to apply it.

It is not within the scope of this book to describe all the considerations which together constitute manipulation skills, training methods, positioning skills, stance, thrust skills, reaction times and joint pre-load tension which together, when performed in unity, result in a smooth synchronized coordinated action; an action which necessitates, as previously stated, a learning process over long years of regular practice. These concepts have been described in great detail in other texts (Schafer and Faye, 1990; Vernon and Grice, 1992; Byfield, 1996) and the reader is referred to them.

Technique limitations in skill or variation may only be overcome by diligent practice accompanied many times by expert instruction. 'No realistic, or for that matter acceptable substitute exists for hard work and regular practice to assimilate the wealth of practical dexterity needed to perform skilled manipulation' (Byfield, 1996).

From the many adjustive approaches possible for peripheral joint technique, five mainstream methods have been chosen on the grounds of practicality, wide application and widespread use in the profession.

In the majority of joint corrections shown in this book, standard chiropractic short lever methods are demonstrated, and on a few, long leverage methods have been used.

Technique types:

1 *Direct thrust technique*
2 *Recoil technique*
3 *Short lever pull technique* } *Short lever*
4 *Clasp technique*
5 *Traction leverage technique* } *Long lever*

1(a) DIRECT THRUST TECHNIQUE.

Direct thrust technique is perhaps the most widely used of all chiropractic manipulative procedures in the manual treatment of the spine and is also used substantially on peripheral biomechanical joint problems. It is significant that Byfield (1996) quotes Bourdillon and Day (1987), Greenman (1989) and Bergman (1992), who have all recorded that the high velocity, low amplitude, single impulse-based short lever thrust technique is one of the oldest and most widely practised of the manipulative procedures in the field of manual medicine. Copland-Griffiths concurrs, describing the technique as 'the core of chiropractic and ... a classically high velocity thrust with a carefully measured force rapidly applied. Actual joint movement is minimal and any slack within the joint must be removed during the build up (joint tension pre-load) to the adjustment. Movement must be sufficient to carry the joint beyond its voluntary range whilst remaining within that range permitted by nature' (Copland-Griffiths, 1991).

When applied to the peripheral joints, the stance adopted for delivery of the thrust must ensure close proximity to the joint to be treated and the trunk is frequently semi-flexed

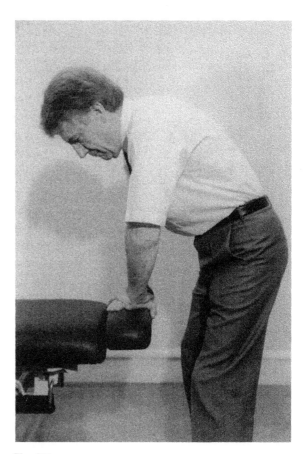

Fig. 2.1

Direct thrust technique

forwards, positioning the episternal notch directly above the contact (see Fig. 2.1). Occasionally, the trunk remains erect (see Acromio-clavicular, joint Chapter 8, technique 2.4). The hands may be linked or placed on contacts apart. The thrust may be unilateral or bilateral; one contact may be required to push and the other to pull (see Sterno-clavicular joint, Chapter 8, technique 1.2). The thrust may be a single impulse or a series of pump-like rapid thrusts of pre-selected varied depth (see Hip joint, Chapter 8, technique 7.6).

A high degree of precision, balance, coordination, dexterity and deftness together with a sound knowledge of biomechanics and a clear understanding of what needs to be achieved remain paramount.

1(b) BODYDROP TECHNIQUE

Body drop technique is a variant of the direct thrust technique and is a method of adding to the power of the impulse. It requires the typical forward semi-flexed trunk position for the direct thrust and the episternal notch to be directly above the contact for the correct body balance point.

The thrust is initiated by a swift, shallow drop of the trunk downwards towards the contact, while the shoulders, elbows and wrists are held rigid.

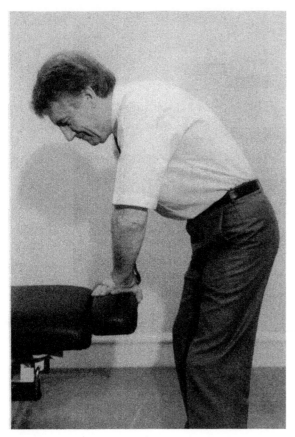

Fig. 2.2

*The chiropractor adopts a forward semi-flexed posture
with the neck flexed. The episternal notch is immediately
above the contact and the balance must remain over or
just ahead of the contact*

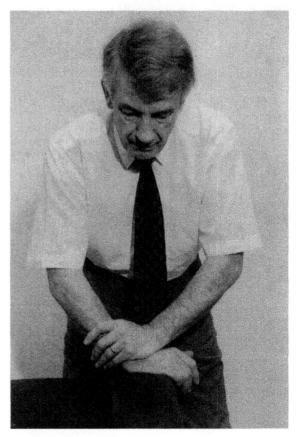

Fig. 2.3

*The lower hand uses a pisiform contact and the wrist is
dorsiflexed to a 'high' or 'low arch' position. The upper
hand is placed over the lower as shown, with the fingers
clasped around the lower forearm*

2 RECOIL TECHNIQUE

It will be clear from the description of recoil technique how
different it is from the direct thrust technique, even if the
initial posture appears similar. It is a technique which is very
widely used throughout the entire chiropractic profession.

Recoil technique was developed and refined by B.J.
Palmer (Dye, 1939). The posture assumed for the delivery of
the thrust is a forward semi-flexion of the trunk with the
episternal notch positioned directly above the joint to be
treated (see Fig. 2.2). No further trunk movement is made at
all during the rapid thrust delivery. The shoulders are held
level and the neck is flexed. The hands are placed one above
the other, the lower one using the pisiform as the contact
point and the wrist is held in varying degrees of extension
(see Fig. 2.3) as required by the variations of angles of thrust
and/or the topical anatomy of the contact.

Palmer (1920) describes the thrust delivery as 'done by
bringing the elbows together with a quick snappy contraction
of the extensor muscles of the arm; also by a sharp
contraction of the pectoralis muscles which serve to draw the

upper arm towards the chest. This combined action suddenly
forces the nail point (see Glossary of Terms, p. 285)
downward and during the action the shoulders should be
held at the same level. In other words, 'the shoulders should
at all times . . . be kept at a given distance from the floor and
should not be raised when the adjusting move is delivered'
(Palmer, 1920). Emphasis is laid upon arm relaxation before
the thrust is initiated and then the procedure is carried out
with great rapidity. To become proficient takes long training
and much practice.

In the field of peripheral joint technique, its use is limited
to the knee and foot, the shoulder, the wrist and the hand.
It is a safe, effective manipulative procedure, perhaps for the
very reason that Byfield (1996) gives when he quotes from
McCarthy (1993) in a personal communication, suggesting
that a thrust which is faster than normal reaction time is not
compressing the tissues for a long enough period to cause
sufficient damage and a nociceptive response.

The patient's joint to be treated with this method can be
placed straight on to a medium density treatment table-top
cushion to help absorb some of the thrust. In the majority of

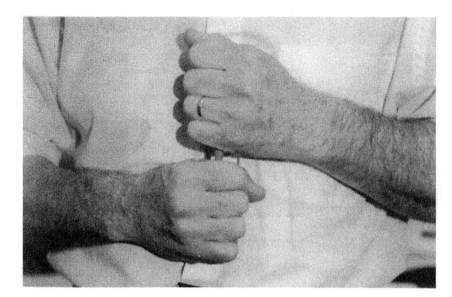

Fig. 2.4

The trunk is erect with the elbows relaxed to the sides. The hands are close up together, placed in opposite directions, shown here holding a pencil

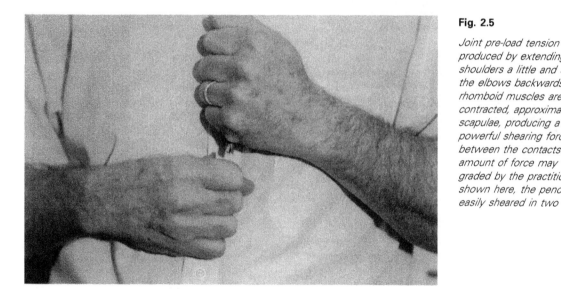

Fig. 2.5

Joint pre-load tension is produced by extending the shoulders a little and drawing the elbows backwards. The rhomboid muscles are rapidly contracted, approximating the scapulae, producing a powerful shearing force between the contacts. The amount of force may be graded by the practitioner. As shown here, the pencil was easily sheared in two

cases, however, this adjustive procedure is employed in conjunction with a drop mechanism (see section 6, Drop technique, p. 11).

As an alternative, or in cases where it would for any reason be unwise to use a standard manual thrust on a peripheral joint, a hand-held spring-loaded centre punch or 'Activator' (Fuhr *et al.*, 1996) can be used to provide a very high velocity low amplitude thrust along the plane line of the affected joint.

3 SHORT LEVER PULL TECHNIQUE

Short lever pull technique (SLPT) is an adaptation of the method described by Schultz (1958) and bears some resemblance to the lock break technique (Janse *et al.*, 1947). It is very versatile, and although opinions concerning its ease

of application differ (Logan, 1995), the clear advantages of SLPT once proficiency is attained make it most often the method of first choice in the treatment of peripheral joints.

Short lever pull technique may be applied to some of the fixations in all of the peripheral joints and the minimal adjustive force needed can be graded by the practitioner for depth of thrust and speed of delivery and is confined to the joint being treated, giving it an added safety value. No specialized equipment is needed and apart from when treating the hip and the knee, the patient may be sitting, standing or reclining, and the chiropractor may sit or stand during the procedure. If through chronicity or the presence of degeneration the joint is extremely stiff, it is sometimes precluded from being the method of first choice. Mobilization and occasionally the use of a longer leverage technique may be necessary initially. Because the chiropractor

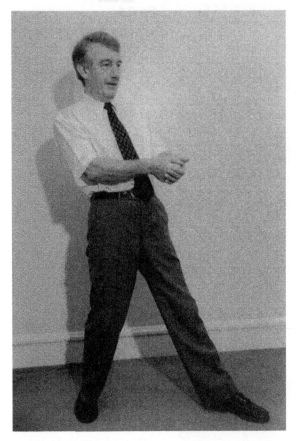

Fig. 2.6

Typically the trunk position for SLPT is erect or with forward semi-flexion. Shown here is one variant where the stance requires the chiropractor to lean straight backwards with the forward leg stiff and straight. The other leg flexes at the knee to remain in balance. This position produces the advantage of minimum traction at the joint concerned (see Talo-crural joint 8.10.50 short lever technique) and minimum trauma to the joint

is either standing erect or seated, operator fatigue is dramatically reduced when using SLPT.

Procedure

Initially the trunk is erect, the elbows are relaxed to the sides and flexed approximately to a right-angle and the hands are placed over the mid-sternal region (see Fig. 2.4). The adjacent bones on each side of the joint to be adjusted are contacted equally and in opposite directions, with the hands held close together and as close to the joint as possible. Frequently, the anterior of the joints between the first and second phalanx of the middle fingers are the contact points. Both thumbs remain uppermost when the hands are on the contacts. By extending the shoulders and by drawing the elbows a little posteriorly, the pre-load tension is produced. This is further enhanced by flexing the trunk a little forwards and by rotating the trunk slightly away from the contact, permitting

a much less vigorous impulse to be needed across the joint where it is applied.

Note: Female chiropractors may opt to use a padded oval-shaped sternal shield placed between the patient's limb and the mid-sternum to protect the breasts or to avoid positional embarrassment with the patient. Alternatively, a lower contact may be taken over the lower sternal region, which is slightly less efficient but still a workable position from which to initiate the adjustment.

Generating the impulse with SLPT

To initiate the adjustment, it is essential first to achieve joint pre-load tension. When joint pre-load tension is felt, the rhomboid muscles are rapidly contracted, the scapulae approximated and a powerful shearing force generated between the two contacts, which are pulled apart in equal and opposite directions across the plane line of the articulation involved (see Figs. 2.4, 2.5.). As with all psychomotor skills, much practice is required to achieve proficiency.

4 CLASP TECHNIQUE

A hitherto little known manipulative/mobilization method, the clasp technique is attributed to Pharoah (1963), and utilizes a shearing force. Its application to the treatment of the peripheral joints is limited but it provides a potent means for adjusting the intercarpal and intermetacarpal joints and of mobilizing and stretching the ligaments between the intermetacarpals and intermetatarsals.

Procedure

The hands are placed with the palms facing each other and the fingers are laced together. The hands are then positioned so that the heel of one hand is adjacent to the palm of the other (see Fig. 2.7). The position of the heels of the hands may be reversed as appropriate. The two adjacent carpals,

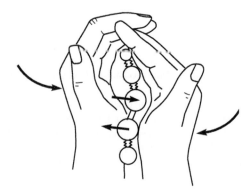

Fig. 2.7

The biased strike on the metacarpals or metatarsals is used to stretch the interosseus ligaments. The bias may be reversed when the mobilization needs to be applied in the opposite direction. The strike action is repeated as often as necessary

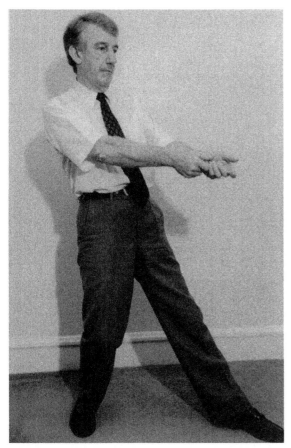

Fig. 2.8

Typical stance for traction leverage technique. The leading leg and the trunk are kept straight and the chiropractor leans back with the arms almost fully extended

intermetacarpals or intermetatarsals to be treated are put in a resting position and placed between the two hands. The palm of one hand is placed against one bone and the heel of the other hand is placed against the adjacent bone. The fingers remain laced together. The wrists are separated and then brought back together very rapidly, producing a biased strike and shearing force at the selected joint, or a stretching of the interosseous ligaments if the strike is mid-way along the metacarpals or intermetacarpals

5 TRACTION LEVERAGE TECHNIQUE

Long lever techniques employ a high velocity low amplitude force which extends across at least two joints to produce the manipulative effect on the joint targeted.

The joint to be treated may be adjacent to the point of contact and the force applied travels through several joints proximal to it before it is dissipated (Reinert, 1972) or the point of contact may be several joints away from the articulation to be treated, as in lumbo-sacral facet imbrication technique (Walther, 1976 quoting Holmes).

Procedure

Typically the practitioner leans the trunk backwards with the spine kept straight and rigid. One leg is placed ahead of the other, the knee on the leading leg is kept fully extended and the knee on the other leg is semi-flexed. The arms are almost straight and held stiffly out ahead of the trunk (see Fig. 2.8). By leaning back a little further, the limb is brought into tension. Without slackening the tension, the impulse is made by bracing the legs and, by rapidly thrusting the rigid trunk backwards, a pull thrust is exerted on the contact.

Great care must be taken when using traction leverage moves. The patient is protected to some extent by the use of a very swift thrust and by minimal depth of thrust. Patient selection is important, eliminating osteoporotic, post-surgical, frail and elderly subjects.

6 DROP TECHNIQUE

Finally we must discuss drop technique, a manipulative procedure commonly encountered in chiropractic practice. Developed as a system of chiropractic treatment by J. Clay Thompson of Davenport, Iowa, and called 'Terminal point technique,' it utilizes either direct thrust or recoil adjusting methods on specialized treatment tables (Pharoah, 1963).

Usually, up to three different sections of the treatment table are designed to be individually raised several millimetres and cocked, either at one end or in their entirety. When cocked, they can be cocked and set for tension both to accommodate the power of the thrust employed and also for the recumbent weight of the patient. The joint to be adjusted is placed over the mechanism and the vectored downward thrust plus drop induce a shearing force across the joint.

It is difficult enough to learn manual skills of such dexterity for practising chiropractic from visually presented material even in a classroom setting. The traditional maxim 'practice makes perfect' is not entirely applicable in learning psychomotor skills. Without instruction or peer correction, practising over and over again is simply not sufficient, because it may be reinforcing technique errors. It is easier to learn new habit patterns than to eradicate old, bad ones. Good instruction can alter the maxim to the required 'perfect practice makes perfect'.

REFERENCES

Byefield, D. (1996) *Chiropractic Manipulative Skills.* Oxford, Butterworth-Heinemann.

Cassidy, J.D., Kirkaldy-Willis, W.H. and Thiel, H. (1983) Manipulation. In *Managing Low Back Pain*, 3rd edn (W.H. Kirkaldy-Willis, ed.) Edinburgh, Churchill Livingstone.

Copland-Griffiths, M. (1991) *Dynamic Chiropractic Today.* Wellingborough, Thorsons Publishing Group.

Droz, J.M. (1971) Indications and contra-indications of vertebral manipulations. *Ann. Swiss Chiro. Assoc.* V, 81.

Dye, A.A. (1939) *The Evolution of Chiropractic.* New York, Richmond Hall.

Fuhr, A., Green, J.R., Colloca, C.J. and Keller, T.S. (1996) *Activator Methods. Chiropractic Technique.* London, Mosby Year Book Inc.

Janse, J., Houser, R.H. and Wells, B.F. (1947) *Chiropractic Principles and Technique*, 2nd edn. Lombard, IL, National College of Chiropractice.

Logan, A.L. (1995) *The Foot and Ankle. Clinical Applications.* Gaithersburg, MD, Aspen Publishers.

Palmer, B.J. (1920) *A Textbook on the Palmer Technique of Chiropractic*, 1st edn. Davenport, IA, Palmer School of Chiropractic.

Pharoah, D. (1963) Personal communication. Davenport, IA, Palmer School of Chiropractic.

Reinert, O.C. (1972) *Chiropractic Procedure and Practice.* Florissant, MO, Marion Press.

Schafer, R.C. and Faye, L.J. (1990) *Motion Palpation and Chiropractic Technique – Principles of Dynamic Chiropractic*, 2nd edn. Huntington Beach, CA, Motion Palpation Institute.

Schultz, A.L. (1958) *Athletic and Industrial Injuries of the Foot and Ankle.* Stickney, SD, Argos Printers.

Vernon, H. and Grice, A. (1992) Basic principles in the performance of chiropractic adjusting: historical review, classification and objectives. In *Principles and Practice of Chiropractic*, 2nd edn (S. Haldeman, ed.) Norwalk, CT, Appleton and Lange.

Walther, D.S. (1976) *Applied Kinesiology.* Abriendo, CO, Systems DC.

3

Peripheral joint kinematics

Christopher J. Good

Most clinicians would probably agree that studying the biomechanics of the peripheral joints is tedious at best. However, upon further consideration gaining knowledge of basic information such as the open- and close-packed positions and the osteokinematic and arthrokinematic motions becomes clinically important when actually attempting to apply the art of chiropractic at the highest level. This chapter is an attempt to simplify the vast amount of information available on the normal biomechanics of the peripheral joints in order to improve understanding by students and field practitioners. There are many far more detailed sources available which contain in-depth analysis of joint biomechanics. Interested individuals are encouraged to use the reference list as a first source if the need arises.

The **open-packed position** of most peripheral joints is the point at which there is the least amount of apposition of the joint surface and the greatest amount of joint capsule slack (Schafer and Faye, 1989). Mechanical forces applied to a joint in the open-packed position have a powerful effect on the capsule, intrinsic ligaments and muscles. This is supported by Lawrence and Bergmann (1993), who maintain that if too large a force is applied to a joint which is in the open-packed position sprain or strain of the soft tissues is likely to occur. Also, it is the author's opinion that the greatest amount of joint gapping (separation) and subsequent cavitation occurs around the open-packed position.

Conversely, the **close-packed position** is the point at which there is the greatest amount of joint surface apposition and the greatest amount of joint tension (Schafer and Faye, 1989). If a very large force is applied to a joint in the close-packed position a fracture or dislocation becomes likely (Lawrence and Bergmann, 1993). Avoiding the close-packed position during manual therapy should prevent or limit aggravation to the hard and soft tissues. It follows that in order to affect the soft tissues and not involve the hard tissues (cartilage and bone) most dysfunctional joints should be mobilized and/or manipulated at the open-packed position initially and then at other positions of restriction which approach the close-packed position. This would be a 'least invasive to most invasive' treatment regime, which is probably safest for all concerned.

Knowledge of joint **osteokinematic motion** (the direction and amount of motion at a joint) allows the examiner to perform active and passive range of motion testing. With this information, the examiner can perform a type of passive motion palpation coined **passive osteokinematic motion**

palpation (POMP). I find this a very useful method of assessing joint dysfunction prior to accessory motion testing or therapeutic treatment. The procedures for POMP are described in the following chapter. The values for the osteokinematic motions which appear in this chapter and the next are compiled from Hoppenfeld (1976), Kapandji (1982, 1987), Bergmann (1993) and Evans (1994). Where significant discrepancies occurred, a best value was chosen.

Arthrokinematic motion is the type of motion at a joint surface. Most joint motion is curvilinear (partly rotational, partly translational), and there is usually one or more recognized arthrokinematic motions for each osteokinematic motion. These are described by how the points on one joint surface move relative to the points on an opposing joint surface. The motion of a structure will be caused by it tilting (rotating) around an axis or gliding (translating) along an axis. This axis of motion of the moving joint surface is usually either parallel or perpendicular to the opposing joint surface. The arthrokinematic motions which occur in the peripheral joints are glide, roll and glide, or some type of rotation (either spin or swing) (Lawrence and Bergmann, 1993).

Glide (translation) is the most common motion in planar joints (also known as gliding or arthrodial joints) like the proximal tibio-fibular joint and the carpal and tarsal joints (Hamill and Knutzen, 1995). This is defined as 'one point on a surface contacting various points on an opposing surface'. In this case, for two relatively flat surfaces the point of interest on one joint surface is simply gliding along multiple points on the opposing surface, usually for a very slight distance (Fig. 3.1).

For larger amounts of motion to occur, the joints generally must exhibit roll and glide and the joint surfaces must be curved (hinge, condylar, ellipsoid, saddle or spheroid joints). Roll is defined as 'various points on one surface contacting various points on an opposing surface at the same interval'. In this case one joint surface is rotating about an axis which is parallel to its opposing joint surface (Fig. 3.2). Glide must also be a component of this joint motion. In this case, the moving surface glides along a plane or series of planes which are also parallel to the opposing joint surface (Fig. 3.3). Whether roll and glide occur in the same direction or in opposite directions is determined by whether a concave surface is moving on a convex surface or a convex surface is moving on a concave surface. In the former case roll and glide are in the same direction and normally there is quite a

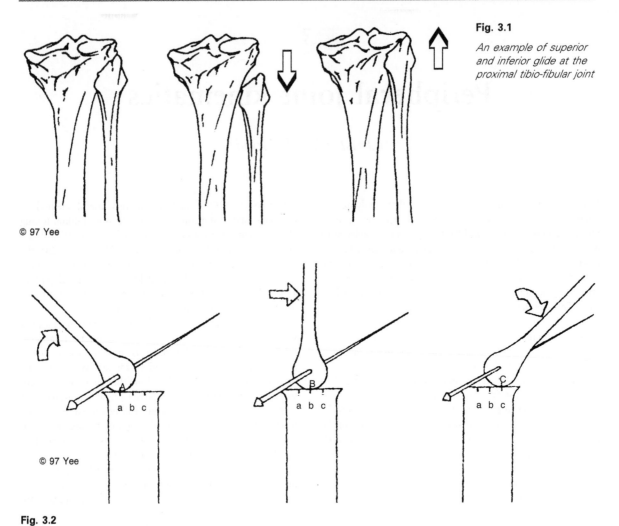

© 97 Yee

Fig. 3.1

An example of superior and inferior glide at the proximal tibio-fibular joint

Fig. 3.2

An example of roll where various points on one surface are contacting various points on an opposing surface at the same interval

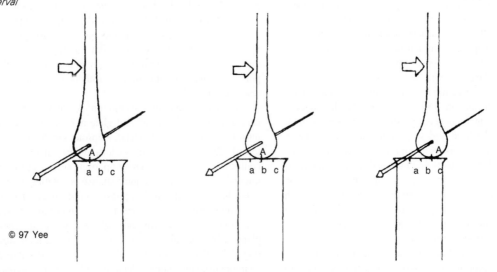

© 97 Yee

Fig. 3.3

An example of glide where the moving surface glides along a plane or series of planes which are parallel to the opposing joint surface

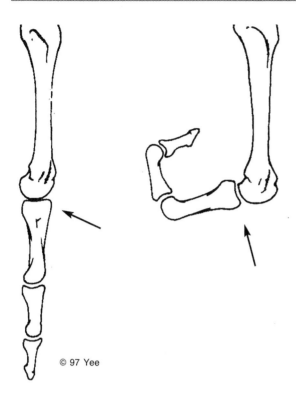

© 97 Yee

Fig. 3.4

When a concave surface moves on a convex surface, roll and glide are in the same direction and a large amount of joint travel occurs

bit of travel along the joint surfaces. An example of this is metacarpal-phalangeal flexion/extension. With metacarpal-phalangeal flexion, the concave surface at the base of the

phalanx glides over the entire face of the relatively convex-shaped metacarpal head. At full extension the proximal phalanx joint surface is facing the inferior joint surface of the metacarpal head and by the end of flexion, it ends up facing the anterior surface of it (Fig. 3.4).

In the case of a convex surface moving on a concave surface, roll and glide are in opposite directions. This can be seen in glenohumeral joint abduction (Fig. 3.5). As the arm is abducted, the spherical head of the humerus rolls in a superior direction, yet also glides inferiorly. This helps to keep the joint surfaces in the same relative juxtaposition within the capsule, unless the amount of glide becomes quite large. If it becomes too large joint dislocation can be observed, which of course is quite common at the glenohumeral joint.

The final arthrokinematic motion is called **rotation** and there are two types: spin and swing. When a joint surface rotates around an axis, it usually does so around an axis which is either perpendicular or parallel to the opposing structure's surface. When the axis of rotation is also its own mechanical axis (the true axial centre of the rotating object) this arthrokinematic motion is called **spin**. If the mechanical axis is perpendicular to the opposing joint surface, one point on the rotating surface will contact various points on the opposing surface and it will circumscribe a circle on the opposing surface (with the exception of a point which is on the mechanical axis itself, in which case it would merely inscribe a point). An example of this is at the radiohumeral joint when the head of the radius spins relative to the capitellum during pronation/supination of the forearm (Fig. 3.6).

If the mechanical axis of rotation runs parallel to the opposing joint surface, various points on the moving surface will contact one point on the opposing surface. The various points will also circumscribe a circle but this circle will be

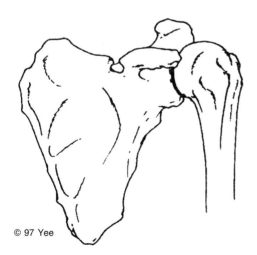

© 97 Yee

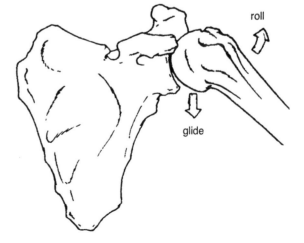

roll

glide

Fig. 3.5

In the case of a convex surface moving on a concave surface, roll and glide are in opposite directions and the joint surfaces do not travel much

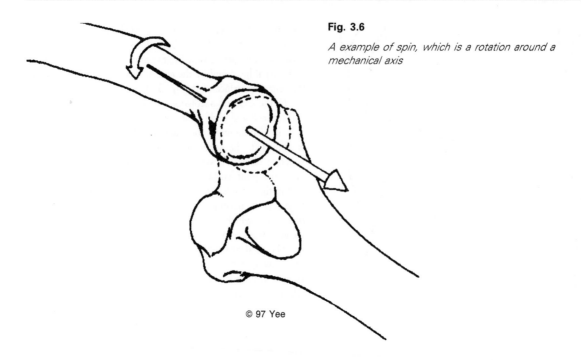

Fig. 3.6

A example of spin, which is a rotation around a mechanical axis

© 97 Yee

perpendicular to the opposing surface. This is one of the arthrokinematic motions which occurs at the tibiofemoral articulation during knee flexion/extension (Fig. 3.7).

When the object which is in motion rotates around an axis perpendicular to the opposing surface but it is not its true mechanical axis, the motion is called **swing**. A point on that rotating surface circumscribes something other than a circle relative to the opposing surface (often an ellipse or egg-shaped figure). This is what occurs at the glenohumeral joint during shoulder flexion/extension (Fig. 3.8).

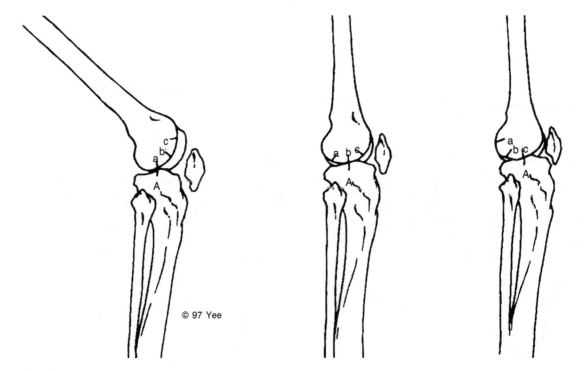

© 97 Yee

Fig. 3.7

When the mechanical axis of rotation runs parallel to the opposing joint surface, various points on the moving surface will contact one point on the opposing surface

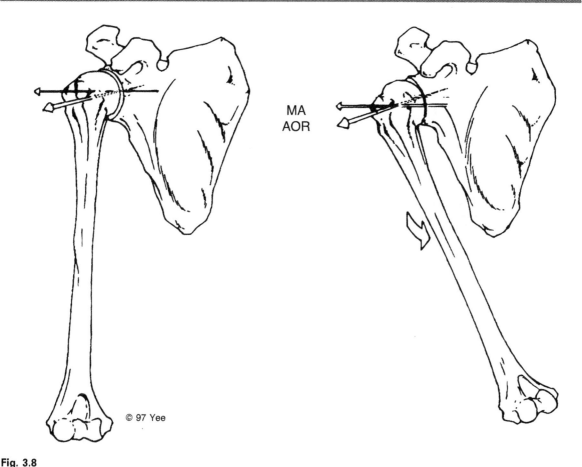

MA
AOR

© 97 Yee

Fig. 3.8

When the object which is in motion rotates around an axis of rotation (AOR) perpendicular to the opposing surface but it is not its true mechanical axis (MA), the motion is described as a swing

Knowing the arthrokinematic motion which should occur for a particular osteokinematic motion can give the practitioner a rationale for the type of treatment which should be applied to a joint. With this information, the practitioner can assess for these motions as well as provide specific treatment for the return of them. For example, because the arthrokinematic motion during pronation/supination at the proximal radioulnar joint is spin, the treatment best applied to return this motion should involve a good deal of spinning of the radial head. Unfortunately, the most common manipulative therapy applied to the radial head is a gliding type of adjustment, which may in fact do little to improve the spin of the joint.

ANKLE REGION

DISTAL TIBIO-FIBULAR JOINT

This is a fibrous joint made from the distal tibia and fibula forming a mortice within which the dome of the talus sits. In fact there are two articulations at this site, the distal tibio-

fibular joint and the talo-fibular joint (Fig. 3.9). However, the distal tibio-fibular joint is far less mobile than the talo-fibular joint (the former joint is designed for stability rather than mobility) and there are no osteokinematic motions listed for it. However, both articulations are probably assessed with the accessory motion tests.

Despite the small amount of movement at the distal tibio-fibular joint, loss of the small accessory motions can lead to very dramatic changes in the function of the entire lower extremity. Hartley (1995) claims than a fibula restricted in a superior malposition could cause ankle overpronation while a fibula restricted in an inferior malposition could cause prolonged ankle supination. Either of these situations would ultimately affect the knee. Most commonly this area is injured by a twisting injury (usually an inversion sprain) (Southmayd and Hoffman, 1981; Evans, 1994) resulting in ligament/capsule damage, or it is injured by a direct trauma resulting in ligamentous/capsule, bony or interosseous membrane damage (Schafer, 1987). Depending on the amount of damage and how the area was rehabilitated, the joint motion will either be normal in quality, hypermobile due to ligamentous laxity or very restricted due to fibrotic infiltration.

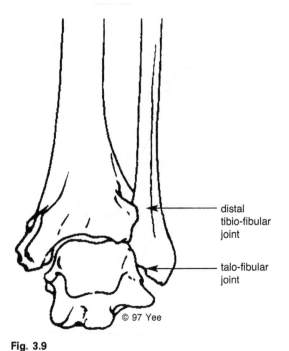

Fig. 3.9

There are two articulations at the lateral malleolus, the distal tibio-fibular joint and the talo-fibular joint

distal tibio-fibular joint

talo-fibular joint

© 97 Yee

Osteokinematic motion
None described for this fibrous joint.

Arthrokinematic motion
Primarily gliding in anterior/posterior or superior/inferior direction.

Open-packed position
Although there is no true open-packed position, with ankle dorsiflexion the distal fibula moves medially, posteriorly and superiorly, and this separates the maleoli (Schafer and Faye, 1989).

Close-packed position
With ankle plantarflexion the distal fibula moves laterally, anteriorly and inferiorly, and this approximates the malleoli (Schafer and Faye, 1989).

ANKLE MORTICE JOINT (TALO-CRURAL JOINT: TIBIO-TALAR AND TALO-FIBULAR JOINTS) AND SUBTALAR JOINT (TALO-CALCANEAL JOINT)

These two articular areas complete the functional ankle region, although technically the subtalar joint is part of the foot region (Kapandji, 1987). Biomechanically there is meant to be well-integrated motion between them. The ankle mortice joint is categorized as a uniplanar hinge joint, suggesting that it moves primarily in one direction. Most authors claim this is where dorsiflexion/plantarflexion of the ankle occurs (Kapandji, 1987; Bergmann, 1993; Thompson and Floyd, 1994; Hartley, 1995).

The subtalar joint is characterized as a multiplanar hinge joint (there are three joint surfaces), but it performs very little dorsiflexion/plantarflexion; instead most of the ankle-foot inversion/eversion occurs here (Fig. 3.10) (Hammer,1991; Evans, 1994; Thompson and Floyd, 1994). Unfortunately, inversion/eversion is sometimes called pronation/supination by some authors (Kapandji, 1987; Logan, 1995). For the purposes of this text, the terms pronation/supination will be used to identify the combined movements discussed below.

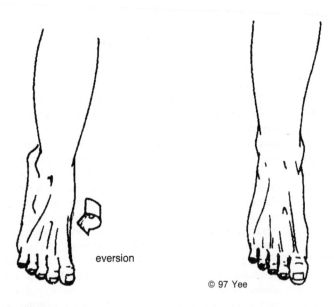
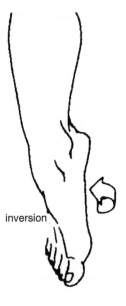

eversion

inversion

© 97 Yee

Fig. 3.10

Inversion and eversion of the ankle–foot region

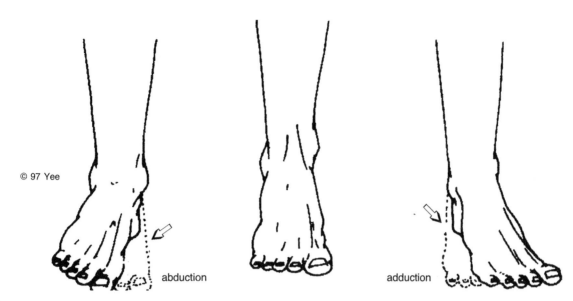

Fig. 3.11

Abduction and adduction of the ankle–foot region

The motions of abduction/adduction are considered a function of the midfoot or forefoot by some authors (Schafer, 1987; Evans, 1994) (Fig. 3.11). Other authors maintain that all three planes of motion occur at the subtalar joint, therefore abduction/adduction is also found here as well (Kapandji, 1987; Bergmann, 1993; Hartley, 1995).

It is my opinion that all three types of motion occur at both the ankle mortice joint and the subtalar joint to some degree and these can readily be felt in normal joints during POMP. However, when inversion/eversion and abduction/adduction become too great at the ankle mortice joint, instability should be suspected. As stated before, the most common cause of increased inversion at the ankle mortice joint would be single or multiple inversion sprains. When this occurs, the subtalar joint gets progressively stiffer as it participates less and less in ankle region motion, while the ankle mortice joint becomes hypermobile for this motion.

The most common cause of increased eversion and abduction of the ankle mortice joint is a chronically pronated ankle–foot region. This is caused by failure of the soft tissue holding elements during the stance phase of gait. Figure 3.12 depicts the phases of gait during both the weight-bearing **stance phase** and the non-weight-bearing **swing phase**. During the initial stance phase of gait (heel strike) the ankle–foot region becomes part of a **closed kinetic chain** (a series of joints stabilized at both ends). Pronation is induced by ground reaction forces against the calcaneus as the lower extremity becomes weight-bearing. At this point pronation is comprised of subtalar joint (calcaneus) eversion and abduction, ankle mortice joint plantarflexion and talar adduction (medial rotation) plus internal rotation of the tibia (Fig. 3.13) (Hartley, 1995). During the foot flat and midstance stage of gait the medial longitudinal arch flattens somewhat and the body weight is transferred to the medial side of the foot (Logan, 1995).

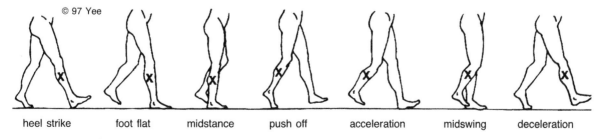

| heel strike | foot flat | midstance | push off | acceleration | midswing | deceleration |

Fig. 3.12

The phases of gait

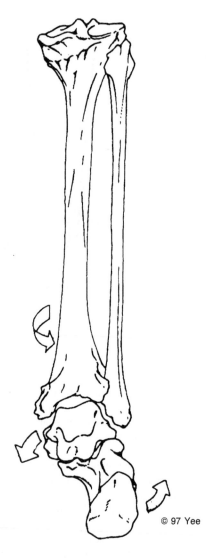

Fig. 3.13

Posterior view of pronation. This is comprised of subtalar joint (calcaneus) eversion and abduction, ankle mortice joint plantarflexion and talar adduction (medial rotation) plus internal rotation of the tibia

By the end of the midstance phase of gait supination occurs and it is comprised of ankle mortice joint dorsiflexion, calcaneal inversion, talar abduction (lateral rotation). It is at this point that the ankle–foot region joints approach their close-packed positions and a rigid lever is created for propulsion (push off). During acceleration (beginning of the swing phase of gait) non-weight-bearing supination is present and is comprised of plantarflexion, calcaneal inversion and adduction. This continues until sometime around midswing when the joints assume a more neutral position and later begin pronation. During the end of the swing phase of gait the ankle region is part of an **open kinetic chain** (a series of joints stabilized at one end and relatively free at the other)

and behaves very predictably: the gross motions observed are calcaneal eversion, abduction and dorsiflexion (Hartley, 1995). This is considered non-weight-bearing pronation.

Severe or prolonged pronation in the stance phase would simply induce greater amounts of talar medial rotation and adduction and subtalar eversion and abduction (Austin, 1994). This would have far reaching effects throughout the lower extremity and lumbo-pelvic area and could cause knee pain, patella tracking problems, pelvic muscle myofascial syndromes, sciatic nerve compression, hip joint, sacro-iliac and/or lumbosacral joint dysfunction as well as possible irritation to the ganglion impar (Innes, 1993; Hamill and Knutzen, 1995).

Lack of pronation (maintained supination) during the initial part of stance phase would be caused by a very rigid series of ankle–foot joints and would inevitably cause a loss of the absorption of ground reaction forces. This would increase the shock waves along the foot and up the lower extremity (Hamill and Knutzen, 1995).

The osteokinematic motions described below are composite values for both joints. It should be understood that the majority of dorsiflexion/plantarflexion occurs at the ankle mortice joint, while in my opinion nearly equal amounts of inversion/eversion and abduction/adduction occur at the ankle mortice and subtalar joints.

Osteokinematic motion
Ankle mortice and subtalar joints combined:
   Dorsiflexion: 20°
   Plantarflexion: 50°
   Inversion: 30°
   Eversion: 20°
   Abduction: 10°
   Adduction: 20°

Arthrokinematic motion
Ankle mortice joint: roll and glide; subtalar joint: roll and glide.

Open-packed position
Ankle mortice joint: slight plantarflexion; subtalar joint: full pronation (eversion and abduction).

Close-packed position
Ankle mortice joint: dorsiflexion; subtalar joint: supination (inversion and adduction).

FOOT REGION

The foot is comprised of the hindfoot (talus and calcaneus), midfoot (cuboid, navicular and medial, middle, and lateral cuneiforms) and the forefoot (metatarsals and phalanges). The subtalar joint is located in the hindfoot and it has been previously discussed in relation to the ankle mortice joint. The midfoot contains the midtarsal joints, which include the calcaneo-cuboid, talo-navicular, naviculo-cuneiforms and naviculo-cuboidal joints. The forefoot joints include the cuneiform-metatarsal, cuboidometatarsal, metatarsal-

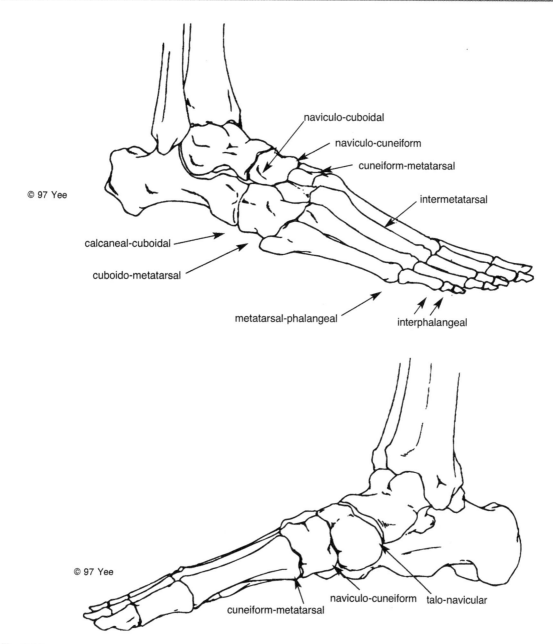

© 97 Yee

naviculo-cuboidal

naviculo-cuneiform

cuneiform-metatarsal

intermetatarsal

calcaneal-cuboidal

cuboido-metatarsal

metatarsal-phalangeal

interphalangeal

© 97 Yee

cuneiform-metatarsal

naviculo-cuneiform

talo-navicular

Fig. 3.14

The midfoot region and forefoot region joints

phalangeal, and interphalangeal joints. Also included as articulations in this region are the intermetatarsal joints (Fig. 3.14). Although these are not true joints, a significant amount of motion must occur between the rays of the metatarsal bones if normal foot function is to occur.

The midtarsal joints are a series of planar joints which allow for small amounts of rolling and gliding during walking and running. These joints also become locked to allow the foot to become a rigid lever during push off in gait. The most important of these clinically is the talo-calcaneonavicular area which is comprised of the medial and anterior facets between the talus and the calcaneus, the talus and spring ligament articulation and the head of the talus-navicular articulation (Hartley, 1995). Normal movement at these sites is important for normal pronation and supination to occur. Overall, the various positions the foot joints take during the phases of gait become important for normal gait mechanics to occur, and the small movements which occur here should not be overlooked.

The metatarsal-phalangeal (MTP) joints are mobile ellipsoid joints which can perform flexion/extension and small amounts of abduction/adduction. In contrast to the hand, extension of the MTP joints is 50–60° while flexion is 30–40° (Kapandji, 1987). The proximal and distal interphalangeal joints are hinge joints which can only perform flexion/extension (Grabiner, 1989). Although joint motion here is important, no measured osteokinematic motion is reported for the foot region with the exception of great toe flexion and extension.

Osteokinematic motion
None described specifically for foot except for first toe:
Metatarsophalangeal flexion: 45°
Metatarsophalangeal extension: 70–90°

Each toe joint should perform flexion and extension. The amounts vary widely but in general motion increases at the metacarpal-phalangeal joints and decreases at the proximal and distal interphalangeal joints as the toes get smaller.

Arthrokinematic motion
All foot joints: roll and glide.

Open-packed position
Midtarsal joints: pronation; forefoot joints: mid-flexion

Close-packed position
Midtarsal joints: supination; forefoot joints: extension

KNEE REGION

The knee region is comprised of the proximal tibio-fibular, the tibio-femoral and the patello-femoral joints (Fig. 3.15). It is a highly stressed joint region primarily because the body's two longest levers come together at a condyloid joint which sometimes is locked to form an even longer lever (Harley, 1995). The capsule and ligaments which maintain the joint are under tremendous compressive, sheer and torsional forces which quite often cause injury.

PROXIMAL TIBIO-FIBULAR JOINT

Like the distal tibio-fibular joint, this articulation is non-weight-bearing and only has small amounts of movement. It is a diarthrodial planar joint and is normally more mobile than its distal counterpart. It is clinically significant due to the soft tissues which attach to its capsule (lateral collateral ligament, biceps femoris tendon). Injuries to either structure or the articulation itself could cause loss of joint motion here or instability (Harley, 1995).

Osteokinematic motion
None described.

Arthrokinematic motion
Primarily glides superior–inferior and anterior–posterior. Some rotation (swing) occurs along an axis parallel to the tibial shaft.

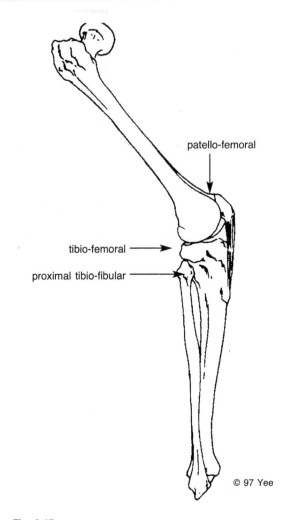

Fig. 3.15

The knee region joints

Open-packed position
None described.

Close-packed position
None described.

TIBIO-FEMORAL JOINT

The tibio-femoral joint is a condyloid joint which most often is presented clinically following trauma. Although the predominant motion is flexion and extension, often it is the rotational movements (internal and external) which become lost or dysfunctional (Schafer, 1987). The small amount of rotation which occurs at this joint is important in normal gait (the tibia internally rotates to unlock it from extension as part of heel strike) (Hartley, 1995). Rotation at this joint also allows a fair amount of torsional load to occur at the articulation without causing tissue damage. It is the lateral side of the joint which is more mobile, and this is primarily due to a very mobile meniscus and the incongruence of the joint surfaces here (Wallace *et al.*, 1985). This is especially important when the foot is planted and a person changes direction during walking or running, and may predispose the medial side of the joint to injury.

Due to the ability of the joint to rotate internally and externally as well translate to a significant degree, subluxations with misalignment are commonly found (Logan, 1994). If present, they would possibly cause patella tracking problems as well as localized pain in the tibio-femoral joint.

Osteokinematic motion
  Flexion: 130°
  Extension: 0–5°
  Internal rotation: 10°
  External rotation: 10°

Arthrokinematic motion
From flexion to extension: roll, glide, spin and external rotation; internal and external rotation: rotation (spin).

Open-packed position
Tibio-femoral joint, 25° flexion.

Close-packed position
Tibio-femoral joint, full extension with external rotation.

PATELLO-FEMORAL JOINT

The action of the patella primarily involves a simple gliding motion over the femoral condyles. It seldom becomes hypomobile; instead, most of the clinical problems are a result of poor tracking of the patella or hypermobility. Because the distance from the tibial tuberosity to the patella is fixed by the infrapatellar tendon, this bone is dragged across the condyles in a very predictable fashion as the tibia is pulled into flexion/extension and internal/external rotation. The articular area becomes troublesome when significant malposition of the tibia and/or femur exists as part of a local misalignment (Schafer, 1987), from the effects of ankle–foot misalignment (Rothbart and Estabrook, 1988) or from abnormal pull of the quadriceps muscles (Grabiner, 1989). These clinical conditions change the tracking of the patella which can then cause increased wear and tear on the undersurface of the patella, or irritation at its medial or lateral borders. Quite often this is the case with genu valgus (knock knees) subsequent to ankle–foot pronation. In this instance the pull of the quadriceps and infrapatella tendon laterally creates a bowstring effect and causes a friction laterally on the underside to the patella (Grabiner, 1989).

The above misalignments are often measured by the Q angle (quadriceps angle). This angle is created by a line simulating the direction of pull of the quadriceps group and a line simulating the direction of pull of the inferior patella tendon (Schafer, 1987; Grabiner, 1989; Bergmann, 1993). Especially important is the role of the vastus medialis which keeps the patella in its groove during motion.

Osteokinematic motion
None described, but the patella must be able to glide along the entire anterior and inferior surface of the femoral condyles during knee flexion, and be able to glide medially and laterally during knee internal and external rotation.

Arthrokinematic motion
When tibio-femoral flexion occurs, the patella glides inferiorly, posteriorly and medially.

Open-packed position
None described, however this joint is most relaxed when the patient is supine and the tibio-femoral joint is in extension.

Close-packed position
None described, however this joint is most tight when the knee is flexed and the patient is weight-bearing.

THE HIP REGION

The femoro-acetabular joint is a multiaxial spheroidal joint which has tremendous freedom of movement (Fig. 3.16).

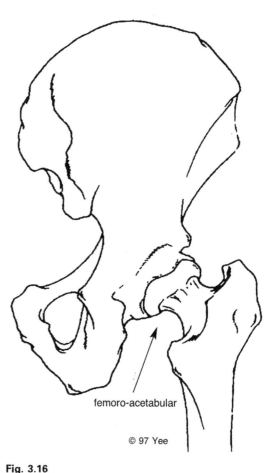

femoro-acetabular

© 97 Yee

Fig. 3.16

The hip region joint

However, the constant tendency for the hamstrings, piriformis and iliopsoas to shorten and tighten (Chaitow, 1985; Janda, 1985), as well as the general inactivity of most patients, allows this joint to become less mobile than it would otherwise be (Hooper and Faye, 1994). Loss of the normal range of motion of the femoro-acetabular joint becomes very apparent during POMP. Other biomechanical changes such as anatomical or functional short leg (Friberg, 1983; Lawrence, 1985), anteversion/retroversion of the femoral head and neck (Hammer, 1991; Bergmann, 1993), chronic ankle–foot pronation/supination (Rothbart and Estabrook, 1988; Lening, 1991), and pelvic malpositions and dysfunctions (Schafer and Faye, 1989) will also affect the mobility of this joint and cause it to become dysfunctional.

Osteokinematic motion
  Flexion: 120°
  Extension: 30°
  Abduction: 45°
  Adduction: 25°
  Internal rotation: 40°
  External rotation: 45°

Arthrokinematic motion
Flexion/extension: rotation (swing); abduction/adduction and internal/external rotation: roll and glide.

Open-packed position
Slight flexion, abduction and external rotation.

Close-packed position
Full extension, abduction and internal rotation.

THE HAND REGION

The joints in this region include the carpo-metacarpal (CMC) joints, the metacarpo-phalangeal (MCP) joints, the proximal interphalangeal (PIP) joints, the distal interphalangeal (DIP) joints and the thumb interphalangeal (IP) joint (Fig. 3.17). With the exception of the 1st and 5th CMC joints, the distal hand is similar to the forefoot; the proximal ends of the metacarpals and all the phalanges are concave in nature and articulate with convex distal surfaces of the preceding bones.

The second, third and fourth digit CMC joints are planar joints which move slightly in flexion/extension. The 1st and 5th CMC (trapezio-metacarpal and hamate-metacarpal joints) are biplanar sellar (saddle) joints which are mobile in flexion/extension and abduction/adduction (Kapandji, 1982).

The MCPs of the fingers are small ellipsoid joints which can flex and extend and abduct and adduct. The thumb MCP joint is a very mobile condyloid joint. It performs flexion/extension, abduction/adduction and some degree of pronation/supination (Kapandji, 1982). The hinge-type finger PIP and DIP joints and thumb interphalangeal (IP) joint primarily flex and extend. Flexion/extension for the hand MCP, PIP, DIP and IP joints exhibit roll and glide in the same direction and there is quite a large amount of travel along

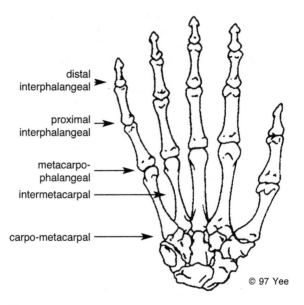

distal
interphalangeal

proximal
interphalangeal

metacarpo-
phalangeal

intermetacarpal

carpo-metacarpal

© 97 Yee

Fig. 3.17

The hand region joints

the joint surfaces (much greater than in the foot). This anatomical design, along with the opposing thumb, allows humans to grasp objects with ease.

Also included as articulations in this region are the intermetacarpal joints. Although these are not true joints, a significant amount of motion must occur between the rays of the metacarpal bones if normal hand function is to occur (Shafer and Faye, 1989).

Osteokinematic motion
Fingers:
  MCP: flexion 90°, extension 30–45°, abduction/adduction 40° total
  PIP: flexion 100°, extension 0°
  DIP: flexion 90°, extension 20°

Thumb:
  Trapezio-metacarpal: abduction/adduction 50° total; flexion/extension 50° total
  MCP: flexion 60°, extension 0°; abduction/adduction 20° total; pronation/supination 25° total
  Interphalangeal: flexion 90°, extension 20°

Arthrokinematic motion for MCP, PIP and DIP joints
Roll and glide

Open-packed position
MCP, PIP, DIP joints: flexion with slight ulnar deviation; intermetacarpal joints: fingers spread apart.

Close-packed position
MCP, PIP, DIP joints: maximum joint extension; intermetacarpal joints: fingers tight together.

WRIST REGION

The wrist region includes the carpal bones and the distal radioulnar joint. Each carpal bone articulates with many of its neighbours by small planar joints which allow small amounts of flexion/extension and abduction/adduction (radial/ulnar deviation). The distal radioulnar joint is not a true joint but must roll and glide properly in order for forearm pronation/supination to occur (Shafer and Faye, 1989).

The carpal bones are aligned in two rows and work as a unit, although individual bones can become subluxated. The proximal row (scaphoid, lunate and triquetrum) have proximal joint surfaces which are convex in shape and their distal joint surfaces are concave. The scaphoid and the lunate articulate proximally with the distal end of the radius in an ellipsoid type joint (Hamill and Knutzen, 1995). The distal row bones (trapezium, trapezoid and hamate) have generally convex proximal surfaces and convex distal surfaces. They articulate proximally at the midcarpal joint area by what are technically considered planar joints (Bergmann, 1993). On the palmar surface of the triquetrum lies the pisiform which is not active in wrist joint motion (Fig. 3.18).

The above wrist joint configurations allow for limited but significant flexion/extension and abduction/adduction at the radiocarpal joint and the midcarpal joint. While there is some controversy as to whether greater amounts of flexion or extension exist at which joint areas, there is no question that significant amounts of both flexion and extension do occur at both sites (Shafer and Faye, 1989; Bergmann, 1993; Hamill and Knutzen, 1995). During abduction/adduction there is reciprocal motion between the rows. The distal row moves as a unit in the direction of movement, while the proximal row moves in the opposite direction (Nordin and Frankel, 1989) (Fig. 3.19).

Osteokinematic motion
  Flexion: 90°
  Extension: 70°
  Adduction (ulnar deviation): 55°
  Abduction (radial deviation): 20°

Arthrokinematic motion for the carpal joints
Roll and glide.

Arthrokinematic motion for the distal radiocarpal joint
Roll and glide.

Open-packed position
Flexion with slight ulnar deviation.

Close-packed position
Extension (and radial deviation for the midcarpal joint).

ELBOW REGION

The elbow region is considered a diathrodial hinge joint, but is actually made of three articulations: the radiohumeral

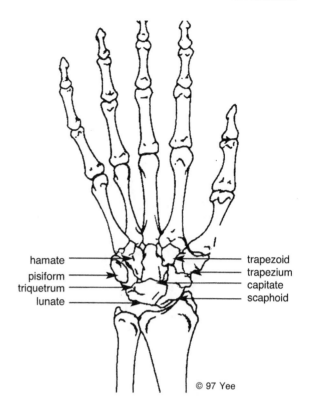

Fig. 3.18

The wrist region joints

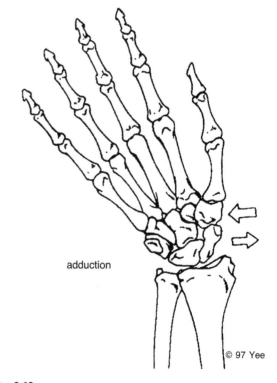

Fig. 3.19

Movement of the carpal rows during adduction

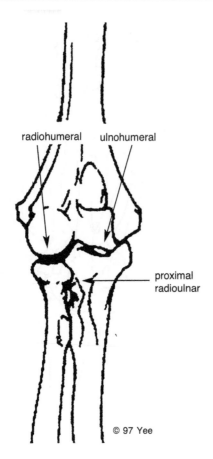

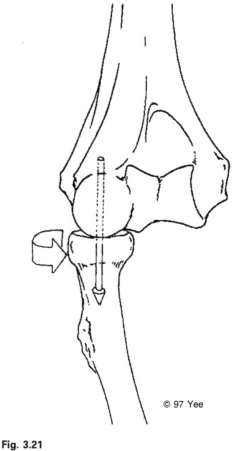

© 97 Yee

Fig. 3.20

The elbow region joints

Fig. 3.21

The radial head spinning around its mechanical axis during pronation

joint, the ulnohumeral joint and the proximal radioulnar joint (Fig. 3.20). Each of these articulations has different physiological capacities, all of which serve to allow the hand to be put into various functional positions for work or play.

The radiohumeral and ulnohumeral joints are active in flexion/extension of the region while the radioulnar joint performs pronation/supination of the forearm. During flexion/extension it is the wedge-shaped humeral trochlea at the ulnohumeral joint that puts the elbow into a valgus position in extension (creating the 'carrying angle' of 15°) and a varus position in flexion (Hamill and Knutzen, 1995). The variation observed between patients in the amount of extension is due either to the length of the olecranon process or laxity of the joint capsule. Also during flexion/extension the concave depression of the meniscus at the superior articulating surface of the radius rolls and glides smoothly over the capitellum. During pronation the proximal head of the radius is held in place by the annular ligament as it spins around its mechanical axis (Fig. 3.21). The somewhat bent midshaft allows the distal end of the radius to roll over the ulna and allows the hand to be turned over.

Overall the region is considered one of the most stable extremity regions (Grabiner, 1989). However, because the

varus and valgus stresses which commonly occur here are not normal motions for this joint region, injuries occur at the medial and lateral aspects of the elbow region. Most often encountered are the tremendous valgus stresses which are applied to the joint region during sporting activities such as throwing or racket swinging (Southmayd and Hoffman, 1981). During valgus stress the radiohumeral joint bears most of the compressive forces as the head of the radius impacts the meniscus and then the capitellum, while at the same time the medial collateral ligament is under very large tensile forces (Hamill and Knutzen, 1995).

It is interesting to note that the radiohumeral and ulnohumeral joints' open- and close-packed positions are nearly opposite of each other (Bowling and Rockar, 1985). Assessing and treating these joints requires the elbow to be put in very different positions so that specificity during the examination is critical.

Osteokinematic motion
 Flexion: 160°
 Extension: 0–5°
 Supination: 90°
 Pronation: 90°

Arthrokinematic motion
Radiohumeral joint:
  flexion/extension: roll and glide
  pronation/supination: spin
Ulnohumeral joint: roll and glide
Radioulnar joint: roll and glide and rotation

Open-packed position
Radiohumeral joint: full extension/supination; ulnohumeral joint: flexed 70°, semi-prone; proximal radioulnar joint: flexed 70°, slight semi-prone.

Close-packed position
Radiohumeral joint: flexed 90°, semi-prone; ulnohumeral joint: full extension/supination; proximal radioulnar joint: semi-prone

SHOULDER REGION

The shoulder region is actually comprised of four articulations, three of which are true diarthrodial joints (the sterno-clavicular joint, the acromio-clavicular joint and the glenohumeral joint) and one physiological joint (the scapulo-thoracic joint) (Fig. 3.22). For normal movement to occur in the joint region all four articulations must be working properly, and therefore all must be assessed.

The glenohumeral joint is the main player in this joint region while the other three articulations form the shoulder girdle and function as a very mobile strut system for the glenohumeral joint (Grabiner, 1989). The glenohumeral joint is the most mobile articulation in the body and this is primarily due to three things: the ball and socket configuration of the joint, the relatively small joint surface area of the glenoid fossa and the very slack joint capsule (Schafer, 1987). The capsule is functionally divided into two halves, with the upper half being tighter and stronger and the lower half being far more lax but prone to the formation of adhesions if no movement is induced there. It is the inability of the head of the humerus to move into the lower joint capsule during flexion or abduction which causes the pain and limitation of motion in adhesive capsulitis.

The scapulo-thoracic articulation is also extremely mobile and can account for up to 33% of shoulder flexion or abduction (Hamill and Knutzen, 1995). However it can only move well if all of the muscles which attach to it are elastic and function in a well-integrated fashion. The sterno-clavicular and acromio-clavicular joints must also be mobile enough to allow the clavicle to elevate/depress, protract/retract and rotate posteriorly during glenohumeral joint and scapulo-thoracic motion (Grabiner, 1989).

There must be synchronous movement of all four articulations for a person to be able to use the shoulder normally. Shoulder abduction will be described but similar movements must occur in flexion as well. Initially in shoulder abduction the glenohumeral joint moves by itself for the first 15–30° of humeral abduction. After this initial movement the scapula begins to rotate laterally at a rate of 4° for every 5°

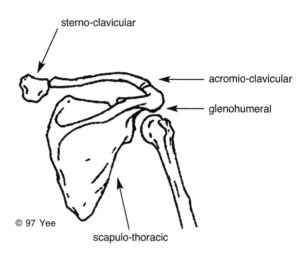

sterno-clavicular

acromio-clavicular

glenohumeral

scapulo-thoracic

© 97 Yee

Fig. 3.22

The shoulder region joints

of humeral abduction (Poppen and Walker, 1976; Soderberg, 1986). The muscular contraction which causes scapular movement forces the clavicle to elevate at a rate of 4° for every 10° of humeral abduction (Kapandji, 1987). The clavicle elevates at a triaxial hinge-type articulation at the sterno-clavicular joint. The movement here is approximately twice as much as the hinge-type motion at the acromio-clavicular joint which is also now occurring (Grabiner, 1989). As the humerus reaches 90° the clavicle rotates posteriorly and protracts slightly to allow further movement at the acromio-clavicular joint as the scapula continues its lateral rotation. All articulations continue their described actions until approximately 145°, at which point the humerus must externally rotate in order to clear the greater tuberosity from the underside of the acromion process. If this is accomplished all joints will continue their movements until endrange is felt at 180° of shoulder region abduction. If there is no external rotation of the humerus, motion of the glenohumeral joint ceases, but the other three joints continue to move until their end-range is obtained, somewhere around 170° of shoulder region abduction (Hamill and Knutzen, 1995) (Fig. 3.23).

Extension and adduction of the shoulder region also require synchronous movement of the four shoulder articulations but internal and external rotation performed with the arm at its side is primarily a rotation of the head of the humerus around an axis running parallel with the shaft of the humerus. This motion is occurring while the head of the humerus is in the upper joint compartment. If internal and external rotation are performed with the shoulder in 90° of abduction, the head of the humerus is forced into the baggy lower joint capsule and greater range of motion can be elicited in a normal joint. Evans (1994) gives 90° for both internal and external rotation (180° total) in the abducted position, however this is contradicted by Halback and Tank (1985), who maintain that only 90° of total internal/external rotation of the humerus occurs when there is 90° of abduction.

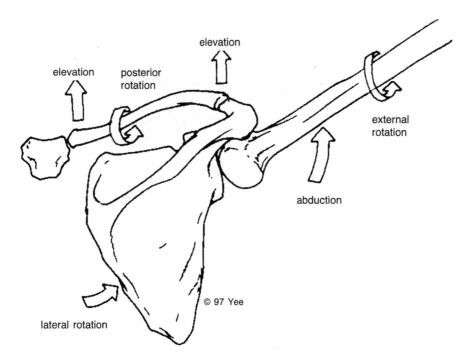

Fig. 3.23

*Individual joint movements
during shoulder region
abduction*

Osteokinematic motion
Glenohumeral joint
    *Flexion: 120° (as part of 180° of shoulder region
flexion)*
    *Abduction: 120° (as part of 180° of shoulder region
abduction)*
    Adduction: 50°
    Internal rotation: 90°
    External rotation: 90°
Sterno-clavicular joint:
    Elevation/depression: 40° total excursion
    Protraction/retraction: 40° total excursion
    *Posterior rotation along the clavicle long axis with
glenohumeral abduction: 10°*
Acromio-clavicular joint:
    Elevation/depression: 20° total excursion
    Protraction/retraction: 20° total excursion
    *Posterior rotation along the clavicle long axis with
glenohumeral abduction: 10°*
Scapulo-thoracic articulation:
    Elevation/depression: 20° total excursion
    Protraction/retraction: 40° total excursion
    Medial/lateral rotation: 60° total excursion

Arthrokinematic motion
Glenohumeral joint:
    Flexion/extension: rotation (swing) and glide (inferior)
    Abduction/adduction: roll and glide
    Internal/external rotation: roll and glide
Sterno-clavicular joint:
    Elevation/depression: roll and glide
    Protraction/retraction: roll and glide
    Posterior rotation: spin

Acromio-clavicular joint:
    Elevation/depression: roll and glide
    Protraction/retraction: roll and glide
    Posterior rotation: spin
Scapulo-thoracic articulation:
    Elevation/depression: roll and glide
    Protraction/retraction: roll and glide
    Medial/lateral rotation: rotation (swing) and glide

Open-packed position
Glenohumeral: 55° abduction, 30° horizontal
                       adduction
Sterno-clavicular: arm at rest
Acromio-clavicular: arm at rest
Scapulo-thoracic: none described
                       (probably arm at rest)

Close-packed position
Glenohumeral: full abduction and external rotation
Sterno-clavicular: full elevation
Acromio-clavicular: 90° abduction
Scapulo-thoracic: none described
                       (probably full lateral rotation)

TEMPOROMANDIBULAR JOINT REGION

The temporomandibular joint (TMJ) region has increasingly become a joint of special interest to chiropractors due to its common involvement with cranio-cervical pain and dysfunction syndromes. Its association with other musculoskeletal conditions such as functional or anatomical short leg, sacroiliac restriction, lumbar restriction, fixed thoracic or rib

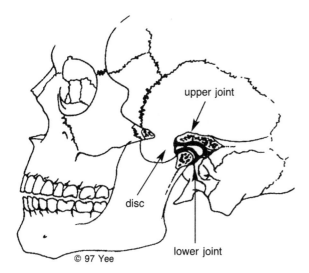

Fig. 3.24

The temporomandibular region joints

cage distortion has also been suggested (Lay, 1977). Postural changes in the body could affect the head and neck region and this invariably affects the resting position of the TMJ. Subsequent changes in the soft tissue holding elements around the joint ultimately cause craniofacial pain (Check and Curl, 1994). For example, the resting position of the TMJ is slight opening. With upper cervical extension the jaw will be drawn open and if held in this position over time the soft tissue holding elements around the joint would lengthen. Similarly acute and chronic pain in the head and neck often causes clenching of the teeth. This could decrease the normal length of the soft tissue holding elements of the TMJ.

When the mandible performs depression (mouth opening) and elevation (mouth closing) the TMJ goes through a complex series of events. It is complex because the TMJ has two joint compartments (upper and lower) which are separated by an intra-articular disc (Fig. 3.24). The first part of mandibular depression occurs in the lower joint compartment of the TMJ as the head of the condyle spins in the joint space. With further depression, the head of the condyle glides anteriorly and this occurs primarily in the upper joint compartment (Bergmann, 1993). For this latter movement to occur there must be disc–condyle synchronicity in which the disc is dragged forward as well. Any disruption of the disc movement will adversely affect the function of the joint and may result in the well-known locked-jaw phenomenon.

Protraction and retraction involve primarily a gliding motion in the upper joint compartment with an associated anterior disc dragging as well. Lateral glide, however, is more complicated. With mandibular lateral glide to the left, the ipsilateral (left) joint simply rotates (spins) in place while the contralateral (right) joint glides inferiorly and left (Bergmann, 1993). This can easily be felt by placing an examiner's fingertips over the joint space and laterally gliding the mandible.

Osteokinematic motion
Depression/elevation: 40–60 mm total excursion
Retraction/protraction: 5–10 mm total excursion
Lateral glide: 5–10 mm total excursion

Arthrokinematic motion
Depression/elevation: inferior joint rotates (spin); superior joint glides
Retraction/protraction: superior joint glides
Lateral glide: ipsilateral joint rotates; contralateral joint glides

Open-packed position:
Mandibular rest position (mouth slightly open).

Close-packed position:
Intercuspal position (teeth clenched).

ACKNOWLEDGEMENTS

I would like to acknowledge my illustrator Will Yee. His persistence and patience were tremendous. He retains the copyright on these illustrations. I would also like to thank my media support person, Herb Sussman, for his excellent work on this project.

REFERENCES

Austin, W. (1994) Orthotic control of biomechanical stress due to motion. *ACA J. Chiro.* Jun, 69–70.

Bergmann, T.F. (1993) Extraspinal technique. In: *Chiropractic Technique* (T.F. Bergmann, D.H. Peterson and D.J. Lawrence, eds), New York, Churchill Livingstone Inc., pp: 523–722.

Bowling, R.W. and Rockar, P. (1985) The elbow complex. In: *Orthopaedics and Sports Physical Therapy* (J. Gould and G.J. Davies, eds), St Louis, MO, Mosby, pp. 476–496.

Chaitow, L. (1985) *Neuro-muscular Technique.* New York, Thorsons Publishers Inc.

Check, P. and Curl, D.D. (1994) Posture and craniofacial pain. In: *Chiropractic Approach to Head Pain* (D.D. Curl, ed.), Baltimore, MD, Williams & Wilkins, pp. 121–162.

Evans, R.C. (1994) *Illustrated Essentials in Orthopedic Physical Assessment.* St Louis, MO, Mosby.

Friberg, O. (1983) Clinical symptoms and biomechanics of lumbar spine and hip joint in leg length inequality. *Spine* 8(6), 643–649.

Grabiner, M.D. (1989) The ankle and the foot. In: *Kinesiology and Applied Anatomy* (P.J. Rasch, ed.), Philadelphia, Lea & Febiger, pp. 208–244.

Halback, J.W. and Tank, R.T. (1985) The shoulder. In: *Orthopaedic and Sports Physical Therapy* (J.A. Gould and G.J. Davies, eds), St Louis, MO, Mosby, pp. 497–517.

Hammer, W.I. (1991) *Functional Soft Tissue Examination and Treatment by Manual Methods*. Gaithersburg, MD, Aspen Publishers.

Hamill, J. and Knutzen, K.M. (1995) *Biomechanical Basis of Human Movement*. Baltimore, MD, Williams & Wilkins.

Hartley, A. (1995) *Practical Joint Assessment: Lower Quadrant*. St Louis, MO, Mosby.

Hoppenfeld, S. (1976) *Physical Examination of the Spine and Extremities*. New York, Appleton–Century–Crofts.

Hooper P.D. and Faye L.J. (1994) The hip as an overlooked cause of low back pain: a case report. *Chiro. Tech.* 6(1): 9–12.

Innes, K. (1993) The pronated foot and the lumbo-pelvic area. *Dynamic Chiropractic* 1 September, p. 22.

Janda, V. (1985) Pain in the locomotor system–a broad approach. In: *Aspects of Manipulative Therapy* (E.F. Glasgow, L.T. Twomey eds), Melbourne, Churchill Livingstone, pp. 148–151.

Kapandji, I.A. (1982) *The Physiology of the Joints*, vol. 1. *Upper Limb*. Edinburgh, Churchill Livingstone.

Kapandji, I.A. (1987) *The Physiology of the Joints,*. vol. 2. *Lower Limb*. Edinburgh, Churchill Livingstone.

Lay, E.M. (1977) The osteopathic management of temporomandibular joint dysfunction. In: *Clinical Management of Head, Neck and TMJ Pain and Dysfunction* (ed. Harold Gelb). Philadelphia, W.B. Saunders.

Lawrence, D.J. (1985) Chiropractic concepts of the short leg: a critical review. *J. Manip. Physiol. Ther.* 8, 157–61.

Lawrence, D.J. and Bergmann, T.F. (1993) Joint anatomy and basic biomechanics. In: *Chiropractic Technique* (T.F.

Bergmann, D.H. Peterson and D.J. Lawrence, eds), New York, Churchill Livingstone Inc., pp. 11–50.

Lening, P.C. (1991) Foot dysfunction and low-back pain: are they related? *ACA J Chiro.* **May**, pp. 71–74.

Logan, A.L. (1994) *The Knee: Clinical Applications*. Gaithersburg, MD, Aspen Publishers.

Logan, A.L. (1995) *The Foot and Ankle: Clinical Applications*. Gaithersburg, MD, Aspen Publishers.

Nordin, M. and Frankel, V.H. (1989) Basic Biomechanics of the Musculoskeletal System. Philadelphia, Lea & Febiger.

Poppen, N.K. and Walker, P.S. (1976) Normal and abnormal motion of the shoulder. *J. Bone Joint Surg.* 58A, 195–200.

Rothbart, B.A. and Estabrook L. (1988) Excessive pronation: a major Biomechanical Determinant in the Development of Chondromalacia and pelvic lists. *J. Man. Phys. Ther.* 11(5), 373–379.

Schafer, R.C. (1987) *Clinical Biomechanics: Musculoskeletal Actions and Reactions*. Baltimore, MD, Williams & Wilkins.

Schafer, R.C. and Faye, L.J. (1989) *Motion Palpation and chiropractic Technique: Principles of Dynamic Chiropractic*. Huntington Beach, CA, Motion Palpation Institute.

Soderberg, G.L. (1986) *Kinesiology: Application to Pathological Motion*. Baltimore, MD, Williams & Wilkins.

Southmayd, W. and Hoffman, M. (1981) *Sports Health: the Complete Book of Athletic Injuries*. New York, Quick Fox.

Thompson, C.W. and Floyd, R.T. (1994) *Manual of Structural Kinesiology*. St Louis, MO, Mosby.

Wallace, L.A., Mangine, R.E. and Malone,T. (1985) The knee. In: *Orthopaedic and Sports Physical Therapy*. (J. Gould and G.J. Davies, eds), St Louis, MO, Mosby, pp. 342–364.

4

Passive osteokinematic motion palpation of the peripheral joints

Christopher J. Good

INTRODUCTION

Passive motion palpation has become one of the most common joint assessment procedures utilized by chiropractic physicians. Motion palpation of the spine was popularized by Gillet and Liekens (1960, 1969, 1984) and their protege L. John Faye (1981), Schafer and Faye (1989). Other notable influences include Gonstead (1980) and his proteges (Heschong, 1997; Cremata, Plaugher and Cox, 1991; Plaugher, 1993) as well as Stierwalt (1977) and more recently Bergmann, Peterson and Lawrence (1993).

Primarily there are two basic types of passive motion palpation: passive osteokinematic motion palpation (POMP) and accessory motion palpation, although these are often confused. POMP is induced by an examiner by placing a patient's joint region through its normal osteokinematic motions while contacting an associated bony landmark and feeling its movement. This is done from the neutral position up to the point of tissue resistance, commonly called the elastic barrier.

Accessory motions include end-feel and joint play, and these are usually performed in directions other than the normal osteokinematics motions (hence the use of the term 'accessory'). End-feel involves springing a joint at the elastic barrier, usually in a translational direction, but sometimes in a rotational fashion. Joint play involves feeling the 'joint slack' when joint surfaces are distracted apart at or near the joint's open-packed position (Bergmann *et al.*, 1993).

Motion palpation of the peripheral joints has been primarily based upon the work of Mennel and his development of end-feel palpation (1964). Subsequent peripheral joint palpation authors (Schafer and Faye, 1989; Bergmann *et al.*, 1993; Logan, 1994,1995) relied heavily on this work and have not applied the same passive osteokinematic motion palpation technique concepts commonly used in spinal motion palpation assessment. It was because of this absence that POMP for the peripheral joints was developed.

POMP of the peripheral joints is a systematic method of assessing the quality and quantity of joint motion. It is performed in the normal osteokinematic directions *and* through the full amount of motion which was discovered during passive range of motion testing. The joint space is *always* palpated during this procedure as well. Besides warming up the joint for further examination and treatment,

this is a relatively non-invasive form of motion palpation which can be well tolerated by patients when accessory motion palpation (end-feel/joint play) is too painful.

The information obtained with these tests includes the following:

1 *The quality of motion can be determined, i.e. is the motion smooth and regular or is it staggered ('catching') with joint crepitus and grinding?*
2 *The quantity of motion can be determined, i.e. for a joint in a kinematic chain do all of the articulations participate in the motions expected to their normal degree?*

It is important to know the normal osteokinematic motions (the direction and amount of motion) for each joint region in order to do POMP. Due to the wide variation in normal range of motion values given by different authors for the peripheral joints, values compiled from Hoppenfeld (1976), Kapandji (1982, 1987), Bergmann (1993) and Evans (1994) are used in this chapter. They are listed at the appropriate points to aid the learning process. It is also important to note that all descriptions are given for contacts on the right side of the patient.

ANKLE REGION

DISTAL TIBIO-FIBULAR JOINT

The osteokinematic motion is not described in the literature for this fibrous joint. Therefore passive osteokinematic motion palpation is not performed and only accessory motions are performed here.

ANKLE MORTICE JOINT (TIBIO-TALAR AND FIBULO-TALAR JOINTS) AND SUBTALAR JOINT (TALO-CALCANEAL JOINT)

These joints are assessed together because these joints move together in their motions. It is important to distinguish the directions and amounts of motion occurring at each articulation. See Chapter 3 on peripheral joint kinematics for further discussion.

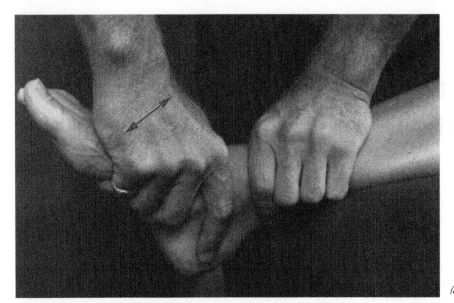

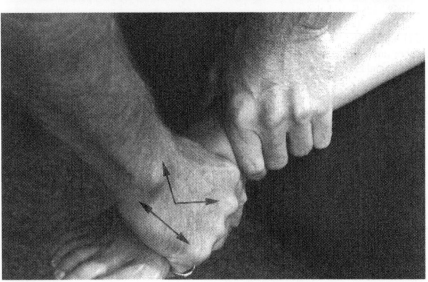

Fig. 4.1

(a) Ankle mortice joint plantar flexion/dorsiflexion. (b) Ankle mortice joint inversion/eversion and abduction/adduction

(a)

(b)

ANKLE MORTICE JOINT

Patient position	Supine, knee straight, foot slightly plantarflexed and off the edge of the foot rest.
Chiropractor's stance	Foot of table, lateral to foot.
Left hand	Left (cephalad) hand with thumb web over anterior distal tibio-fibular joint in the joint space and under the malleoli.
Right hand	Hands facing back to back, right (caudal) hand grasping distal talus area from foot dorsal surface with a thumb web grip.
Procedure	The right hand induces dorsiflexion (20°), plantarflexion (50°), inversion (varus tilt) (30°), eversion (valgus tilt) (20°), adduction (20°), and abduction (10°). Palpate the joint space with the left hand thumb web area as the motions are induced (Figs 4.1(a) and 4.1(b)).

SUBTALAR JOINT

Patient position	Supine, knee straight, foot slightly dorsiflexed, everted and abducted and off the edge of the footrest.
Chiropractor's stance	Foot of table, lateral to foot.
Left hand	Left (cephalad) hand with thumb web over ankle mortice joint just inferior to the malleoli and around the dome of the talus holding it firmly. The thumb and index finger

joint should perform flexion and extension. The amounts vary widely but in general motion increases at the metacarpal-phalangeal joints and decreases at the proximal and distal interphalangeal joints as the toes get smaller. The tarsal joints have no defined osteokinematic motion and therefore no POMP is performed. The small amount of gliding which occurs at the tarsal joints is very important however, and is assessed during accessory motion testing.

METATARSO-PHALANGEAL (MTP), PROXIMAL INTERPHALANGEAL (PIP), DISTAL INTERPHALANGEAL JOINTS (DIP) JOINTS

Patient position	Supine, lower extremity straight.
Chiropractor's stance	Lateral to foot.
Left hand	Left (cephalad) hand with a pincher grip over the joint space on the dorsal and plantar surface.
Right hand	Right (caudal) hand with a pincher grip just distal to joint on the dorsal and plantar surface
Procedure	Flex and extend the toe with the right hand and palpate the joint space with the left hand. First toe metatarso-phalangeal flexion is 45°, metatarso-phalangeal extension is 70–90°. The other toes can flex (to 50° in total) and extend (varying amounts) at each articulation (Fig. 4.3).

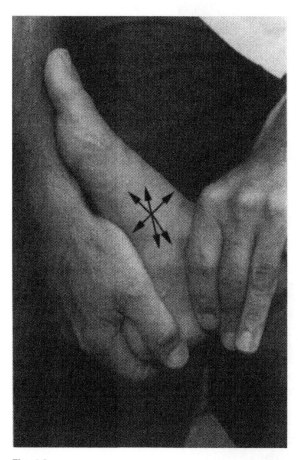

Fig. 4.2

Subtalar joint dorsiflexion/plantarflexion, inversion/eversion, abduction/adduction

	should be over the talocalcaneal joint space.
Right hand	Right (caudal) hand grasping the calcaneus from the plantar surface with the thumb pointing posteriorly and the forearm along the plantar surface helping to move the foot
Procedure	The right hand induces subtalar dorsiflexion (5°), plantarflexion (5°), inversion (varus tilt) (15°), eversion (valgus tilt) (10°), adduction (10°) and abduction (5°). Palpate the subtalar joint space with the thumb and index finger of the left hand as the motions are induced (Fig. 4.2).

FOOT REGION

There are no osteokinematic motions described specifically for the foot except for the first toe MCP joint. Each toe joint

KNEE REGION

PROXIMAL TIBIO-FIBULAR JOINT

Although this joint does not have any recognized osteokinematic motions, the following motion palpation test provides good information about its ability to move freely.

Patient position	Supine, knee straight.
Chiropractor's stance	Foot of table, side of table
Left hand	The left (cephalad) hand palpates over the fibular head with the index finger (2nd digit) and over the neck with the middle finger (3rd digit).
Right hand	The right (caudal) hand holds the foot from the plantar surface with the doctor's forearm along the plantar surface.
Procedure	The right (caudal) hand pulls the foot into dorsiflexion and eversion. Tension on the peroneal tendons at the inferior aspect of the fibula will force the fibula to glide superiorward. This gliding motion can be palpated at the superior aspect of the fibula with the cephalad hand (Fig. 4.4).

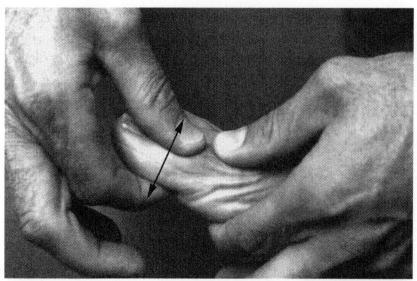

Fig. 4.3

Second toe DIP joint flexion/extension

(a)

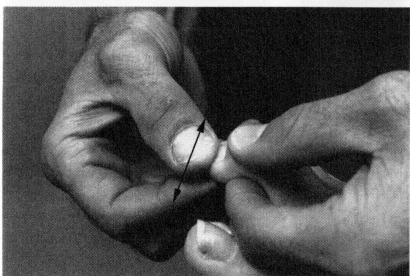

(b)

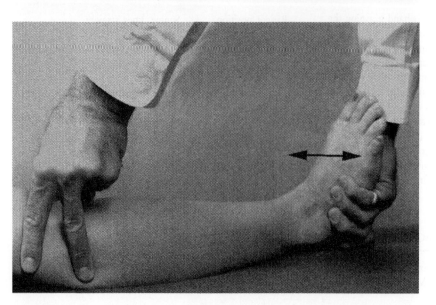

Fig. 4.4

Proximal tibio-fibular joint superior glide

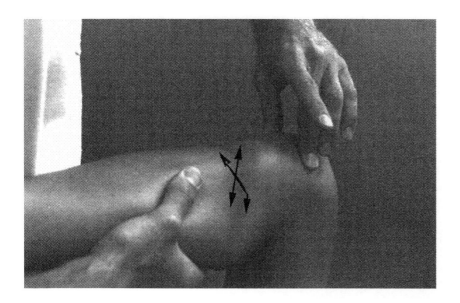

Fig. 4.5

Tibio-femoral joint flexion/extension and internal/external rotation

TIBIO-FEMORAL JOINT

Patient position	Supine, thigh slightly abducted.
Chiropractor's stance	Side of table.
Right hand	Right (caudal) hand grasping around the ankle (can be done with the doctor's axilla holding the ankle area and caudal hand grasping the calf).
Left hand	Left (cephalad) hand fingers and thumb in joint space at the knee.
Procedure	Palpate the joint space while flexing (130°), extending (0–5°), internally (10°) and externally (10°) rotating the knee joint with the caudal hand (Fig. 4.5).

PATELLO-FEMORAL JOINT

There is no osteokinematic motion described in the literature, but the patella must be able to glide along the entire anterior and inferior surface of the femoral condyles during knee flexion, and be able to glide medial and laterally during knee internal and external rotation.

Patient position	Supine, thigh straight on table.
Chiropractor's stance	At the side of the knee.
Right and left hands	Bilateral pincher grip contact.
Procedure	Glide the patella in superior/inferior and medial/lateral directions (Fig. 4.6).

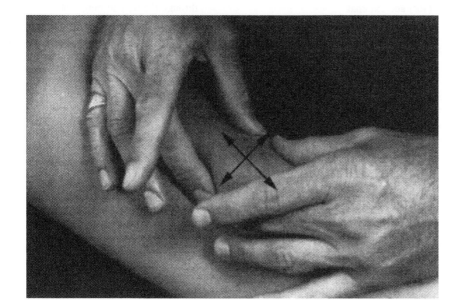

Fig. 4.6

Patello-femoral joint superior/inferior glide and medial/lateral glide

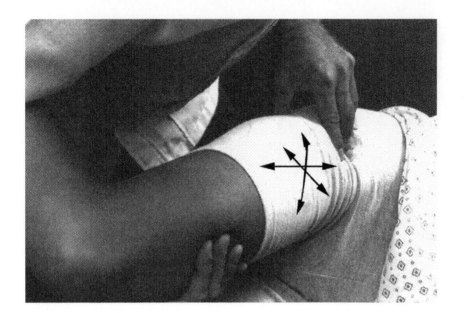

Fig. 4.7

*Femoro-acetabular joint
flexion/extension,
abduction/adduction and
internal/external rotation*

HIP REGION

The femoro-acetabular joint is not easily palpated in one patient position, but the side-lying position appears to be the easiest position to obtain all motions.

Patient position	Side-lying, thigh slightly abducted.
Chiropractor's stance	Behind patient.
Right hand	Caudal arm grasping around bent knee.
Left hand	Cephalad hand fingers in the joint area, just anterior to the greater trochanter.
Procedure	Induce hip flexion (120°), extension (30°), abduction (45°), adduction (25°), internal (40°) and external rotation (45°) with the right hand as the left hand palpates the joint area (Fig. 4.7).

HAND REGION

The finger joints' osteokinematic motions are as follows:
Metacarpo-phalangeal (MCP): flexion 90°, extension 30–45°, abduction/adduction 20°.
Proximal Interphalangeal joint (PIP): flexion 100°, extension 0°.
Distal interphalangeal joint (DIP): flexion 90°, extension 20°.

The thumb joints' osteokinematic motions are as follows:
Trapezio-metacarpal (TMC): abduction/adduction 50° total, flexon/extension 50° total.
MCP: flexion 60°, extension 0°; abduction/adduction 20°
total, pronation/supination 25° total
Interphalangeal (IP): flexion 90°, extension 20°.

For each digit (MCP, PIP, DIP, IP, TMC joints) the following can be performed:

Patient position	Seated, pronated hand presented in front of body.
Chiropractor's stance	Standing in front of patient.
Left hand	Pincher grip over the joint space, dorsal and palmar surface.
Right hand	Pincher grip on the mid-ray just distal to joint, dorsal and plantar surface.
Procedure	Move the ray of the distal bone through the normal ranges of motion as described above with the right hand while palpating the joint space with the left hand (Fig. 4.8).

WRIST REGION

Patient position	Seated, elbow flexed, hand pronated.
Chiropractor's stance	Lateral to arm.
Left hand	Grip around radial and ulnar styloid processes.
Right hand	Grip around proximal and distal rows of the carpal bones.
Procedure	Flex (90°), extend (70°), abduct (20°) and adduct (55°) wrist with the right hand while palpating the motion of the carpal bones (Fig. 4.9).

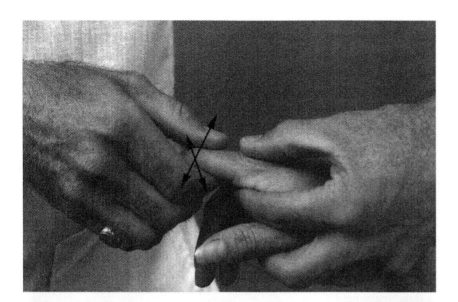

Fig. 4.8

Second digit MCP joint flexion/extension and abduction/adduction

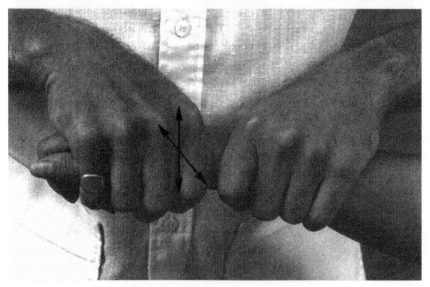

Fig. 4.9

Wrist joints flexion/extension and abduction/adduction

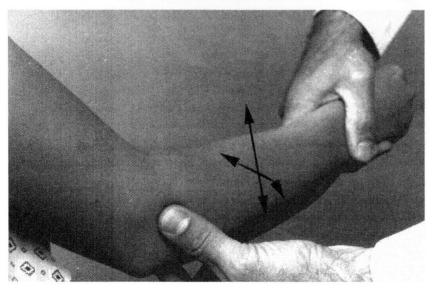

Fig. 4.10

Elbow joint region flexion/extension and pronation/supination

ELBOW REGION

The radiohumeral and ulnohumeral joints are palpated together for flexion and extension. The same contacts are then used for pronation/supination of the radioulnar joint.

Patient position	Seated, elbow flexed to 90° to find landmarks.
Chiropractor's stance	Lateral to arm.
Right hand	Chiropractor's anterior hand thumb web over patient's radial styloid area as though shaking hands (this is known as a 'wrist shake' grip).
Left hand	Chiropractor's thumb and middle digit is in the joint spaces at radiohumeral and ulnohumeral joints.
Procedure	The chiropractor flexes (160°) and extends (0–5°) the patient's elbow with the 'wrist shake' (right) hand and palpates the joint space with the left hand as doing so. Then with the patient's elbow at 90° the chiropractor places his/her left thumb over the radial head and pronates (90°) and supinates (90°) the patient's forearm (Fig. 4.10).

SHOULDER REGION

GLENOHUMERAL JOINT

Patient position	Seated, arm slightly abducted.
Chiropractor's stance	Posterior and lateral to patient.
Left hand	Posterior hand fingers under acromion process on humeral head.
Right hand	Anterior hand just below elbow inducing all motions.

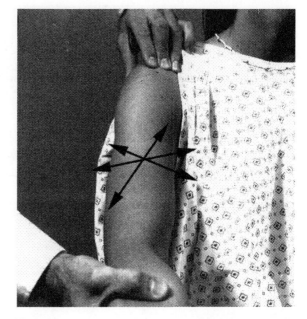

Fig. 4.11

Glenohumeral joint flexion/extension, abduction/adduction and internal/external rotation

Procedure	The chiropractor uses his/her stabilization hand to induce flexion (120°), extension (50°), abduction (120°), adduction (50°) (reaching in front of the patient's body), internal rotation (90°) and external rotation (90°). For internal/external rotation the patient's elbow is flexed to 90° (the humerus can remain at the patient's side or be brought to 90° of abduction). In the latter case the

Fig. 4.12

Sterno-clavicular joint elevation/depression, protraction/retraction and posterior rotation (not shown)

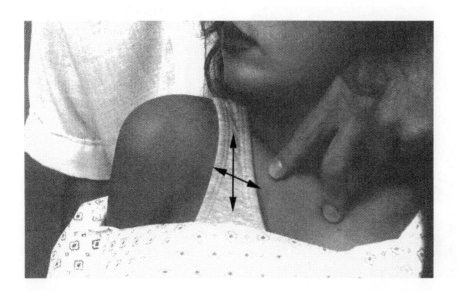

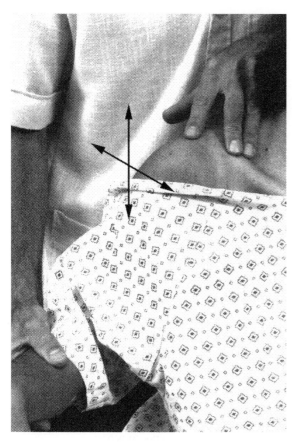

Fig. 4.13

Acromio-clavicular joint elevation/depression,
protraction/retraction and posterior rotation (not shown)

humeral head is brought into the lower joint compartment where there is more freedom of motion, particularly in external rotation (Fig. 4.11).

STERNOCLAVICULAR JOINT

Patient position	Seated, arm slightly abducted.
Chiropractor's stance	Behind patient.
Left hand	Medial hand around patient's neck, one finger on sternum, one on clavicle (2 inches lateral to joint).
Right hand	Lateral hand at mid humerus.
Procedure	The lateral hand moves the patient's humerus inducing elevation/depression (40°), protraction/retraction (40°), and glenohumeral abduction which causes posterior rotation of the clavicle (10°) (Fig. 4.12).

ACROMIO-CLAVICULAR JOINT

Patient position	Seated, arm slightly abducted.
Chiropractor's stance	Behind patient.
Left hand	Medial hand contacting the acromio-clavicular joint, one finger on acromion, one on clavicle (1 inch medial to joint).
Right hand	Lateral hand at mid humerus.
Procedure	The lateral hand moves the patient's humerus inducing elevation/depression (20°), protraction/retraction (20°), and glenohumeral abduction which causes posterior rotation of the clavicle (10°) (Fig. 4.13).

Fig. 4.14

Scapulo-thoracic articulation
elevation/depression,
protraction/retraction and
medial/lateral rotation

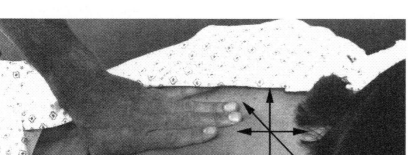

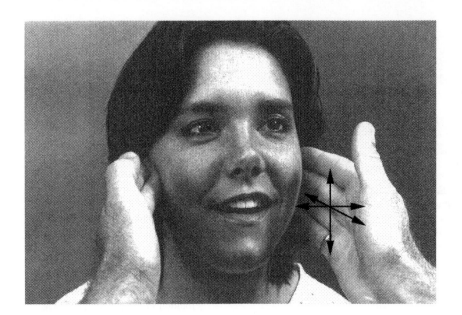

Fig. 4.15

Temporomandibular joint elevation/depression, lateral deviation and protraction/retraction

SCAPULO-THORACIC ARTICULATION

Patient position	Prone, patient's arm under their ipsilateral ASIS.
Chiropractor's stance	Ipsilateral two line stance.
Left hand	Caudal hand thumb web contacts the scapular inferior angle.
Right hand	Cephalad hand contacts around the patient's anterior shoulder.
Procedure	Both hands help induce the following scapular motions: elevation/depression (20°), protraction/retraction (40°), medial/lateral rotation (abduction/adduction) (60°). The left hand should be moved around the scapular inferior angle in order to obtain the best mechanical advantage to move the scapula (Fig. 4.14).

TEMPOROMANDIBULAR REGION

This is the only time that the patient actively moves the articulation being palpated and therefore this is actually a form of active kinematic motion palpation.

Patient position	Seated.
Chiropractor's stance	Anterior to patient.
Right and left hands	Chiropractor places one or two fingers over the joint space which is anterior and inferior to the external auditory meatus.
Procedure	Ask the patient to elevate/depress (40–60 mm), laterally deviate (5–10 mm) and protract/retract (5–10 mm) the mouth while palpating the joint space (Fig. 4.15).

ACKNOWLEDGEMENTS

I should like to thank my models, Emyln Munger, Kristin Jacobsen and Lisa Francey, and my media support person, Herb Sussman.

REFERENCES

Bergmann, T.F. (1993) Extraspinal technique. In: *Chiropractic Technique* (T.F. Bergmann, D.H. Peterson and D.J. Lawrence, eds) New York, Churchill Livingstone Inc., pp: 523–722.

Bergmann, T.F., Peterson, D.H. and Lawrence, D.J (1993) *Chiropractic Technique*. New York, Churchill Livingstone Inc.

Cremata, E.E., Plaugher, G. and Cox, W.A. (1991) Technique system application: the Gonstead approach. *Chiro.Tech.* 3(1), 19–25.

Evans, R.C. (1994) *Illustrated Essentials in Orthopedic Physical Assessment.* St Louis, MO, Mosby.

Faye, L.J. (1981) Motion palpation of the spine. *Motion Palpation Institute Notes.* Huntington Beach, CA, Motion Palpation Institute.

Gillet, H. (1960) Vertebral fixations, an introduction to movement palpation. *Ann. Swiss Chiro. Assoc.* 1, 30–33.

Gillet, H. and Liekens, M. (1969) A further study of spinal fixations. *Ann. Swiss Chiro. Assoc.* 4, 41–46.

Gillet, H. and Liekens, M. (1984) *Belgian Chiropractic Research Notes.* Huntington Beach, CA, Motion Palpation Institute.

Gonstead, C.S. (1980) *Gonstead Chiropractic Science and Art.* Mt Hareb, WI, SCI-CHI Publications.

Heschong, R.S. (1997) The Gonstead System. *Chiro. Prod.* October, pp. 36–37.

Hoppenfeld, S. (1976) *Physical Examination of the Spine and Extremities.* New York, Appleton–Century–Crofts.

Kapandji, I.A. (1982) *The Physiology of the Joints*, vol. 1. *Upper Limb.* Edinburgh, Churchill Livingstone.

Kapandji, I.A. (1987) *The Physiology of the Joints*, vol. 2. *Upper Limb.* Edinburgh, Churchill Livingstone.

Logan, A.L. (1994) *The Knee: Clinical Applications.* Gaithersburg, MD, Aspen Publishers.

Logan, A.L. (1995) *The Foot and Ankle: Clinical Applications.* Gaithersburg, MD, Aspen Publishers.

Mennel, J. McM. (1964) *Joint Pain: Diagnosis and Treatment Using Manipulative Techniques.* Boston, MA, Little, Brown & Co.

Plaugher, G. (1993) *Textbook of Clinical Chiropractic: a Specific Biomechanical Approach.* Baltimore, MD, Williams & Wilkins.

Schafer, R.C. and Faye, L.J. (1989) *Motion Palpation and Chiropractic Technique: Principles of Dynamic Chiropractic.* Huntington Beach, CA, Motion Palpation Institute.

Stierwalt D.D. (1977) *Fundamentals of Motion Palpation.* Self published.

5

Neurological implications of biomechanical disorders of the peripheral joints

Peter McCarthy and Susan Hill

Initially, we will look at the types of nerve present, passing quickly over a resume of the joint itself. Following this, the reflex will be introduced in its many guises as will the confounding element of neuroplasticity. The subjects closest to the hearts of the practitioner – namely disorders and their repair, with respect to rehabilitation of the patient – will be the focus of this chapter.

PERIPHERAL INNERVATION

GENERATION

To start at the beginning, with embryology of the nervous system, leads us into a complex subject area. At this juncture, it may suffice to say that there are two elements to the peripheral nervous system from this perspective: those nerves with cell bodies (somata) outside the central nervous system (CNS) and those whose cell bodies are inside it. The neurones whose cell bodies are outside the CNS derive from the neural crest cells and include both the dorsal root ganglion and autonomic chain cells, whereas the spinal cord cells and other cell bodies inside the CNS derive from the neural tube after closure and separation of the neural crest.

GROWTH AND GROWTH FACTORS

The growth of the peripheral nerve fibres into the limb buds appears to be dependent on the presence of chemical agents, which attract in the nerve fibres. These agents are referred to as growth factors. Growth factor secretion is continually required to maintain the presence of the nervous system: even after development has stopped! Too little growth factor and nerves recede from the area or die; too much growth factor and nerves will grow into the area or branch further.

Growth of the two components of the neural crest component of the peripheral nervous system (the autonomic motor and the primary afferent neurones) into the limbs appears to be competitive. The growing nerve fibres appear to compete for the same growth factors. A lack of either the primary afferent or sympathetic efferent component could lead to a greater degree of innervation by the other (Hill *et al.*, 1988; Anand *et al.*, 1996; Apfel and Kessler, 1996).

The somatic motor component also has a requirement for growth factor, but, this type appears to derive from the skeletal muscle fibres. Initially there are more nerve fibres and synapses formed than are required. This is obvious in skeletal muscle, where muscle fibres are initially polyneuronally innervated. Later, excess neurones are lost, ostensibly due to their being unsuccessful in obtaining a supply of 'growth factor' sufficient for their survival. Again this is more obvious in skeletal muscle, where the end product is a mononeuronally innervated muscle fibre. This loss of cells follows the activation of a standard pattern of programmed cell death (apoptosis) which arises because of the overall imbalance, i.e., relative lack of supportive 'growth' factors for all the nerves present (Henderson *et al.*, 1994)

The over-innervation of tissue, initially, is a protective feature. It ensures that all structures requiring an innervation have one. At the same time, this system results in balanced proportions of the three main neuronal populations in the periphery. These three types of neurone can be roughly categorized as:

1 *Somatic motoneurones*
2 *Autonomic motoneurones*
3 *Primary afferent sensory neurones.*

All of these neuronal types are represented in joint and muscle tissue, although their roles may not be unequivocal. The nerve growth agents are being investigated with respect to their use in degenerative nerve disorders such as motoneurone disease and diabetic neuropathy (Riaz and Tomlinson, 1996).

As is becoming evident, this subject area cannot be discussed properly unless reference is made to the nerves and their sub-groupings. To this end, it is appropriate at this point to introduce, with some detail, the important components of this system.

NOMENCLATURE

Over the years, study into the workings of the nervous system has produced a number of methods capable of resolving the neuronal components present. However, the result is a potentially confusing series of names, which are often used simultaneously to differentiate the nerve fibres present. In order to dispel some of this confusion, the following text will endeavour to outline and compare the naming systems most commonly encountered.

The obvious delineation is that of sensory and motor, however, it is not always possible to differentiate these two populations (in say an *in vitro* isolated nerve preparation). As a result, those nerve fibres present may be differentiated on the basis of their conduction velocity. The basic delineation is whether they are myelinated or not. Further groupings are based on the conduction velocities of the natural groups of fibres present in the nerve bundle, in some instances also relating this to receptors. With respect to the myelinated nerves, the vagus has a large preganglionic autonomic population, whose stimulation results in a distinctive waveform not found in the other long nerves, the so-called B-wave.

The designation A, B and C fibre is based on the conduction velocity of the axons of long nerves such as the sciatic and vagus nerves. This designation **does not** directly relate to the motor or sensory nature of the fibre.

Grossly:

- *A **fibres** are sensory and somatic motor.*
- *B **fibres** are preganglionic autonomic.*
- *C **fibres** are unmyelinated sensory and postganglionic autonomic motor.*

The A fibre group has been resolved into subgroups each given a Greek suffix:

- *Aα-fibres represent the α-motoneurones for skeletal muscle, and some faster sensory fibres.*
- *Aβ-fibres represent the fast conducting sensory fibres.*
- *Aγ-represents the γ-motoneurones to the intrafusal muscle fibres.*
- *Aδ-fibres represent the slow conducting, yet myelinated sensory fibres.*

The other popular method of classification takes its information from studies of muscle afferents. This system, therefore, relates to the conduction velocity and receptor properties of sensory neurones.

- *Type I fibres are rapidly conducting, associated with the bag fibres (stretch receptors) of the muscle spindle and the Golgi-tendon organs (GTO). There are subdivisions; i.e., type Ia (stretch receptors), type Ib (GTO).*
- *Type II fibres are slightly slower conducting than type I, associated with the flower spray endings in the intrafusal fibres.*
- *Type III, these are akin to the sensory Aδ-fibres, they*

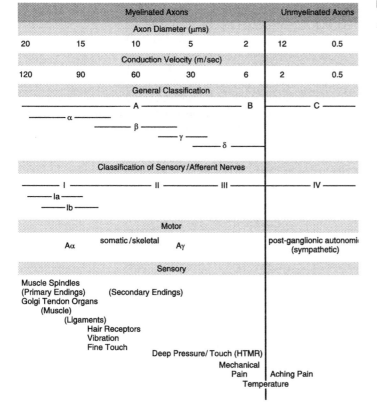

Fig. 5.1

Peripheral nerve nomenclature

*have free nerve endings and tend to require high
threshold mechanical stimulation.*

- *Type IV fibres are the unmyelinated component,
associated with noxious stimuli reception. Many of
these are nociceptors.*

Figure 5.1 shows how these systems of nomenclature overlap. As mentioned above, these are grossly simplified descriptions.

THE PRIMARY AFFERENT, SENSORY NERVES

Classification of the primary afferents can be made on the basis of receptor types and the conduction velocity of the peripheral axon. Grossly, primary afferents can also be divided with respect to the size of stimulus required. Those requiring large amounts of mechanical stimuli are referred to as High Threshold Mechano-Receptors (HTMRs), conversely, those requiring small amounts of stimuli are referred to as being Low Threshold Mechano-Receptors (LTMRs). The LTMRs tend to be encapsulated receptors whereas the HTMRs are on the whole unencapsulated or free nerve endings.

Receptor types

Receptors can detect stimuli based on mechanical, chemical and or electromagnetic properties. The electromagnetic properties include heat (infra-red), or lack of it (cold) and radiation of a shorter wavelength such as UV (sunburn) or beyond. The types of receptor found in peripheral tissues relate to movement, mainly responsive to mechanical distortion; i.e., having such names as mechanoreceptors, proprioceptors, kinesthioceptors. These receptors may give information on rate of movement, degree of movement and other forms of distortion, such as vibration. The name tends to be more related to function and position rather than the morphology and electrical characteristics.

It must also be stated that even though receptors may be specific to a particular form of stimulus (or stimuli), this is not absolute. Receptor potentials are graded within the range of sensitivity, and are not propagated along the fibre. Large, potentially damaging stimuli can also 'non-specifically' stimulate receptors. The sensation perceived by the conscious would still reflect the receptors' specific characteristics, however. An easy example of this is the 'bright light' which is perceived when you push your finger against your closed eye.

Proprioception

This term was first coined by Sherrington at the beginning of this century (Sherrington, 1906). It referred to the conscious or unconscious sense of limb position and movement. The receptor responsible for transducing this information was called the proprioceptor. Since those days the term has been used in reference to conscious awareness of position (limbs, etc.) and also, more contentiously, to describe the automatic or unconscious reflexes. It would appear that, currently, its use is becoming more aligned to the conscious control mechanisms.

A further method of defining a receptor is based on its rate of adaptation to a constantly applied stimulus. There are roughly two categories – rapid and slowly adapting, however, the slow group can be further differentiated into two subgroups. Adaptation of receptors can be demonstrated easily by placing your finger on a flat featureless surface and holding it there. The initial contact is palpable, due to a burst of fast conducted information. This train of activity is generated in the dynamic receptors of the LTMR population, which are rapidly adapting. The sensation is, therefore, short lived, in some cases only one or two action potentials. Consequently, the surface contact quickly becomes almost imperceptible. The rapidly adapting (probably Pacinian, Merkel and Meissener) receptors indicate the change in deformation of the skin. As well as the rate of adaptation, the speed of conduction is also high, therefore the information reaches the brain quickly. This information is highly conserved along the pathway to the brain and so is capable of being used to produce a high resolution 'image'. The receptors stop firing once the change has stopped, even though contact is maintained. The next burst of activity from these receptors will be when the finger is taken off the surface.

Joint receptors and deeper skin receptors, probably type II or III mechanoreceptors (Ruffini and free nerve endings), tend to register the contact for longer. These give the proprioceptive sensations required for body position sense and, therefore, are required to give 'constant' feedback with respect to degree of distortion. Of course this is relative, the receptors will adapt if the stimulus is sufficiently prolonged.

Both these types of receptors are necessary for the brain to 'know' what is happening with the body and for it to react with an appropriate motor response. Anybody having the unfortunate loss of the LTMR population would need to relearn use of the musculoskeletal system with a greater dependence on visual feedback.

The information in Table 5.1 will now be used to describe the functional innervation to the peripheral joints. Remember, a name associated with a particular receptor does not always relate to its stimulus; it usually refers to what it looks like! The type and size of stimulus required will depend on numerous factors such as the properties of the tissue in which it is embedded, the proteins present in the receptor and the local biochemistry as well as the accessory structures present!

Innervation of specialized structures: joints and associated tissues

In the extremities there are a number of complex joints with respect to their use, structure or both: e.g., knee, wrist or shoulder. The majority of innervation studies in these specialized peripheral joints have been performed in animal models. In the knee, this information is derived from work performed mainly on cats, with a little confirmatory work on humans. These studies have revealed that the patella is, like other dense packed cartilaginous structures, essentially without an innervation, hence the lack of sensation from this structure. The superficial layer of the joint capsule, the inner and outer surfaces of the ligamentum patellae and ligamentum collat-

Table 5.1   Joint, ligament and muscle receptors

Name	Location	Adaptability	Stimulus	Type
Ruffini	Fibrous joint capsules	Slow; static or dynamic depends on location	Movement amplitude and velocity, joint position sense, intra-articular pressure	I or II, dependent on source.
Golgi-tendon organ-like	Intrinsic ligaments of the joint capsule	Slow	Joint position	I or II
Golgi–Mazzoni	Loose pericapsular tissue	Fast	Rapid acceleration, movement	I
Free-nerve endings	Fibrous joint capsules	Slow	Nociception	III–IV
Pacinian	Near tendons and joints	Fast	Acceleration, movement and vibration	II
Pacinian	Ligaments	Fast	Acceleration, movement and vibration	II
Nuclear bag	Intrafusal fibres	Fast	Rapid acceleration, movement	Ia
Chain	Intrafusal fibres	Fast	Rapid acceleration, movement	II
Chain	Intrafusal fibres	Slow	Stretch, tension and length	II
Golgi-tendon organ (GTO)	Tendon	Slow	Tension 'Muscle work'	Ib
Ergoceptor	Between muscle fibres	Slow	Nociception	III/IV

erale mediale, are all innervated structures. The innervation is roughly 50:50 autonomic:sensory nerve fibres, the balanced proportions of which may be illustrative of the competition by each for similar growth factors. The sensory nerve fibres are mainly type IV (approx. 65%), with representation from all of the other grades (type III, approx. 18%; type II, approx. 15%; type I, approx. 2%) (Schaible and Schmidt, 1996). Many different neuropeptides have been immunohistochemically located in nerve fibres associated with these structures. These include substance P (SP), calcitonin gene-related peptide (CGRP), neurokinin A and a variety of the less common neuropeptides, the list of which is still growing.

Functional interpretation of an innervation

Many studies of synovial joint innervation have reported a similar picture with respect to both the types of afferent present and their relative proportions. When interpreting the data one needs to consider the emphasis of any study, as this can tend to bias the discussion. One should also consider all the receptor types present, as well as how often each could expect to be used.

There appears to be a greater proportion of type III and IV fibres present than type I and II fibres. However, the relative importance is dependent on function and may be different from the apparent importance derived from weight of numbers. In this, the relatively few type I and II fibres have a greater role in motor control, relative to the types III and IV. The latter tend to be of use (become activated) towards the end of a joint's range of motion.

The type III and IV fibres may also have a peripheral trophic role in the maintenance and production of the joint matrix components. The relatively large proportion of the type III and IV fibres may be a compensation for both the small size of these fibres individually, and the large area they would be required to cover in order to perform this role.

The cruciate ligaments appear to be innervated by both encapsulated (primarily types I, II) and unencapsulated (i.e., free nerve endings: types III and IV) sensory nerves. The presence of encapsulation suggests the nerve ending to be a LTMR. In this category, the types found have been Ruffini, Pacini and GTO-like receptors. This variety of receptors suggests the afferents from the ligament would be capable of relaying information about both dynamic and static stretch. Although the position and composition of the structure in which the receptor is embedded is important in determining the final receptor properties, it is still possible to suggest a relationship between receptor structure and stimulus modality. To this end, a brief outline of each receptor type for the knee cruciate ligaments is listed below.

STRUCTURE OF A SYNOVIAL JOINT: WITH AN EMPHASIS ON INNERVATION

Most joints in the extremities are synovial (apart from one or two exceptional structures such as the inferior tibio-fibula joint). Figure 5.2, shows a schematic representation of such a joint. Synovial joints are points of articulation between two (diarthroidal) or more bones. The interface between each bone is smooth and relatively frictionless. This is due mainly to the presence of a hyaline cartilage layer over the articulating surface of each bone. Synovial joints have a space between the articulating surfaces, which is filled with a lubricating layer of synovial fluid (the joint space). These joints are surrounded by a synovial membrane, which is a specialized, highly vascular secretory membrane. The synovial membrane is the only part of the interface which has a significant innervation. Nutrition for the hyaline cartilage layer derives from synovial fluid (therefore indirectly from the blood vessels in synovial membrane), as well as from the blood supply to the subjacent bone. The deeper vascular

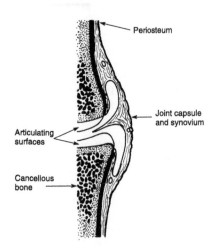

Fig. 5.2

Schematic representation of a synovial joint

structures, underlying the hyaline cartilage, are a further point of sensory and autonomic motor innervation.

These joints are also surrounded by series of ligaments, which appear to have the role of intrinsic stabilizers. These ligaments are also a major source of sensory feedback to the CNS. This role has been underplayed, especially in repair and rehabilitation, therefore, this area needs further discussion. However, before this is possible one needs to appreciate the complexity of the joint in its entirety.

SPECIALIZATIONS TO TENDONS AND LIGAMENTS NEAR JOINTS

Due to the requirements of movement and joint mechanics, there are many specializations to the simplified 'synovial joint' and 'muscle tendon.' As many of these structures have roles other than simply structural support, they will be mentioned here. Most of these structures probably have some neurological function, be it in the normal or 'pathological' functioning of the limbs.

Where tendon sheaths pass close to, or over, a joint capsule there is a need for some degree of protection of the former. This protection usually is in the form of a lubricated sheath or cover, which prevents direct contact and subsequent abrasion. The main type of structure used is the bursa. These structures are innervated at both the capsule and the tendon. The innervation to this region appears to be mainly slowly conducting sensory neurones (the so-called type III and IV), with free nerve endings. The innervation by these afferents become most noticeable when, due to abnormal wear, or injury, an inflammatory reaction takes place (bursitis). Swelling and pain are the main problem from the patient's perspective. However, neurologically this can generate abnormal movement (dyskinesia). If left unattended, the inflammation can develop into fibrosis between the sheath and tendon, which may result in the need for surgical intervention. Inflammation is most probably assisted, if not initi-

ated, by the presence of the type III and IV fibres and the neuropeptides they contain.

Ligaments are fibrous, and occasionally elastic structures which have roles as restraints and reinforcers. Most importantly, yet often ignored, ligaments act as adjuncts to the sensory receptor systems for feedback control of joint position, movement and force. The importance of such structures in proprioceptive feedback can be seen in any sports person who has had a cruciate ligament tear or prosthetic replacement of such. In these people, their knee stability is compromised, usually leading to continually recurring knee injuries. The only way of preventing this would be either by relinquishing their sporting activity or re-educating the use of the leg (with respect to muscle use: i.e., comprehensive rehabilitation) with the possible inclusion of a support during times of stressful use.

JOINT RECEPTORS AND THEIR PROPERTIES (E.G. THE KNEE)

A number of basic sensory receptor types have been described in or around the synovial joint capsule, meniscus and associated ligamentous structures. The predominant types of receptor are listed below. Although other types have occasionally been implicated elsewhere, for simplicity, these will not be included.

- *Ruffini are slowly adapting LTMRs with both a dynamic and static component. They are capable of signalling intra-articular pressure, static joint position as well as amplitude and velocity of joint movement: dependent upon location.*
- *Pacinian corpuscles are classically rapidly adapting LTMRs, with a low threshold to mechanical stress. They are inactive in an immobile joint or when the joint is moved at a constant speed; becoming active on acceleration or deceleration.*
- *GTO-like receptors: those associated with knee ligaments are slowly adapting receptors which have a higher mechanical stress threshold. They are completely inactive at rest and in immobile joints. It has been suggested that these organs best measure the tension in the ligament at, or towards, the extremes of its range; i.e., extremes of the movement range for the joint.*
- *Free nerve endings include the nociceptor population. Normally inactive, they become active either when subjected to abnormal mechanical stresses/deformation, or following introduction to chemical agents such as those found in an inflammatory response: e.g., bradykinin, prostaglandins, certain neuropeptides*
- *NB: These are all represented in the anterior cruciate (Johansson et al., 1991).*

The majority of the receptors present are found close to the ligament–bone interface, rarely in the deep connective tissue of the ligament, more often sub-synovially and in the more superficial fibrous layer.

FUNCTION OF THE DIFFERENT AFFERENTS

The type I and II joint afferents (fast conducting fibres) tend to have no resting discharge, and therefore would not be involved with signalling angle or position of the joint. They can be activated by low threshold mechanical changes such as gentle probing, touching and movement of the joint within its working range. The output from these receptors is related to the direction of the movement more than its intensity. They encode for intensity up to the noxious range, but are not 'nociceptors' *per se*. Instead, they may be described as being proprioceptive (relating to deep pressure sensation) and kinesthetic (relating to motion).

Type Ia muscle afferents tend to have no resting discharge, however, the type Ib and some type II do. The type Ia receptors signal dynamic change in length, whereas type Ib (GTOs) signal tension and type II muscle afferents signal length (therefore, position). The latter group also has a dynamic component, which could be interpreted as signalling rate of change (therefore, also speed of change).

About a third of the type III and IV afferents (slow conducting fibres) have resting discharges, usually below 0.5 Hz. They can be grossly divided into four groups based on their mechanical sensitivity:

- *easily, activated by non-noxious mechanical stimuli;*
- *marginally, activated by non-noxious mechanical stimuli; or*
- *not activated by non-noxious mechanical stimuli (two groups).*

The latter ones were either activated by noxious stimuli or not activated by noxious stimuli.

- *Only the ones activated by noxious stimuli alone can be accurately referred to as* **true nociceptors**.
- *The group of afferents showing mechano-insensitivity fall into the category of 'silent' or 'sleeping' nociceptors. These appear to be of great importance in inflammatory disorders, where they become active due to the presence of the chemicals, in the periphery.*
- *They appear to be involved in mediating the inflammatory state (Schaible and Grubb, 1993).*

A similar profile of afferents has been reported for the rat ankle joint, indicating a potential similarity between the control mechanisms in existence for feedback of proprioceptive, kinesthetic and nociceptive information. This also suggests a similarity of control for complex peripheral joints in general.

It is only fair to say, at this juncture, that the absolute presence of receptors means little without consideration of the results of activating them. Therefore, the next section will attempt to describe how sensory information can influence motor control.

THE MOTOR RESPONSE

For this part of the discussion, we need to introduce the motoneurone and its connections at the spinal level. A basic form of interaction between the sensory and motor systems is the reflex. The shortest reflex is the so-called 'monosynaptic' reflex Fig. 5.3.

A dynamic Ia stretch receptor forms part of the intrafusal fibre system found in all skeletal muscles. These Ia receptors can be activated by either a slight overload of the muscle during contraction, a sharp stretch of the muscle during rest (e.g., tendon tap), or by the shortening of the contractile element of the intrafusal fibre (during pre-programmed movement). The impulses generated by the Ia stretch receptor are rapidly conducted along its Ia afferent fibres to the spinal cord, where they cause neurotransmitter to be released from their terminals. The important synapses, with respect to this reflex, are around dendrites of the homonymous α-motoneurones in the ventral horn of the spinal cord. These motoneurones then discharge action potentials, which then travel along their Aα axon to the extrafusal fibres of the homonymous muscle. At the terminals of the motoneurone the action potential releases acetylcholine which crosses the neuromuscular junction and initiates the production of an action potential in the muscle fibre's cell membrane leading to contraction.

This reflex is idealistic and overly simplistic, in as much as there are many stretch receptors affected by any stimulus and many motoneurones affected even by a single stretch receptor afferent! Each motoneurone, when activated, will

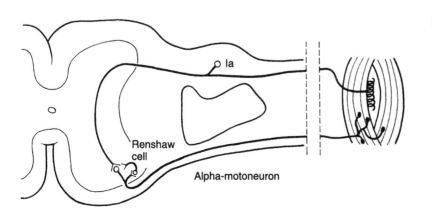

Fig. 5.3

The stretch reflex

la

Renshaw cell

Alpha-motoneuron

stimulate more than one extrafusal fibre. In fact, the ratio varies from one α-motoneurone to four extrafusal fibres in some proximal muscles (finger movement), to 1:4000 muscle fibres in postural muscles such as soleus. The number of motoneurones excited by the Ia afferent impulse and the number stimulated 'sufficiently' to produce an action potential are not the same. This depends on **inhibition**.

MOTONEURONES

The cellular component of the spinal grey matter is highly organized into columns, dictated by the genetic and embryological canalization of the pathways; even though this may not be immediately apparent. This organization allows for the processing of information to be performed efficiently and reliably. With respect to the motoneurones in the ventral cord, there are a number of features of interest:

- *Adjacent pools tend to perform similar functions.*
- *The gross arrangement consists of the flexor pools in the medial ventral cord and the extensor pools in the lateral ventral cord.*
- *A fusiform arrangement of motoneurones in each motoneurone pool (Burke et al., 1977).*

Each motoneurone innervates a different number of skeletal muscle fibres. The ratio of motoneurones to muscle fibres varies quite dramatically, approximately averaging 1:300 in the dorsal interosseous muscle and 1:2000 for the gastrocnemius muscles in humans.

These features may be functionally important with respect to input both from the segmentally related afferent neurones and the upper motoneurones from higher centres. A small proportion of Ia afferents innervate heteronymous motoneurone pools, furthermore, upper motoneurones also appear to innervate motoneurones from pools of muscles with a similar function. These overlaps may only be small, probably becoming significant only during high force requirements. However, this system would allow smooth recruitment of adjacent muscles as and when the need arises, such as when extra force is required. Use of this system becomes apparent when somebody attempts to lift a mass close to their maximum capacity.

α:γ RATIOS

As with the ratio of motoneurones to muscle fibres, this ratio is very much related to the degree of refinement in muscle control required. The muscles of the hands are more densely supplied with motoneurones than those of our limbs. The following example is given to allow an appreciation of the level of innervation: the soleus (cat) contains about 25,000 muscle fibres and only 50 muscle spindles, however, there were only 100 α-motoneurones to 50 γ-motoneurones (Matthews, 1972).

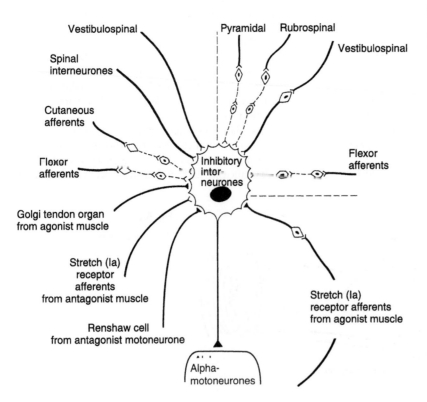

Fig. 5.4

Influences on the inhibitory interneurone

INHIBITION AND MOTONEURONES

Motoneurones are large, fast-conducting and highly excitable neurones with a propensity for discharging high frequency volleys of action potentials. At first glance, this would not appear to be an ideal cell to have controlling your motor system. However, these characteristics are prerequisites, with an obvious need for a strong modulating influence. Therefore, it is obvious there is a need for motoneurones to be under a 'firm controlling hand'. This is the role of the inhibitory interneurones found alongside the motoneurone pools in the ventral horn (see Fig. 5.4 for outline).

It has been roughly estimated that 90% of the neurones in the CNS have an inhibitory function. Indeed, a number of inhibitory neurones exist, which are primarily related to motoneurone function.

The two main examples are:

* *The Renshaw cell: helps control (moderate) the output frequency of the motoneurone.*
* *The Ia inhibitory interneurones: help coordinate those inputs, which suppress motoneurone activity (normally motoneurones are under tonic inhibition).*

Direct input from upper motoneurones or muscle spindle receptors can lead to excitation of the required motoneurones and subsequent muscle contraction. Indirect input from upper motoneurones, Golgi-tendon organs, joint receptors, skin receptors, antagonist muscle stretch receptors, etc. can lead to increased inhibitory tone and suppression of muscle activity. The inhibitory interneurone acts as a focal point for these inputs. The ceasing of muscle activity due to lack of 'interest' or increased negative feedback may work through this route. Indeed, the inhibitory interneurone is one point at which a central fatigue mechanism may reside.

SPILLOVER BETWEEN MOTONEURONE POOLS

These effects are most probably actioned via changes in inhibitory interneurone activity as well as direct stimulation of the motoneurone. The spillover between pools can be demonstrated by linking your hands and attempting to pull them apart. As the force applied is slowly increased, you should notice the sequential recruitment of those muscles not directly involved initially. The sequence of recruitment runs distal to proximal. If you really work at it, the legs and neck musculature will also become involved. Part of this action is the result of a release from 'descending' inhibitory tone. This effect can be used clinically when patients have weak reflexes, undertaking what is referred to as the Jendrassik manoeuvre (clenching teeth to facilitate reflexes in the limbs) can reinforce the reflexes to allow a more appropriate and informative assessment of the patient.

So far, only unilateral reflexes have been considered. In the real world of movement, it is easy to demonstrate that this is not the case. In one sense muscle activation may follow the third law of mechanics, namely every action has an equal and opposite reaction. For every agonist muscle contraction there will be a degree of spinal inhibition onto other motoneurones, innervating the ipsilateral antagonist muscles. In addition, however, there also appears to be a contralateral effect: the equivalent agonist muscles' motoneurones would be inhibited, whereas their antagonist muscles' motoneurones will be excited. Such a mirror image can be seen when you have to withdraw your hand or foot from an unpleasant stimulus. Simultaneous to the withdrawal of the limb, there is an extension of the contralateral limb (crossed extension reflex). In dysfunction of one limb, these reflex pathways will probably be involved in altering the use of the normal contralateral limb.

ARTHROKINETIC (OR JOINT AND LIGAMENT RECEPTOR MEDIATED) REFLEX

The previous text has centred on the role of stretch (and other muscle) receptors, tendon organs and skin afferents in modulation of muscle activity. This is not the full story, however. To more fully understand motor control and joint stability, we also need to consider the ligamentous receptors (the arthrokinetic reflex) and the autonomic nervous system.

It is obvious from the above text, that ligaments associated with the knee (and most probably other synovial joints) have a significant innervation and appear to have a real functional significance with respect to muscle activity. From their classic experiments on cat ankle and knee joints Freeman and Wyke (1966, 1967a,b) concluded that there was a considerable contribution from joint receptors in the normal coordination of muscle activity in both posture and movement. As one well-researched example, the anterior cruciate has a definite effect on the activity of the hamstrings. Recent studies have shown that tensioning of the ACL causes an increase in hamstring tension. It has been suggested that this has a protective role, preventing anterior tibial translation (Sjolander and Johansson, 1997). The ACL is also integral in the accuracy of proprioception around the knee joint in human subjects. There was an increase in inaccuracy from approximately 4° in people with intact ACLs to 10° in those without an ACL (Barrett, 1991). These ligament receptors are not omnipotent, however. It is now reasonably well accepted that, at least with respect to the ACL, ligament receptor stimulation does not normally affect the α-motoneurone (skeleto-motoneurone) directly. However, under heavy stretch there does appear to be a direct effect. **Instead the ligament receptors appear to exert their effects via changes in γ-efferent activity.** These efferents alter the intrafusal muscle components' degree of contraction and thus the tension of the stretch receptor. By applying tension to the stretch receptors, there is an increase in sensitivity of these receptors to further stretch. There is also, and arguably more importantly, an increased resting discharge from the stretch receptors onto the motoneurone pool for that muscle. This may manifest itself in an increased motor activity, i.e., muscle tension. The importance of these relatively few ligamentous afferents to conscious proprioception and potentially also to motor control was recently shown indirectly. Stimulation of the mid-ACL during knee surgery resulted in a consistent somatosensory evoked potential in the cortex (Pitman *et al.*, 1992). This reinforces the statement made earlier concerning the relative number of afferent types and their apparent significance.

NUMBER OF RECEPTORS IN RELATION TO FUNCTION

There are very few LTMRs in the ACL, yet their information is capable of reaching the cortex. One may infer from this that the information they carry is important with respect to conscious aspects of proprioception. There is also the suggestion that it is not the number of receptors, but the type of information they carry which determines the degree of cortical activation. It also may be reasoned that if there are more than enough receptors to perform the task at hand then there may be some other 'more local' role, which we are as yet not privy to.

A further sign of the relative importance of these ligaments and their receptors derives from observations of the effects of injury. Chronic knee injuries relate to atrophy and weakness of the knee extensors particularly, but the flexors are by no means unaffected. It has been suggested that the muscle atrophy, and consequent decrease in diameter, were primarily the result of a decreased type 2 (fast contracting, force generating, fatiguable) skeletal muscle fibre volume or numbers. This is as yet to be resolved, however, the muscles' capacity to produce force when there is ligamentous damage does appear to be less than normal. This change in force output is not simply due to the decrease in muscle mass. When the mass of the muscle was taken into account and the damaged knee compared to the contralateral 'undamaged' knee, there was still a disparity with the lower force being produced by the muscles of the damaged leg (Sjolander and Johansson, 1997).

THE ROLE OF ARTHROKINETIC REFLEXES: CONCLUSION

Ligament receptors of the same structure to those in muscle (the so-called GTO-like receptors of the ACL) produce a different response from those associated with the musculature. Stimulation of the anterior cruciate indirectly causes (via the γ-loop) an increase in tension produced by muscles, which stabilize or reinforce the knee joint. A similar mechanism appears to exist for the ankle joint. It would appear that, instead of inhibiting motoneurone activity, the ligament receptors promote it. In addition, the ligament receptors do not recognize 'agonist' and 'antagonist' muscles on the basis of flexion and extension. Instead, they lead to an increase in tone of both, thus leading to a greater rigidity in the system and safeguarding against abnormal displacement of the joint.

DAMAGE AND REHABILITATION

The best form of recovery from ligamentous of damage does not involve simply trying to strengthen the muscle: the system would tend to fail at sub-maximal loads anyhow. Instead, **successful rehabilitation appears to follow strengthening of**

the proprioceptive feedback system and the use (coordination) of those muscles involved in normal movement patterns.

Again using the ACL as an example: with an intact ligament, the treatment would attempt to strengthen the structures and develop a greater appreciation of proprioception in the area. If the ligament is damaged, then strengthening alone may be inappropriate, instead the emphasis should be on developing the proprioception of the adjacent muscles and ligaments which remain intact. Only when this is optimally achieved should one concentrate on strengthening the muscles further.

In neither case should the strength training be based on single muscle repeated exercises. Coordination of the muscle into normal movement should instead form the basis of the strengthening exercises.

AUTONOMIC INVOLVEMENT

It is important to consider this motor outflow for many reasons, not least its role in peripheral vascular regulation, digestive system (nutritive supply) and temperature regulation. The majority of these actions are relatively unfocused, widespread effects; however, if the disorder is distal to the ganglion (sympathetic nervous system) it may produce a focal change. There are a number of disorders related to hyper- or hypo-activity in the sympathetic nervous system. These disorders can have vascular, hydrotic and pain components (e.g., reflex sympathetic dystrophy). In addition to the disorders associated with the peripheral autonomic nervous system, histological studies have found potential autonomic nerve fibres in and around the intrafusal fibres near to the sensory receptors (Desaki, 1990). As a consequence, one must also consider the possibility that there is a role for the autonomic nervous system in modulating spindle activity and muscle function. This activity is a potentially more subtle effect, which may go unnoticed by the practitioner.

There are two ways in which the autonomic nervous system may affect muscle function, directly:
- *Alteration (vasoconstriction) of the muscle blood flow.*
- *Alteration of muscle nerve activity: depression of the spindle receptors, excitation of the type III receptors.*

In man, the main vascular effect of the sympathetic nervous system is vasoconstriction. Thus, initiating exercise will lead to a potential reduction in blood flow initially. Any vasoconstriction will obviously affect the function, potentially leading to hypoxia, cramping and pain: hypoxia has been shown to alter both LTMR and HTMR sensitivity. However, the normal reaction would be offset by a resultant increase in blood flow, following the waste product build-up. Other potential vasodilators could be released from sensory nerves sensitive to the waste products (including heat) and the increased muscle activity. These sensory nerves appear to be type III, CGRP containing, afferents. CGRP release, as a consequence of their increased activity, has been postulated as a potential source of vasodilator activity within muscle. Acupuncture and trigger point literature has begun to implicate these afferents to explain the mechanisms underlying aspects of their treatment.

The direct effects of adrenergic compounds on intrafusal sensory receptor activity has also been the subject of study. Adrenaline was shown to **depress** the activity of muscle spindle receptors of type I and II. In contrast, type III and IV receptors were apparently **excited** in the presence of catecholamines and hypoxia. The latter effect was developed if these receptors were irritated by a constant mechanical stimulus at a noxious intensity (Kieschke *et al.*, 1988). This may not only have a consequence with respect to pain, it may also affect feedback control. The depression of type I and II fibre activity could allow the muscle to reach either a greater degree of, or a greater rate of stretch during exercise. The type III fibre excitation could potentiate the spasm in a muscle following damage! The excitation of type III fibres may also facilitate vasodilation within the muscle during times of increased activity, however, the concomitant increase in sympathetic mediated vascular tone may negate this change.

INFLAMMATION AND THE PRIMARY AFFERENT RECEPTOR

In **inflammation**, the activity of the afferents themselves changes. Again the knee has been the subject of extensive study and, therefore, data from the knee will be used to support the following text; however the changes observed are probably also manifest in other structures.

Abnormal or excessive wear causes irritation, and thus stimulation, of some afferents with free nerve endings (type III and IV). Apart from signalling discomfort, which can result in gait disturbance, etc., such irritation can cause a peripheral release of the neuropeptides contained in the afferents. Two of the most extensively studied neuropeptides are SP and CGRP.

Neuropeptides such as SP and CGRP have various actions in mammals. In normal tissue the release is minimal, but it may be sufficient for the neuropeptides to have a role in the trophic maintenance of the tissue matrix components. Following irritation of these nerves, the neuropeptides are released in greater quantities. This has been associated with the initiation and actual production of an inflammatory reaction. More specifically, CGRP can induce a local vasodilatation, whereas SP can lead to extravasation of plasma proteins (from the vascular system) leading to an oedema. The two together have had such actions as neutrophil attraction, macrophage/monocyte activation and numerous tissue stimulatory effects ascribed to them. The combined action results in the formation of a neurogenic inflammation.

Apart from the oedema and other vascular changes, a noticeable feature of an inflammatory reaction is that of the change in resting neuronal traffic from the region. To some degree this would be expected due to the damage. However, microneurographic recording reveals that the increase in neuronal traffic is not specifically nociceptive, in that:

- *Resting activity (measured as total activity in the nerves) increased six-fold.*
- *There was, apparently, a two-fold increase in the number of LTMRs (more nerves excited by weak mechanical stimuli).*

- *The number of action potentials per unit time in response to knee joint movement increased seven-fold (Schaible and Schmidt, 1996).*

All in all, these changes, as a response to an acute inflammatory reaction, lead to an enormous amplification of the afferent signals reaching the CNS. These changes were primarily ascribed to the **peripheral sensitization** of nociceptors (either the HTMRs, true nociceptors or the 'silent' variety). The aspirin-like drugs (the non-steroidal anti-inflammatory drugs; NSAIDs) have been shown to reduce both the increases in spontaneous and mechanically-induced activity.

Further stages in nociceptive amplification, and therefore altered function, comes with **central sensitization**. In addition, there are also neuroplastic changes associated with use of the afferent pathways. Some of these changes are associated with altered genetic expression of neurones in the pathways. Whether the sensitization occurs centrally or peripherally, it will still lead to an amplification of the sensory stimuli from the affected site. These changes will, of course, affect the output through both the motor systems (autonomic and somatic). In a patient suffering pain in their hand, there may be a state of partial flexion (withdrawal response) to protect the hand from further damage, along with signs of increased autonomic activity. The latter will not necessarily be localized to the limb unless there is some peripheral compromise to the autonomic component of the nerve bundle.

The altered motor function should regress as the pain subsides. However, if the dysfunction alters a joint's activity, all the muscles crossing that joint will also be affected. These activity changes will be wide-ranging, probably affecting other muscle groups in the limb and, via reflex pathways, muscle activity in other limbs and more proximal structures. Programming for the recruitment of muscles resides in the spinal cord and above (higher CNS centres). These centres will attempt to adapt to the weakening muscles and the relatively large bombardment of afferent activity from the damaged region. The adaptation in the CNS will be minimal at first, merely re-routing signals and adapting other less commonly used motor pathways. However, with time, those systems used to facilitate the damaged one will supplant them as the predominant pathway. The continual use will consolidate their place as the primary system for that movement, with programmes being designed around the changed priorities. These changes rely on the nervous system's ability to adapt, this ability is known as **neuroplasticity**. Reversal of these changes will depend on re-instituting the original pattern of use. This will need to be rehearsed just as with any 'new' movement pattern.

THE CONSEQUENCES OF DAMAGE

As mentioned above, afferent input from the LTMRs in periarticular tissue affects efferent activity (muscle tone). Inappropriate afferent impulses may cause aberrant activation of the muscles. This would be apparent in those 'postural' muscles proximal to the spine as an inappropriate change in tone. This can be detected using manual palpation methods. In the more distal, 'phasic' musculature, the aberrance may be manifest as a greater difficulty in controlling fine movement and force generation.

Normal activation and use of the muscular system relies on continual, reliable, input from the LTMRs. The rate of LTMR discharge is affected by both damage to the periarticular tissue (i.e., inflammation, muscle/tendon strain, ligament sprain) and degeneration of the articular tissue. Damage or degeneration will impair the use of a joint and, therefore, also affect the postural and kinesthetic input. A result of this would be altered use and can be the generation of new motor patterns. The new patterns will affect the sequence of muscle activation, strength and force generation properties of the affected muscles. All the structures involved would undergo some degree of structural remodelling in compensation. These changes are easy to initiate, especially where a high demand is put on a young and still excessively plastic system: i.e., young athletes (Cosgarea and Schatzke, 1997)

DEVELOPMENT AND MAINTENANCE OF THE CENTRAL NEURONAL PATHWAYS (NEUROPLASTICITY)

Plasticity is not just a capability of muscle, ligament, joint surfaces and bone, it can also occur in the nervous system. The extent of connections and ease of activation of any neuronal pathway appears to be use-dependent: i.e., has a competitive element. The firing of a neurone can cause gene expression change. The production of new proteins maintains the viability of the cell and, with an adequate nutrition supply and metabolism, allows for increased synaptogenesis. This means that neuronal systems can become triggered more easily and consistently with practice. There appears to be a creation and 'strengthening' of synapses within the functional pathways.

There is, of course, a 'down side' to everything. Those neuronal systems not used regularly will degrade, with their extra synapses and facilitated pathways being reduced to the 'default' minimum! Therefore, if there is damage to either the peripheral nerve, or the motor system, it can lead to altered priorities. These will change the bias with respect to which synapses are strengthened or weakened, even lost. The subsequent remodelling will take time, however, as the changes will have to be 'unlearned' before full (and appropriate, i.e., 'normal') use of the system returns. Therefore, the rehabilitative process will need to take into account the 'relearning' of the original motor patterns after the damage has healed (or better, concomitant with the healing process). This process could take as long again as the injury has been in existence. Indeed, as well as simply addressing the rehabilitation of the injured region, one should also perforce be considering the rehabilitation of the adjacent and other associated musculature (remember the kinematic chain!).

Age and use of the motor systems are only two of the factors affecting plasticity. Arguably more important is the frequency with which the injured individual has been required to learn new motor patterns. The ability of any system to react to imposed change appears to be dependent (to some extent) on use and the external pressures causing a need for adaptation to change. These are components that are not always assessed by rehabilitative practitioners, and which may allow some patients to be 'fast-tracked' through a rehabilitation programme.

FACILITATING CHANGE

Neuroplasticity can also be related to changes in facilitation of neuronal pathways following a noxious stimulus. In this case, there are changed priorities in the second order (spinal) neurones and higher centres caused by a short period of 'high' activity in nociceptors. This makes it easier to activate some second order neurones (especially those which sample a wide variety of sensory modalities from LTMRs to nociceptors), namely those with a wide dynamic range (WDR). Once sensitized, these neurones can easily be excited by LTMR activity alone. This is then interpreted as being nociceptive (or painful) by the higher brain centres. Such a change equates with the generation of a secondary zone of high sensitivity to touch, which is perceived as pain (hyperalgesia), around the main site of damage (the primary site). Other sequelae are related to increased inhibition onto associated motoneurones (preventing voluntary use) and increased sensitivity to stimuli leading to hyperactive withdrawal reflexes. The whole picture is one of protection. One such change in central processing of primary afferent information is referred to as the *wind-up* phenomenon. This is a form of learning akin to that seen in many other brain areas. It can be initiated by a short duration high frequency burst of nociceptor activity. Wind-up can be a relatively short-term facilitation (hours to days), but can lead to those pathways becoming used predominantly.

Wind-up can alter movement patterns by changing the weighting of the inputs and outputs through the spinal cord. If reinforced, this can lead to more permanent change because, as mentioned above, synapse development is use-dependent: nerve fibre terminals appears to migrate from inactive synapses and stay with functional synapses. Therefore, the trend is always towards the formation of functional connections.

The element of plasticity allows the easy building and rebuilding of recruitment patterns for slightly differing tasks. The importance of a use-dependency of muscle recruitment has only recently been recognized and utilized in both training and rehabilitation regimes. The days of single muscle development in isolation of the task it will be called on to perform are now passing. Training and rehabilitation requires rehearsal of the use as well as, or even instead of, simply lifting a mass repetitively.

GREATER DEGREES OF PERIPHERAL NERVE TRAUMA

CONTRIBUTING FACTORS AND CAUSES

Changes to neuronal firing within the periphery may be as a result of injury to the axons themselves, independent of the receptor site. This could be as a consequence of many forms of disorder, which will either directly or indirectly affect the nerve, i.e.:

- *Direct trauma to other adjacent tissue.*
- *Over- or misuse of muscles/ligaments.*
- *Altered or compromised blood flow to the nerve.*
- *Inflammatory disorders.*
- *Space-occupying lesions.*
- *Autoimmune reactions.*
- *Hormonal disorders.*
- *Altered biochemistry/nutrition.*
- *Altered or deficient nutrition.*

Usual scenarios include direct trauma or compression/traction as the nerve root passes over, under, around or through ligaments, muscles or bone. Areas of focal demyelination (see this more as a breakdown in the integrity of the myelin sheath than a total removal) can occur which will not damage the axon as such. The result is an area where the action potential can only be conducted along the axon in the same way as it would along an unmyelinated axon. This method is slower than the normal saltatory conduction possible along myelinated axons, and hence the conduction velocity across this region is reduced. These reductions in conduction velocity are often used as a diagnostic confirmation in entrapment neuropathies; they can also be used to locate the sites of entrapment, or to determine if there is involvement of more than one joint, i.e., sites of multiple compromise, a.k.a. double or triple crush injury.

Obvious sequelae of such complaints are dependent on the degree of compression or damage as well as the time from the initial injury. There is a relationship between the vulnerability of an axon to the effects of nerve compression and the axon's diameter and degree of myelination, as well as its position in the nerve bundle. However, it is difficult to determine these characteristics without dissecting your patient. Fortunately, there is a relationship between these characteristics, conduction velocity and to some extent type of sensation, which can be employed in such situations. The most quickly conducting fibres are the Ia afferents and α-motoneurones (Fig. 5.2). These are also some of the earliest fibres incapacitated by a decrease in their blood flow, as would be found in nerve compression. The most obvious signs of this include muscle weakness and atrophy in the myotome affected. The next largest sensory fibres carry information of use in proprioception, vibration and fine touch: it is these sensations which are next affected. To compound the problem, the degree of damage can be from total loss to barely affected. The latter can sometimes be more irritating, as the nerve will exhibit characteristics of an amplifier to sensations such as vibration.

THE ENTRAPPED NERVE AS AN AMPLIFIER

Any area of nerve that is only occasionally compromised will not necessarily 'demyelinate'. Instead it may have a slightly depolarized membrane potential, due to lack of nutrients/O_2

or local inflammation. This will cause it to be more excitable in that region, but it will also be more difficult for it to repolarize quickly after an action potential has passed. The phenomenon which results from this change in character is known as reverberation: the nerve membrane potential will oscillate in response to the first action potential and thus produce some more. As the strength of the signal at the receptor is coded in both the number of action potentials and their frequency, this effectively will amplify the original signal.

Such phenomena can easily be exhibited on any peripheral nerve by occluding its blood supply for a short while (sitting cross-legged on a hard surface, or placing your arm over the back of a chair (compressing the radial nerve on the humerus) for around 10–20 minutes). Induction is slow and usually not noticeable until proprioception is required. At this point, people attempt to move the limb and exhibit many of the signs of a peripheral nerve sensory-motor deficit. The limb is immobile and there will be spontaneous sensations of temperature change and tingling, which can become uncomfortable. If recovery is hindered, vibration sensation can be amplified and the muscle contractions uncontrollable, the latter due either to poor feedback or too few motoneurones available for activating the muscle. As a rule of thumb, the fine afferent (small diameter: HTMR) input is usually less affected than that of the large fibres (LTMRs) by a decreased blood flow due to vascular damage, nerve compression or inflammation. The presence of normal pain sensation (nociception) without fine sensation would suggest the existence of this type of neuropathy. During recovery, the types of fibre affected and the sequence of their involvement is reversed and the change **most noticeable**. This can be therefore the most effective method of demonstration.

PAIN RELIEF, LARGE FIBRES AND THE GATE THEORY

Manipulative therapists often use this mechanism to explain some of the effects of manipulation. Apart from the sensory deficit, a consequence of loss of fine sensation is also a reduction of competing input into the spinal cord. Dynamic sensations from LTMRs are usually deemed to be of higher importance because they give information about change. The need for the higher centres to be kept aware of change has caused this input to be given priority. In real terms this means that the more dynamic LTMR input prevents the more static HTMR input from exciting its second order neurone. Therefore, HTMR information, such as nociception, is prevented from reaching the higher centres and, thus, conscious awareness.

DEGENERATION OF AXONS

If the damage to the nerve is more extensive (vascular occlusion, physical trauma, or myelin degeneration), then the area of nerve affected will start to degenerate. The part of the axon proximal to the site of damage tends to survive (at least for a time). However, the distal section will no longer be obtaining nutrients and replacement proteins from the cell

soma and thus degeneration occurs. This type of degeneration is termed **Wallerian degeneration** and follows a specific
pattern. The site of damage will be the earliest to exhibit
change, which includes fragmentation of the axon and myelin
sheath and formation of lipid droplets (this can occur very
shortly after damage: i.e., within 24 hours). Soon after,
phagocytes appear (dependent on the degree of inflammation
present) and undertake phagocytosis of the axon remnants
(within a week).

Proximal to the site of injury there may be no initial
indication of change. However, occasionally some axons
shown signs of retrograde chromatolysis (a reduction in
staining due to the decrease in Nissl substance, swelling of
the cell body with eccentricity of the nucleus and a decreased
mitochondrial presence). It is highly possible that these cells
will not survive the insult. The repair of such damage is made
less likely if the axon and myelin sheath are interrupted
(broken and displaced: i.e., axontmesis). Although Wallerian
degeneration may take place distally, there remains the possibility of repair if the basal lamina remains intact. If,
however, there is complete transection of the connective
tissue components of the basal lamina around the nerve as
well as the nerve fibre itself (neurontmesis), then the pos-
sibilities for repair become severely impaired.

REGROWTH AND REPAIR

The rate of peripheral nerve regrowth depends on many
factors, however, as a rule of thumb an axonal growth of
approximately 1–2 mm/day is not unreasonable. A major
factor is age: the older you are, the slower the nerves regrow.

Regrowth of axons through the myelin sheath (if intact)
has been shown to be sensitive to those antibodies selective
to cell surface markers expressed by the Schwann cells
(specifically the cell adhesion molecules, CAMs). These
CAMs act as markers for the regenerating axon so it 'knows'
where to go next. In addition to this, there is also evidence
indicating that growth factors, released from the denervated
areas and Schwann cells, attract the axons during regrowth.
A major limiting factor to regrowth is that of collagen formation (scar tissue), however, nerves will still attempt to find
their way around or through. Those axons not successfully
regenerating, or intact yet under constant irritation, may
produce a local ball of entangled neurites which can become
excitable (an example of the latter being Morton's neuroma).
This type of structure will create a sensitive region capable
of referring pain, or another sensation, to the dermatome,
which the affected nerve originally supplied.

The changes in expression of proteins required for
regrowth or repair are not specifically targeting those lost or
in need of replacement. The increase in production also
appears to include many other relatively redundant proteins.
In the latter group may be receptors which, if exhibited in
the membrane, could alter both the nerve's normal stimulus
and its sensitivity. In addition, any changes will not be specifically aimed at the damaged site. All other regions of the
nerve would be supplied with the new complement of
proteins. A consequence of this may be to stimulate the

primary afferent nerve to re-grow in the spinal cord as well
as at the peripheral site of damage. This may be made more
likely by the parallel loss of the fine afferents following nerve
injury. This latter change leaves the second order neurones
producing 'unclaimed' growth factors which will attract any
sensitive terminals. Such changes may make a fine touch
receptor connect to second order afferents of nociceptors

Such changes in growth do not require complete nerve
rupture. In some patients, the reaction to long-term irritation,
or poorly healed trauma in which the nerve root is tethered,
can be severe and debilitating even in an intact nerve, possibly as a consequence of altered gene-expression in nerves
that have reduced contact with the peripheral sites. **Sudex**
atrophy or reflex sympathetic dystrophy results from altered
sensitivity and excitability of the affected nerves: both sympathetic motor and primary afferent. Although not fully understood, it appears that the excessive sympathetic nervous
activity promotes the hypersensitivity of the fine afferents. It
is thought that the fine afferents may express new receptors,
which are directly or indirectly stimulated by the
catecholaminergic or peptidergic compounds released by the
sympathetic efferents. In their part, the sympathetic fibres
tend to become hyperactive giving the diagnostic signs of
vasoconstriction and hyperhidrosis distal from the trauma
site. The increased activity in both afferent and efferent are
compounded (if not caused) by the ongoing nerve trauma,
amplifying the activity as it passes through.

Clinical aside

In cases of reflex sympathetic dystrophy, manipulative treatment may help relieve sites of additional nerve compromise.
This is important as, in multiple nerve bundle compromise,
the outcome of the insult tends to be greater than that
expected from simply adding together the individual effects.
Patients with this type of disorder do not like to move the
affected limb. Therefore, it may be appropriate to address the
contralateral limb initially to gain their confidence and
redress the input from the contralateral receptors.

DIAGNOSTIC AND THERAPEUTIC CONSIDERATIONS

When considering the PNS, differential diagnosis must be
made through careful history-taking, observation and examination of the specific nerve functions (Morgenlander, 1997).
This regime is necessary in order to ascertain the type and
degree of loss, the probable cause and duration as well as the
site of insult. It is essential to recall that the largest diameter
nerves are the most vulnerable to compression, reductions in
temperature and, of course, as with any end organ, suffer the
consequences of reduced vascular supply. With this in mind
diagnosis of a peripheral lesion must look towards finding
evidence of reduced function of both large diameter sensory
and motor axons. Examination of the sensory system is beset
with problems, especially when it requires the patient to
respond with perceptual comparison of applied cutaneous
sensory stimuli. Examples of such problems would include
the overlap of sensory supply to a region (especially in the
upper extremity), and the 'alertness' and understanding of the

patient in their reply. Comparison is a necessary tool, often helping the patient and practitioner determine the 'normal' values for comparison with the 'abnormal'. With respect to the pain, which often associates with the 'abnormal,' there are a number of definitions which might help in clarification and comparison of the situation as well as increasing the practitioner's own appreciation of the situation.

- **Spontaneous pain**
  Burning, shooting, lancinating in quality
- **Paraesthesia**
  Spontaneous or evoked non-painful sensation which is abnormal (e.g. tingling)
- **Dysaesthesia**
  Spontaneous or evoked painful sensation which is abnormal
- **Hyperalgesia**
  Exaggerated painful response to a normally painful stimulus
- **Hyperpathia**
  Exaggerated painful response generated by painful or non-painful stimuli
- **Allodynia**
  Painful response to a normally non-painful stimulus (Elliott, 1994)

The examination of the extremity should be capable of determining the cause of a problem. The basic delineation needs to resolve whether the problem is a consequence of:

- *direct trauma;*
- *a compensatory mechanism;*
- *a peripheral or central neuropathy; or*
- *a systemic effect (e.g., inflammatory/hormonal).*

At this point, consideration should be given to the neurological scenario that may have allowed for the complaint to occur and any ramifications from its effects on the neuraxis.

Observing for differences in any accompanying motor response may aid your assessment. Motor examination can be considered to have two aspects, that of somato-motor and that of viscero-motor. However, it should be remembered that these functions are linked and subserve each other. The largest diameter axons are those of the α-motoneurones, so careful examination of muscle function is of prime importance by assessment and comparison of motor strength, fatiguability and by palpation, observation and questioning as to the presence of fasciculations or fibrillations within the muscle(s). Signs of electrical activity within fibril or fascicle of a muscle at rest would indicate peripheral axonopathy and would be expected to occur approximately 7 days post insult. Alternatively, a similar pattern may suggest ventral horn disease or a lesion at the neuromuscular junction. Definitive diagnosis, may require the use of electrodiagnostic studies (electromyography) of peripheral nerve function. However

the distribution of muscles involved will be a key to making an appropriate diagnosis, i.e., is a single muscle involved? If a number of muscles are involved the question must include location; are they all distal to a single nerve branch? If a root lesion is suspected, are all the compartments for that level involved (anterior, posterior and postural)?

Therapeutically, the choice of treatment would then be to direct healing in a manner that promotes a permanency and is not detrimental to the function of another body part. Chiropractic manipulation of any joint is performed with the intent of restoring 'normal' movement patterns. It is important to realize that such an intervention can have an effect both locally, segmentally and both supra- and infra-segmentally. The changes in relationship of joint angulation following manipulation can have a profound effect on the afferent input. Part of this will result from changing the sensitivity of the muscle spindles, the rest will manifest through changes in the ligamentous and joint capsule receptors described above.

If aware of the above effects, one may decide, on a therapeutic basis, to reduce the impact of treatment on the rest of the body. This can be done by modifying treatment to include facilitation or enhancement of either a cross-cord mechanism or an ipsilateral motoneuronal pool, in order to strengthen or weaken a muscle's functional activity. One should also consider that these mechanisms may well have been involved in the origin of a complaint. This principle may also be of use if there is the need to immobilize an area due to instability whilst still wishing to increase muscle tone and normal vascular supply. Examples of this could include:

- *the exercising of a hand and wrist whilst the elbow is immobilized; or*
- *flexion of a contralateral elbow, to facilitate treatment about an elbow restricted in flexion.*

Consideration should always be given to cerebellar involvement, as any reduction in cerebellar afferent input will have consequences in both vestibulospinal output and thalamocortical and basal ganglionic loops. Loss of type I firing from dynamic joint afferents will especially reduce cerebellar modulation; furthermore, it should be remembered that vestibulospinal output to the spinal intrinsic musculature is essential for spinal column stability. Having a stable spinal column is integral to the stabilization of all extremity movement, not to mention the dynamics of the intervertebral spaces.

The ability of chiropractic treatment to facilitate the controlling influences of motor control, via complex feedback loops (involving thalamus, cortex, palleocortex, neostriatum and subthalamic nuclei etc.), should not be overlooked. Lesions to any of the control regions can result in a variety of obvious movement disorders; athetosis, ballismus, tics, rigidity and tremors for example. However, it should also be noted that more subtle disorders may also result from a minor change in afferent or efferent feedback.

REFERENCES

Anand, P., Terenghi, G., Warner, G., Kopelman, P., Williams-Chestnut, R.E. and Sinicropi, D.V. (1996) The role of endogenous nerve growth factor in human diabetic neuropathy. *Nat. Med.* **2**, 703–707.

Apfel, S.C. and Kessler, J.A. (1996) Neurotrophic factors in the treatment of peripheral neuropathy. *Ciba Found. Symp.* **196**, 98–108; discussion, 108–112.

Barrett, D.S. (1991) Proprioception and function after anterior cruciate reconstruction. *J. Bone Joint Surg.* **73B**, 53–56.

Burke, R.E. *et al.* (1977) Anatomy of medial gastrocnemius and soleus motor nuclei in cat spinal cord. *J. Neurophysiol.* **40**, 667–673.

Cosgarea, A.J. and Schatzke, M.D. (1997) Knee problems in the young athlete: a clinical overview. *J. Musculoskeletal Med.* **14**, 96–109.

Desaki, J. (1990) A reexamination of multiaxonal nerve endings innervating intrafusal muscle fibers of the Chinese Hamster. *Arch. Histol. Cytol.* **53**, 449–454.

Elliott (1994) Taxonomy and mechanisms of neuropathic pain. *Sem. Neurol.* **14**, 195–205.

Freeman, M.A.R. and Wyke, B. (1966) Articular contributions to limb muscle reflexes. The effects of partial neurectomy of the knee joint on postural reflexes. *Br. J. Surg.* **53**, 61–69.

Freeman, M.A.R. and Wyke, B. (1967) Articular reflexes at the ankle joint: an electromyographic study of normal and abnormal influences of ankle joint mechanoreceptors upon reflex activity in the leg muscles. *Br. J. Surg.* **54**, 990–1001.

Freeman, M.A.R. and Wyke, B. (1967) The innervation of the knee joint. An anatomical and histological study in the cat. *J. Anat.* **101**, 505–532.

Henderson, C.E., Phillips, H.S., Pollock, R.A. *et al.* (1994) GDNF: a potent survival factor for motorneurons present in peripheral nerve and muscle (see comments) [published erratum appears in *Science* 1995, **267**, 777]. *Science* **266**, 1062–4.

Hill, C.E., Jelinek, H., Hendry, I.A., McLennan, I.S. and Rush, R.A. (1988) Destruction by anti-NGF of autonomic, sudomotor neurones and subsequent hyperinnervation of the foot pad by sensory fibres. *J. Neurosci. Res.* **19**, 474–482.

Johansson, H., Sjolander, P. and Sojka, P. (1991) A sensory role for the cruciate ligaments. *Clin Orthop*, 161–178.

Kieschke, J., Mense, S. and Prabhakar, N.R. (1988) Influence of adrenaline and hypoxia on rat muscle receptors in vitro. In: *Progress in Brain Research* (W. Harmann and A. Iggo, eds), Amsterdam, Elsevier Science, pp. 91–97.

Matthews, P.B.C. (1972) *Mammalian Muscle Receptors and Their Central Action.* London: Edward Arnold.

Morgenlander, J.C. (1997) Recognising peripheral neuropathy. How to read the clues to an underlying cause. *Postgrad. Med.* **102**, 71–72.

Pitman, M.I., Nainzadeh, N., Menche, D., Gasalberti, R. and Song, E.K. (1992). The intraoperative evaluation of the neurosensory function of the anterior cruciate ligament in humans using somatosensory evoked potentials. *Arthroscopy* **8**, 442–447.

Riaz, S.S. and Tomlinson, D.R. (1996) Neurotrophic factors in peripheral neuropathies: pharmacological strategies. *Progr. Neurobiol.* **49**, 125–143.

Schaible, H.G. and Grubb, B.D. (1993) Afferent and spinal mechanism of joint pain. *Pain* **55**, 5–54.

Schaible, H.G. and Schmidt, R.F. (1996) Neurobiology of articular receptors. In: *Neurobiology of Nociceptors* (C. and F. Belmonte ed.), New York, Oxford University Press, pp. 202–219.

Sherrington C.S. (1906) *The Integrative Action of the Nervous System.* London, Constable.

Sjolander, P. and Johansson, H. (1997) Sensory endings in ligaments: response properties and effects on proprioception and motor control. In: *Ligaments and Ligamentoplasties* (L.H. Yahia, eds), Heidelberg, Springer-Verlag, pp. 39–83.

6

Rehabilitation: the role of exercises as supportive therapy in the treatment of the peripheral joints

Daniel Lane

INTRODUCTION

In its most general sense, rehabilitation can be said to be concerned with the restoration of normal form and function after injury or illness (*Dorland's Medical Dictionary* 24th edn). Within the musculoskeletal field of health care, it follows that rehabilitation is concerned with restoring musculoskeletal function (Liebenson, 1990). Increasingly, there is a shift to more vocational-style rehabilitative programmes, with emphasis placed upon attaining and maintaining specific skills.

As far as spinal rehabilitation is concerned, it is now generally accepted that effective management should no longer consist of rest and passive therapies, but instead should be concerned with early exercise and functional restoration. As a result of this paradigm shift, there has been an explosion in the number of spinal rehabilitation facilities. These 'high-tech' centres can fulfil an important role for some chronically disabled, but they are frequently expensive and considered inappropriate for most patients (Liebenson, 1990), including those with peripheral joint problems. Instead, it is recognized that 'low tech' assessment and management is the cost-effective modern management of choice for the great majority of neuro-musculoskeletal disorders. Practitioners in small private practices are ideally suited to providing this type of health care, and it is predicted that they will come to dominate the management of neuro-musculoskeletal disorders.

Therapeutic exercise plays a major role in rehabilitation. Indeed, Liebenson (1990) writes that manipulation and exercise are the two methods that have become the standard of care in the delivery of high quality neuro-musculoskeletal health care. He advocates an approach to rehabilitation that encompasses biopsychosocial considerations, primary conservative care, secondary functional restoration, and tertiary multidisciplinary functional restoration, where indicated, for those who are chronically disabled. It is accepted that improving muscular flexibility, coordination, strength and endurance, stretching soft tissues, and proprioversory re-

education form an integral part of functional restoration. This is the role of therapeutic exercise.

EFFECTS OF THERAPEUTIC EXERCISE

Therapeutic exercise is directly concerned primarily with the prevention of dysfunction, and the development and maintenance of strength, mobility and flexibility, stability, coordination and balance, and functional skills (Kisner and Colby, 1996). It also assists with the promotion of local vascular dynamics, including the production and movement of synovial fluid which is required for cartilage nutrition and maintenance and hence joint function.

TYPES OF THERAPEUTIC EXERCISE: AN OVERVIEW

Open versus closed kinetic chain exercise
The kinetic chain deals with the anatomical–functional relationship in the upper and lower extremities. Open kinetic chains refer to a series of joints in which the distal segment is free. A closed kinetic chain is a series of joints in which the distal segment is fixed or weight-bearing. Because the extremities, particularly the lower extremity, function in a closed-chain mode most of the time, it follows that closed-chain exercises are more likely to lead to a faster functional recovery. Indeed, closed-chain exercises have become the treatment of choice in the field of sports injury rehabilitation.

Isotonic exercise
This may be defined as exercise with constant resistance. It usually involves the use of free weights, pulleys, or weight-stations. Some of this apparatus may be complex and expensive. Isotonic muscle contraction is not common in day-to-day life, and for this reason its role in functional restoration is limited.

Isometric exercise
Isometric exercise involves muscular contraction performed without movement or a change in length of the muscle. The

vast majority of muscle action is accompanied by joint movement. For this reason isometric exercise also has limited application in functional restoration. However, it is not infrequently utilized in the early stages of a rehabilitative regimen, where joint movements would be likely to aggravate the early stages of recovery.

Concentric exercise
Concentric exercise occurs when a muscle contracts and shortens at the same time. Concentric activity is common, and concentric exercises lend themselves well to effective rehabilitation programmes.

Eccentric exercise
When a muscle contracts but lengthens at the same time eccentric exercise occurs. It is accepted that muscles develop more tension, require less energy and are more efficient when contracting eccentrically than either concentrically or isometrically. Eccentric activity is also common, and eccentric exercises also lend themselves well to effective rehabilitation programmes.

Plyometric exercise
This form of exercise, also known as 'stretch–shortening' drills, is an approach to isotonic exercise that combines speed, strength and functional activities. It is considered appropriate only in the later stages of rehabilitation of young active individuals who must achieve a high level of physical performance in a specific activity.

CONTRAINDICATIONS TO THERAPEUTIC EXERCISE

The presence of joint inflammation and effusion, joint hypermobility, malignancy, bone disease, unhealed fractures, pain, prosthetics, weakened connective tissue (e.g. post-injury, surgery, disuse, medication, e.g. corticosteroids), or systemic connective tissue disease are recognized as relative and in some cases, total contraindications to therapeutic exercise. Caution should be exercised if any doubt exists.

APPLICATION OF THERAPEUTIC EXERCISE

It is generally accepted that for best results, patients should follow a graduated pain-free exercise plan, advancing from one exercise to another as progress is achieved, and to continue at least until optimum functional recovery is attained. It is recommended that both subjective and objective assessments are used in order to monitor the patient's status and progress. Patients should also be encouraged to perform the exercises frequently, particularly in the early stages of rehabilitation. The exact numbers of repetitions and sets, and the weights involved, are of course dependent upon the patient's exact problem, stage of recovery, physical status and general health. Practitioners are encouraged to modify the procedures as required.

SPECIFIC REHABILITATIVE PROCEDURES

There follows an extensive, but not exhaustive, programme for the rehabilitation of peripheral joints. It is not intended to be a step-by-step guide, but a source of reference from which the practitioner may select and modify the most appropriate rehabilitative procedures. A 'low-tech' approach has been taken wherever possible, using the minimal of apparatus. Many of the exercises listed may also be performed in water, with the obvious advantages that a non-weight-bearing environment bestows.

THE TEMPOROMANDIBULAR JOINT

RELAXATION

General whole body relaxation techniques
These are often of benefit to patients with temporomandibular joint problems (Kessler and Hertling, 1983). Practitioners are directed to texts dedicated to such techniques, including biofeedback and stress management.

Local relaxation techniques
The patient is instructed to regularly clench the jaw firmly for a few seconds and then relax, allowing the jaw to fall open. The patient should try to concentrate on the sensation of tightness over the temples as well as the jaw itself.

PASSIVE RANGE OF MOTION

Finger stretch
The patient may be able to gently passively increase the range of motion by gently stretching the mouth open using the fingers and/or thumb on the upper and lower incisors.

Proprioceptive neuromuscular facilitative stretching techniques
These are particularly useful in helping to rehabilitative hypermobile and/or unstable temporomandibular joint problems. The patient should place a number of spatulus (or similar spacing object) just inside the mouth, between the teeth. Then the patient gently bites down onto them, holding the bite for a few seconds and then relaxing, repeating a number of times. This procedure can then be repeated with increasing numbers of spacers, to gently increase the range of motion.

Variation
A variation of this exercise negates the need for separate spacers. The patient should place their tongue on the back of the hard palette, with the mouth held gently open. The patient than gently performs isometric contraction to depress the palette, against the resistance of the tongue. The patient may provide additional resistance by applying gentle pressure to the chin.

ACTIVE RANGE OF MOTION/STRENGTHENING

Corrective digital pressure

Whilst watching in a mirror, the patient should open and close the jaw with his/her fingers positioned over the temporomandibular joints. The patient should try to gently correct any abnormal movements using digital pressure. This will provide both visual and tactile corrective biofeedback.

Corrective molar pressure

As stability increases the patient may perform additional exercises to improve function. The patient should place the tip of the tongue on the palatal contralateral maxillary molars. The patient then slowly opens and closes the mouth whilst pressing the tongue into the molars.

Note

Neck rotation facilitates motion of the ipsilateral temporo-mandibular joint. The practitioner may wish to consider this when prescribing and/or adapting the above exercises.

PROPRIOCEPTIVE EXERCISES

Both passive and active range of motion exercises should provide excellent proprioceptive training.

FUNCTIONAL RESTORATION

To include activities of daily living (ADL) e.g. chewing and specific functioning skills as required.

THE GLENOHUMERAL JOINT

PASSIVE RANGE OF MOTION

'Codman's' pendular exercises

The patient stands or sits, bending forward at the waist, such that the upper body is flexed forwards by approximately 45°. The affected upper limb is allowed to 'hang free'. The patient may gain support by holding onto a chair or table, etc. with the contralateral hand. The patient is instructed to gently swing the upper body so that passive movement occurs at the affected glenohumeral joint. Flexion, extension, abduction, adduction and clockwise and anti-clockwise movements should be performed by altering upper body movements. This exercise may be repeated with small weights in order to increase joint traction if required.

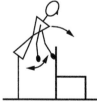

ACTIVE RANGE OF MOTION/STRENGTHENING

Finger-walking, supine

The patient lies supine, with arms laid next to their body.

The affected arm is internally rotated such that the palm faces the floor. The patient slowly abducts the arm by 'walking' it with their fingers along the ground.

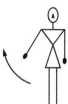

Finger-walking, standing

The patient stands facing a wall, about 10–12 inches away from it, and rests the hand of the affected limb against the wall. The patient then slowly takes the arm into forward flexion by 'walking' it with his/her fingers, within the active pain-free range of motion. This may be modified to include varying degrees of abduction, if the patient repeats the exercise and turns away from the wall, taking the shoulder gradually into abduction.

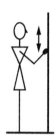

Finger-walking, sitting

The patient sits facing a table at approximately elbow height, with the hand of the affected limb resting palm-down on the table-top. The patient then slowly 'finger-walks' along the table-top taking the shoulder into flexion. This may be modified to include varying degress of abduction, if the patient repeats the exercise and turns away from the table, taking the shoulder gradually into abduction.

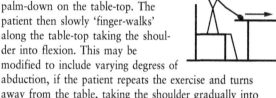

Active range of motion

The patient either sits or stands and gently moves the affected arm within the pain-free active range of motion. The patient may draw different figures in the air to help maintain interest and compliance. This may be modified by using weights to increase resistance, or squeezing an object such as a tennis ball which helps to stimulate the rotator cuff musculature.

CAPSULAR/SOFT-TISSUE STRETCHES

Self-traction

The patient may sit or stand, and gently holds onto an appropriate fixed object (e.g. door handle). The patient then slowly leans away, applying gentle traction to the glenohumeral joint. This may be performed with altered upper body positions (e.g. rotation of the trunk away), to create traction stress.

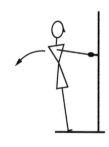

Anterior glide

The patient lies supine, leaning on the elbows and forearms. Next the patient gently relaxes,

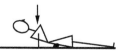

allowing their body weight to stretch the joint capsule and surrounding tissues.

Posterior glide
The patient lies prone, propped up on the elbows and forearms. Next the patient gently relaxes, allowing their body weight to stretch the joint capsule and surrounding tissues.

Adduction stretch
The patient flexes the arm to 90° and with the contralateral hand pulls the elbow into adduction, to stretch the posterior capsule.

Overhead stretch
The patient holds the affected arm overhead, whilst flexing the elbow. The contralateral hand applies gentle adductive and slight extension pressure.

Dumb-bell stretches
The patient lies supine on a table or bench holding a light weight, with the elbow flexed to 90° and the shoulder abducted to 90°. The patient then slowly externally and/or internally rotates the arm.

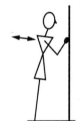

Standing press-ups
The patient stands at arms length from a wall, with their hands at shoulder height, resting against the wall. The patient then performs gentle 'press-ups'.

PROPRIOCEPTIVE EXERCISES

All joint movement will provide excellent proprioceptive feedback; however, the practitioner may consider additional exercises.

Wobble-board proprioception
The patient kneels with the hand of the affected shoulder or both hands resting on a wobble board, with the elbows locked into extension. The goal of this exercise is to maintain balance whilst performing small movements, created by moving the upper body.

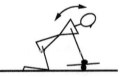

Oversized ball proprioception
The patient kneels alongside an oversized ball (e.g. gymnastic balls), with the hand of the affected shoulder resting on top. The patient gently rolls the ball around, whilst maintaining contact and balance with the hand.

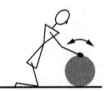

Normalizing scapulo-thoracic motion

The patient retracts the scapulae, then flexes the elbows to 90° and then slowly abducts the arms to 90°.

Functional restoration
The patient is encouraged to perform ADLS e.g. driving and specific functional skills as required.

THE ACROMIO-CLAVICULAR JOINT

Considering the proximity of the acromio-clavicular joint to the glenohumeral joint, and its role as part of the shoulder joint complex, most glenohumeral joint exercises will also benefit the acromio-clavicular joint. However, it should be noted that traction may tend to place excessive strain on the joint, and the practitioner should consider this when prescribing and/or modifying the exercises.

PASSIVE RANGE OF MOTION

'Codman's' pendular exercises
The patient stands or sits, bending forward at the waist, such that the upper body is flexed forwards by approximately 45°. The affected upper limb is allowed to 'hang free'. The patient may gain support by holding onto a chair or table, etc. with the contralateral hand. The patient is instructed to gently swing the upper body so that passive movement occurs at the ipsilateral glenohumeral joint; this will also create gentle movement at the affected acromio-clavicular joint. Flexion, extension, abduction, adduction and clockwise and anti-clockwise movements should be performed by altering upper body movements. This exercise should not be performed using weights.

ACTIVE RANGE OF MOTION/STRENGTHENING

Exercises given for the glenohumeral joint are suitable.

Resistance shrugs
The patient performs gentle shoulder shrugs with a light resistance (approx 1–2 kg). The weights should not be allowed to hang freely, as this may place strain on the acromio-clavicular joint.

PROPRIOCEPTIVE EXERCISES

Exercises given for the glenohumeral joint are suitable.

FUNCTIONAL RESTORATION

Exercises given for the glenohumeral joint are suitable.

THE STERNO-CLAVICULAR JOINT

Considering the proximity of the sterno-clavicular joint to the glenohumeral joint, and its role as part of the shoulder joint complex, most glenohumeral joint exercises will also benefit the sterno-clavicular joint. However, it should be noted that traction may tend to place excessive strain on the joint, and the practitioner should consider this when prescribing and/or modifying the exercises.

PASSIVE/ACTIVE RANGE OF MOTION/STRENGTHENING

Exercises given for the glenohumeral joint are suitable.

Shoulder rolling The patient gently rolls their shoulders backward and forwards. This may also be performed using light hand weights. The weights should not be allowed to hang freely, as this may place strain on the sternoclavicular joint.

Standing press-ups
The patient stands at arms length from a wall, resting the palms of hands against the wall at shoulder height. The patient then slowly leans forwards, performing 'standing press-ups', and then gently returns to the upright position.

FUNCTIONAL RESTORATION

Exercises given for the glenohumeral joint are suitable.

THE WRIST AND HAND

PASSIVE RANGE OF MOTION

Hand-shake
The patient should hold the affected hand in a loose grip with the contralateral hand, and gently guide the affected wrist and hand into all ranges of motion.

Rolling pin or tennis ball
The patient gently rests the affected hand, palm-down, on a rolling-pin or tennis ball. The patient then slowly encourages passive movement of the wrist or hand by guiding movement from the ipsilateral elbow, shoulder and upper body.

Digits
The patient gently holds the affected digit and moves the affected joint within a passive range of motion.

ACTIVE RANGE OF MOTION/STRENGTHENING

Gross movement
The patient simply moves the affected wrist or hand within the active range of motion. This may be repeated using a light weight to provide added resistance.

Exercise putty or tennis ball
The patient gently squeezes exercise putty or a tennis ball.

Functional restoration
In addition to ADLs the patient is instructed to perform intricate tasks, such as tieing and untieing knots, or transferring matches from one box to another, using grips created by the thumb and different fingers.

CAPSULAR/SOFT-TISSUE STRETCHING

'Hand-shake'
The patient should hold the affected hand in a firm grip with the contralateral hand, and apply gentle traction. This may be combined with small passive movements.

Digits
The patient gently holds the affected digit and applies gentle traction. This may be combined with small passive movements.

PROPRIOCEPTIVE EXERCISES

The active and passive range of motion exercises detailed earlier will provide excellent proprioceptive training.

FUNCTIONAL RESTORATION

The patient is encouraged to perform ADLs and specific functional skills as required.

THE ELBOW

PASSIVE RANGE OF MOTION

Table-top
The patient rests the affected elbow and forearm on top of a stable surface and encourages passive joint movement by moving the shoulder and upper body forwards, backwards, and leaning or turning from side to side. This may be performed with the hand of the affected limb resting either supinated or pronated.

Door handle
The patient stands gently holding a door handle with the hand of the affected limb. The patient then encourages passive joint movement by moving the ipsilateral shoulder and upper body forwards and backwards.

Hand-shake
The patient should hold the hand of the affected limb in a gentle grip with the contralateral hand. The patient then slowly encourages flexion, extension, supination and pronation of the elbow by controlled movements of the unaffected limb. This exercise may be performed with the affected limb either suspended or resting on a stable surface.

ACTIVE RANGE OF MOTION/STRENGTHENING

Gross movement
The patient simply moves the affected elbow within the active range of motion. This may be performed using a light hand-held weight to provide added resistance.

CAPSULAR/SOFT-TISSUE STRETCHING

Self-traction
Whilst performing passive range of motion exercises, the patient applies gentle traction to the elbow joint complex, e.g. during door handle or hand-shake exercises.

PROPRIOCEPTIVE EXERCISES

The active and passive range of motion exercises detailed earlier will provide excellent proprioceptive training.

FUNCTIONAL RESTORATION

The patient is encouraged to perform ADLs and specific functional skills as required.

THE HIP

PASSIVE RANGE OF MOTION

Standing
The patient stands on a lightly elevated stable surface (e.g. telephone directory) on the unaffected leg, such that the affected leg is suspended from the floor. The patient may require additional support, which may be provided by stabilizing themselves against a wall or chair. The patient then gently produces passive movement at the affected hip by slowly moving their upper body forwards, backwards, leaning and turning from side to side. This exercise produces gentle traction.

Kneeling
The patient is standing, with the knee of affected side flexed to 90° and resting on a chair alongside, which will also provide additional support. The patient then gently produces passive movement at the affected hip by slowly moving forwards, backwards, leaning left and right and turning from side to side.

ACTIVE RANGE OF MOTION/STRENGTHENING

Standing
The patient stands on a slightly elevated stable surface (e.g. telephone directory) on the unaffected leg, such that the affected leg is suspended from the floor. The patient may require some additional support, which may be provided by stabilizing themselves against a wall or chair. The patient then slowly moves the affected hip into its active range of motion. Additional resistance may be provided with the use of small ankle weights.

Isometrics
The patient either sits or lies supine or prone on a comfortable surface and performs isometric contraction of the muscle groups required.

Mini-squats
The patient performs 'mini-squats' by squatting to no more than 90° knee flexion. This may be performed with various amounts of hip rotation and/or abduction. The patient may require support from a chair or wall.

CAPSULAR/SOFT-TISSUE STRETCHING

Refer to standing passive range of motion.

Supine
The patient lies supine, with a towel wrapped around the ankle of the affected leg, which 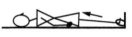 is secured to a stable object (e.g. large piece of furniture). The patient may thereby create traction at the affected hip joint by gently pulling on the towel with the affected leg. This may be combined with internal and external rotation.

PROPRIOCEPTIVE EXERCISE

The active and passive range of motion exercises detailed earlier will provide excellent proprioceptive training.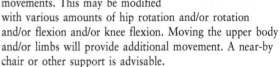

Wobble board training
The patient stands with both feet on a wobble-board, and maintains their balance whilst performing gentle movements. This may be modified with various amounts of hip rotation and/or rotation and/or flexion and/or knee flexion. Moving the upper body and/or limbs will provide additional movement. A near-by chair or other support is advisable.

FUNCTIONAL RESTORATION

The patient is encouraged to perform ADLs (e.g. cycling, walking) and specific functional skills as required.

THE KNEE

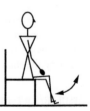

PASSIVE RANGE OF MOTION

Sitting
The patient sits such that their feet do not reach the ground. The foot of the

unaffected limb is hooked under the ankle of the affected limb. The patient then passively flexes and extends the affected knee by actively flexing and extending the unaffected knee.

ACTIVE RANGE OF MOTION/STRENGTHENING

Sitting
The patient sits such that their feet do not reach the ground, and then slowly moves the affected knee within the active range of motion. Additional resistance may be added with the use of ankle weights.

Squats
The patient performs gentle squats.

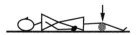

Supine extension
The patient lies supine with a small roll under the affected knee. The patient then performs gentle extension of the knee, against the resistance of the roll.

CAPSULAR/SOFT-TISSUE STRETCHING

Sitting
The patient sits such that their feet do not reach the ground, with small weights fastened around the ankle of the affected knee. Gentle traction is created, and small active or passive movements of the knee may be added.

Supine
The patient lies supine. A towel is wrapped around the ankle of the affected leg, which is secured to a stable

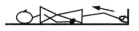

object (e.g. large piece of furniture). The patient creates traction at the affected knee joint by gently pulling on the towel with the affected leg. This may be performed with various amounts of knee flexion.

PROPRIOCEPTIVE EXERCISE

The active and passive range of motion exercises detailed earlier will provide excellent proprioceptive training.

FUNCTIONAL RESTORATION

The patient is encouraged to perform ADLs (e.g. cycling) and specific functional skills as required.

THE FOOT AND ANKLE

PASSIVE RANGE OF MOTION

The patient holds the affected foot/ankle and gently moves it within the passive range of motion.

Sitting
The patient sits comfortably, resting the affected foot on a rolling-pin or ball. The patient then encourages passive movement at the foot and ankle by moving the ipsilateral knee and hip.

ACTIVE RANGE OF MOTION/STRENGTHENING

Sitting/supine
The patient moves the affected foot/ankle within the active range of motion, either sitting or supine. This may be repeated using the added resistance of shoes or other foot weights. Drawing figures in the air helps to maintain interest.

Intricate tasks
The patient performs intricate tasks such as picking up objects (e.g. marbles, towels) with their toes.

CAPSULAR/SOFT-TISSUE STRETCHING

Supine
The patient lies supine. A towel is secured to a stable object, and also wrapped around the affected foot. The patient creates traction at the affected foot and/or ankle joint by gently pulling on the towel with the affected leg.

PROPRIOCEPTIVE EXERCISE

The active and passive range of motion exercise detailed earlier will provide excellent proprioceptive training.

Standing
The patient stands on both feet, and maintains their balance whilst performing gentle general body movements. Additional movement may be obtained by moving their upper body/limbs. This may be performed with the eyes closed, and also standing on the affected foot/ankle only.

Wobble-board training
The patient stands with both feet on a wobble-board, and maintains their balance whilst performing gentle movements. Additional movement may be obtained by moving the upper body/limbs. This may be performed with the eyes closed, and/or standing on the affected foot/ankle only.

FUNCTIONAL RESTORATION

The patient is encouraged to perform ADLs (e.g. walking) and specific functional skills as required.

CONCLUSION

REFERENCES

Kisner, C. and Colby, L. (1996) *Therapeutic Exercise – Foundations and Techniques*, 3rd edn. Philadelphia, PA, F.A. Davis.

Liebenson, C. (ed.) (1990) *Rehabilitation of the Spine – a Practitioner's Manual*. Baltimore, MD, Williams & Wilkins.

FURTHER READING

It is intended that the exercises that have been outlined, modified where necessary, will form part of an integral treatment and management regimen, directed towards safe and fast functional restoration.

Cailliet, R. (1991) *Shoulder Pain*. Philadelphia, F.A. Davis.

Codman, E.A. (1934) *The Shoulder*. Boston, MA, Thomas Todd Co.

Cookson, J.C. and Kent, B.E. (1979) Orthopaedic manual therapy: an overview. Part I: The extremities. *Phys. Ther.* 59, 136.

Cyriax, J. (1982) *Textbook of Orthopaedic Medicine*, vol I: *The Diagnosis of Soft Tissue Lesions*, 8th edn. London, Baillière Tindall.

Deusinger, R. (1984) Biomechanics in clinical practice. *Phys. Ther.* **64**, 1860–8.

Dontigny, R. (1970) Passive shoulder exercises. *Phys. Ther.* 50, 1707.

Gray, G.W. (1993) Understanding closed chain exercise. *Rehab. Ther. Prod. Rev.* Nov/Dec, pp. 16–17.

Hawkins, R.J. and Mohtadi, G.H. (1991) Controversy in anterior shoulder instability. *Clin. Orthop. Rel. Res.* **272**, 152–161.

Jobe, F.W. and Pink, M. (1993) Classification and treatment of shoulder dysfunction in the overhead athlete. *J. Orthop. Sports Phys. Ther.* **18**(2), 427–432.

Kaltenborn, F. (1989) *Manual Mobilisation of the Extremity Joints: Basic Examination and Treatment Techniques*, 4th edn. Oslo, Odas Norlis Bokhandel.

Kamm, K, Thelen, E. and Jensen J.L. (1990) A dynamical systems approach to motor development. *Phys. Ther.* **70**, 763–775.

Keshner, E.A. (1990) Controlling stability of a complex movement system. *Phys. Ther.* **70**, 844–854.

Kesseler, R. and Hertling, D. (1983) *Management of Common Musculoskeletal Disorders*. Philadelphia, Harper & Row.

Lewit, K. (1985) The muscular and articular factor in movement restriction. *Manual Med.* 1, 83–85.

Magee, D. (1992) *Orthopaedic Physical Assessment*, 2nd edn. Philadelphia, W.B. Saunders.

Margery, M. and Jones, M. (1992) Clinical diagnosis and management of minor shoulder instability. *Aust. J. Physiother.* **38**(4), 269–280.

Mulligan, B.R. (1993) Mobilisations with movement. *J. Manual Manip. Therp.* **1**(4), 154–156.

Payton, O., Hirt, S. and Newton, R. (1977) *Scientific Basis for Neurophysiological Approaches to Therapeutic Exercise*. Philadelphia, F.A. Davis.

Wadworth, C. (1988) *Manual Examination of the Spine and Extremities*. Baltimore, MD, Williams & Wilkins.

Joint Manipulation

7

Temporomandibular joint examination and techniques

Daniel J. Proctor

INTRODUCTION

Head and neck pain are virtually epidemic in our society. It is commonly known that 86 per cent of the population experience some level of lower back pain in their lives and 25 per cent may be disabled with this condition. A lesser known fact is that 40 per cent of the population are afflicted with disabling head and neck pain. Almost three times as many people seek care for their disabling headaches as compared to lower back pain (20 million versus 7 million respectively) at a cost of 3 billion US dollars per year relative to 20 billion US dollars per year for lower back care (circa 1990) (White and Gordon, 1982; Kelsey, 1982). So many of our patients suffer from head and neck pain yet so little of our education focuses on this problem. The subsequent cost to the population in productivity, enjoyment of life and psychological strain has never been fully estimated (Schurr *et al.*, 1990).

The relevance of these facts to this chapter is most apparent when one considers the estimate that about 30 per cent of headache problems are caused by the temporomandibular joint (Reik and Hale, 1981). It is further estimated that 85–90 per cent of the population exhibit some aspect of temporomandibular joint pain dysfunction syndrome (TMJ–PDS) throughout their life (Saghafi and Curl, 1995).

Temporomandibular joint pain dysfunction syndrome (TMJ–PDS) is the subject of considerable debate due to its varied aetiological theories and variety of both successes and failures in treatment. The reports that so many different types of treatment have some efficacy relates to the reality that the condition is multifactorial (Marotta, 1993). As will be illustrated, the condition has a number of specific subcategories which are collected under one diagnostic label. Each component has a unique presentation and requires a different clinical approach.

Chiropractic management and specifically chiropractic treatment have proven to be an effective form of therapy for many aspects of this condition. In patients showing at least one sign or symptom, studies demonstrate that 3–40 per cent benefit from treatment (Saghafi and Curl, 1995). The greatest success of this profession's treatment comes from proper recognition of the condition and appropriate, timely intervention directed to the components of the syndrome.

Among all the health disciplines, TMJ–PDS is poorly understood, incompletely examined and often inappropriately treated. For the chiropractor, as important as knowing when to manipulate and how to perform the manipulation, is an understanding of when not to manipulate. If a course of manipulation has been provided, the practitioner should not assume that chiropractic involvement in the case is complete. This is too simplistic a view, suggesting that we only have one tool with which to assist a patient. Rather, it is important for the clinician to be as complete and comprehensive as possible.

There are few good examples in the literature of a complete description of the diagnoses and differential considerations for TMJ–PDS and its subcategories. As well, simple, 'low tech' examination procedures for daily practice are difficult to find. Lastly, the sort of treatment(s) and prognosis for each condition type needs to be presented in a collected format. The goals and objectives for this chapter follow these ideas. It is designed to be used by chiropractors with many levels of experience. It is also meant to provide information to other professional groups as we all work toward a better understanding of this condition.

ANATOMY, BIOMECHANICS AND PATHOLOGY

The TMJ–PDS can be managed with clinical efficacy and cost-effectiveness. However, the condition is multifactorial and therefore requires a multifactorial approach. Chiropractic management includes a unique assessment, manual methods including mobilization and manipulation, as well as adjunctive physiotherapy, exercise and clinical advice. While chiropractic treatment is both important and integral, it is not a stock approach or recipe. The clinician must fully understand the specific problem in order to discern the appropriate treatment. The goals of treatment are to decrease pain, tenderness and adverse loading within the joint and thereby limit disc degeneration. Intervention should restore normal function, return the patient to activities of daily living and manage aetiological factors to prevent recurrence (Saghafi and Curl, 1995). In respect of these comments it is important that a brief review of the anatomy, biomechanics

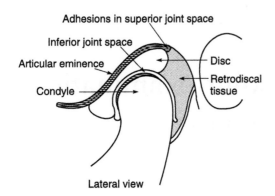

Fig. 7.1

Anatomy of the TMJ from the lateral aspect showing normal structures and the site of adhesion formation (adapted from Curl, 1995)

and pathology of the temporomandibular joint be presented to define principles and provide a rationale for the examination and treatments to follow.

The temporomandibular joint is a ginglymoarthrodial synovial joint with the capsule of the joint being well vascularized and innervated (Fig. 7.1). Synovial membrane lines both the inferior and larger superior compartments of the joint. The articular surfaces are lined with fibrous connective tissue rather than the typical hyaline cartilage of synovial joints, hence making the TMJ less vulnerable to degenerative changes and more apt to regenerate. This recovery is important because of the demands put upon the joint by repetitive compressive forces (Brand and Isselhard, 1986; Curl, 1995).

The articular disc is dense, fibrous collagen tissue and has two articulating surfaces. The superior surface (upper joint) articulates with the temporal bone, allowing linear articulation (translatory or sliding movement) with the mandibular condyle. The inferior surface (lower joint) permits rotary movement of the condyle around a horizontal axis (Helland, 1986).

The articular capsule and the temporomandibular ligament together are known as the true TMJ ligaments. Synovium lines the capsule and provides lubrication, nutrition, phagocytosis and immune functions. The capsule is composed of loose areolar connective tissue. It is loose anteriorly thus providing little stability to the joint as it translates forward. Clinically, this is significant in cases of whiplash or while performing a manipulation, since the anterior aspect is the weakest point of the capsule. It is reinforced laterally by the TM ligament and merges with the disc posteriorly where it is thicker. The TM ligament is the most important ligament conferring stability to the TMJ (Helland, 1986).

The retrodiscal tissue (RDT) is a continuation of the disc posteriorly which, unlike the disc itself, is highly vascularized and innervated. Functions of the RDT are that it produces a pseudodisc and more importantly synovial fluid. The pseudodisc occurs following a chronic dysfunctional state where the condyle no longer articulates on the disc but rather at its posterior margin. Once formed, the pseudodisc is functionally and histologically indistinct from the original disc except for its relative disordered matrix structure. The pseudodisc takes about one year to form (Saghafi and Curl, 1995).

As mentioned, the retrodiscal tissue is highly vascularized. If traumatized it will haemorrhage and this will lead to adhesion formation in the upper joint (Fig. 7.1). Treatment should be initiated early to minimize both the extent of the bleeding and the degree of adhesion formation. Encroachment of the condyle into the fossa (at the RDT) alters the production of synovial fluid (Fig. 7.2). Poor synovial fluid production decreases disc lubrication and joint nourishment. If this occurs simultaneously with disc malposition, the likelihood of subsequent degenerative changes and perforation is increased. While no firm proof of the cause of degenerative joint disease exists, it is suspected that it is caused by impact loading rather than by shearing stresses (Reik and Hale, 1981).

Collateral discal ligaments attach the lateral and medial poles of the condyle to the articular disc. These non-elastic ligaments are composed of collagenous connective tissue which, if intact and functional, prevent posterior and anterior displacement of the disc (Fig. 7.3) (Saghafi and Curl, 1995).

Recurrent dislocations of the disc decrease or change both the biconcave shape and the collateral ligament

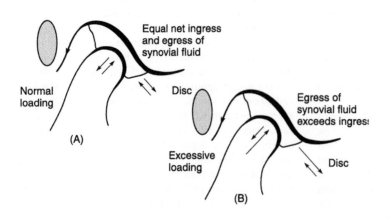

Fig. 7.2

Encroachment of the condyle into the articular fossa in (a) a healthy and in (b) an impact-loaded joint (adapted from Curl, 1990)

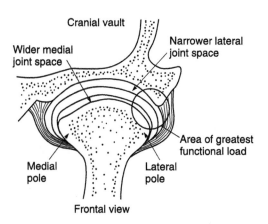

Fig. 7.3

Frontal view of the TMJ illustrating collateral ligaments stabilizing the disc and the site of greatest functional load (adapted from Curl and Saghafi, 1995)

Table 7.1

Muscle function in the TMJ illustrating the combination of muscles used in normal jaw movement

Muscle	O	C	P	R	LD
Masseter		+	+		
Temporalis		+		+	+
Medial pterygoid		+	+		+
Inferior lateral pterygoid	+		+		+
Digastric	+			+	
Superior lateral pterygoid		+			+

Opening (O), closing (C), protrusion (P), retrusion (R), lateral deviation (LD). (+) means the muscle is active in that movement.

function. Therefore, even if the disc is relocated following dislocation, the stabilizing structures are compromised or possibly absent (Curl, 1995).

Anterior displacement of the disc occurs: (1) when the collateral ligaments become deteriorated or damaged; (2) with significant wearing of the posterior portion of the disc; (3) following a whiplash injury; or (4) after a prolonged or difficult dental procedure, endotracheal intubation or wide-mouth yawning (Curl and Saghafi, 1995).

The disc most often dislocates anteromedially because of aberrant lateral pterygoid muscle function. This causes increased lateral collateral ligament stress, compromising joint stability. Other muscles involved in the TMJ are listed with their functions in Table 7.1 (Curl, 1995).

Adjacent structures include the tympanic artery, the cordi tympani nerve and the anterior malleolar ligaments. Tinnitus and altered auditory acuity are common in most cases of TMJ-PDS (Guralnick et al., 1978).

The discussion of TMJ-related anatomy would not be complete without some mention of the teeth. The most important teeth are the premolars to the molars. Improper occlusion during mastication or abusive habits (e.g. gum chewing) leads to aberrant loads being transmitted across the joint posterosuperiorly. This again may increase impact loading, microtrauma and accelerate degenerative joint changes (Curl, 1991).

Intercuspal position (ICP), when the teeth are in contact, is dependent upon the dentition. Presence or absence of teeth, height or loss of height of teeth, presence of prostheses and tooth alignment all may increase condylar movement and therefore increase intradiscal pressure and stress TMJ ligaments. Increased intradiscal pressure decreases discal nourishment. ICP also influences mandibular posture by disturbing the action of the surrounding muscles. The status of the dentition should also not be ignored in the evaluation of chronic neck pain (Curl, 1993).

Biomechanics of the TMJ must be considered at rest and during motion. Both ICP and mandibular postural rest position (MPRP) influence the health of the TMJ. Mandibular postural rest position (Fig. 7.4) is the result of muscle tone of the anterior and posterior cervical muscles, head posture and inherent elasticity of the muscles. Normally there is no occlusal contact between the teeth during MPRP. This space is usually 3–5 mm. This dimension is increased in mouth breathers and decreased in people who brux or clench. The importance of the MPRP is that it is a time for the TMJ system to rest, repair and allow ingress of synovial fluid (see Fig. 7.2). The condyle is disengaged from the fossa decompressing the RDT. Disturbances in the MPRP impact upon the remodelling and reparative processes and, therefore, interfere with the adaptive capacity of the joint (Curl, 1991).

Mandibular postural resting position will change throughout the day and throughout a person's life. Variance in this position is dependent upon emotional tension, parafunctional habits etc., as well as changes in posture, head

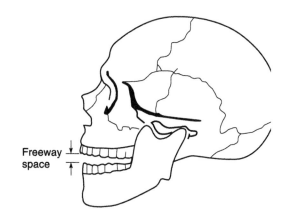

Fig. 7.4

Mandibular postural resting position exhibiting a freeway space of 3–5 mm (adapted from Curl, 1995)

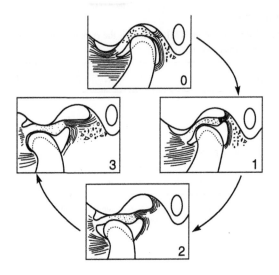

Fig. 7.5

Normal opening cycle showing the relationship of hard and soft tissues from mouth closed position (0) through 1, 2 and 3 finger widths to full mouth opening (adapted from Solberg and Blaschke, 1980)

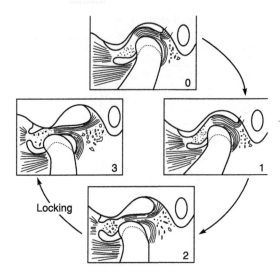

Fig. 7.6

Severe disc derangement illustrating a discal lock limiting full mouth opening (adapted from Solberg and Blaschke, 1980)

carriage, dentition, occlusal harmony, systemic disease (e.g. myasthenia gravis) or even psychological states.

Since MPRP influences the health of the TM joint it must be considered in TM joint assessment, treatment and prognosis. Factors that influence MPRP, specifically the cervical spine and posture, must also be considered (Curl, 1989).

There is a reciprocal relationship between the posterior neck muscles, anterior neck muscles and the muscles of the jaw. Any change in the tension in one group is experienced in the other two groups owing to the many postural reflexes that control head and jaw position. Furthermore, there is a distinct interdependence of function of the TMJ and upper cervical segments from occiput to the third cervical vertebra that can be seen in clinical examination of both areas. Mandibular retrusion and an altered closing trajectory are associated with an anterior head carriage and accentuated cervical lordosis. This can be observed in any patient where a forward head position and an increased cervical lordosis is adopted. A relaxed jaw spontaneously moves superoposteriorly. Head posture is probably the single most important factor controlling MPRP (Rocabado, 1983; Curl, 1995).

Patients with TMJ dysfunction often present with other spinal or postural problems such as scoliosis, lordosis, kyphosis, abnormal head carriage and leg length discrepancy. A laterality of the first cervical segment is often ipsilateral to malocclusion of the TMJ while a short leg is ipsilateral to TMJ malposition (Curl, 1989).

Malocclusion is one of the most common causes of TMJ dysfunction. The consequences of malocclusion include:

1   *disharmony between MPRP and ICP leading to a shift in the jaw and a change in shear and compressive*

forces. The symptoms of this include pain while clenching the teeth that is relieved when biting on tongue depressors or with use of a bite plate or night splint. Subjectively, the malocclused patient may experience joint noise, clicking or a feeling of stress while clenching (Curl, 1989).

2   *secondary muscle spasm or bruxism causing muscle fatigue, trigger points and spasm (Solberg and Clark, 1980).*

Two basic movements occur in the TMJ: rotation and translation. The entire normal opening cycle is represented in the cycle depicted in Fig. 7.5. **Rotation** is the motion observed in the lower joint. Disturbances of this motion are seen by the disc blocking condylar movement causing an inability to open more than 15 mm. This is an 'opening lock' (Fig. 7.6). **Translation** is a function of the superior joint where the disc and condyle slide or translate down the articular eminence in an anterior, inferior and medial direction. Disturbance of translation typically results in limited opening (generally 25–30 mm) or decreased laterotrusion. Often there is an 'opening click' as the condyle rides over the disc (Rocabado, 1983). Adhesions in the superior joint space would have the greatest effect during this motion (Fig. 7.7) (Curl and Saghafi, 1995).

Lateral shifting is an abnormal motion that contributes to shear and compressive forces. Laterotrusion movement involves a unilateral translatory cycle. The disc–condyle complex moves medially on the opposite or 'non-working' joint which is moving medially. On the non-working side, the articular eminence displaces the disc and condyle inferiorly. The disc and condyle on the 'working side' pivot until posterior motion is arrested by the TM ligament. This motion is particularly stressful to the ligaments and is believed to

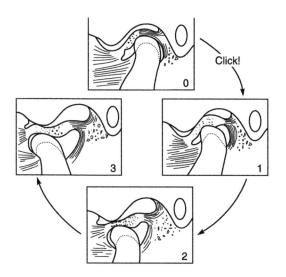

Fig. 7.7

Disc derangement or dislocation illustrating an opening click (adapted from Solberg and Blaschke, 1980)

accelerate TMJ joint breakdown (Saghafi and Curl, 1995).

The most common result of muscle hypertonicity, contracture and spasm is that the condyle is held posterosuperiorly behind the disc instead of on it. As the jaw starts to open, the condyle slides onto the disc with a resultant click (Fig. 7.7).

If the RDT becomes scarred (with its resultant loss of elasticity), if the disc is torn or perforated, or if the musculature, especially the superior lateral pterygoid, is very hypertonic and contractured, the condyle bunches up behind the disc and cannot ride over the edge. This is known as discal lock (Fig. 7.6). This problem is also associated with adhesion formation.

Adhesions (or fibrous ankylosis) begin to form in less than 24 hours after a trauma. Inability to control joint inflammation also causes adhesion formation. This fibrosis is clinically significant in 3 days and by 4–6 weeks it is in a phase where it is increasingly difficult to treat. Early treatment is necessary (Curl and Saghafi, 1995).

The final consideration amongst the common conditions encountered and treated by chiropractors is osteoarthritis (OA) of the TMJ. OA in this joint is often less symptomatic than expected. Studies illustrate that radiographic features of osteoarthritis are observed in the TMJ more often than symptoms are reported. Radiographic features of OA are seen in 8 per cent of patients with pain due to TMJ–PDS (Toller, 1974). However, it has been shown that OA is present in 40 per cent of cadavers over 40 years of age (Evan, 1990). Furthermore, X-ray features were seen frequently in asymptomatic individuals less than 40 years of age but were often absent in the predisposed patient (Guralnick *et al.*, 1978).

In summary, standard functioning of the TMJ is essential for normal chewing, swallowing and vocalization. Normal function depends on the smooth symmetrical alignment of

Table 7.2
Classification of temporomandibular joint conditions

Developmental abnormalities
including hypoplasia, hyperplasia, impingement of the coronoid process and chondromas

Diseases
intracapsular diseases including degenerative arthrosis, osteochondritis, rheumatoid arthritis, psoriatic arthritis, synovial chondromatosis, infections, necrosis, gout and metastatic disease

Dysfunctions
seen as impaired functional conditions and/or bruxism as a result of an increased psychomotor activity

the complex joint surfaces and on the congruency of an equally complex intra-articular disc-condyle mechanism. Subtle dysfunction in any specialized component may precipitate overall joint dysfunction.

AETIOLOGIES OF TMJ–PDS

A thorough review of all the aetiological factors and theories is beyond the scope of this chapter, however, a summary of the most relevant theories is important since it impacts on the comprehensive management theme presented herein.

Temporomandibular joint (TMJ) conditions can be classed as developmental abnormalities, diseases and dysfunctions (Table 7.2). Dysfunction is the most commonly accepted aetiology (Royder, 1981). Within this group, there is extreme disagreement as to whether temporomandibular joint pain dysfunction syndrome (TMJ–PDS) is a myofascial pain syndrome, articular dysfunction, dental malocclusion or psychological problem. The true aetiology is unknown. No investigator has ever attributed TMJ–PDS to only one aetiological factor (Marbach *et al.*, 1988). Most logically there are three major points of view: muscular-mechanical, psychophysiological and occlusal. In the literature of the past 15–20 years, different specialties were observed to have favourite interpretations. A multidisciplinary approach is most prevalent, and as will be shown, most pragmatic to understand this complex condition.

1 MUSCULAR-MECHANICAL THEORY

Long-standing mechanical structural imbalances lead to strain of the masticatory apparatus. The syndrome is insidious in onset, occurring over several years. The dysfunction and imbalance of the chewing mechanism are usually present for many years before there is enough discomfort to prompt the patient to seek professional help (Guralnick *et al.*, 1978).

At present the muscular theory is the most common. Supporting evidence includes the following:

- *Infiltration of surrounding muscles relieves pain although it may not control clicking.*

- *Electromyography supports the clinical finding of increased masseter muscle activity in TMJ patients.*
- *Excessive masticatory function produces pain (normal subjects can grind their teeth for half an hour without pain).*
- *Bruxism is associated with overuse of these muscles and is a common aspect of the syndrome. The muscles most commonly implicated are: lateral pterygoid (36%), medial pterygoid (17%), masseter and temporalis (0–3%). (Ieremia et al., 1990)*

2 PSYCHOPHYSIOLOGICAL THEORY

Psychophysiological theories suggest a patient's behaviour initiates the TMJ condition by creating a functional disturbance followed first by muscular changes and then dentition changes much later. When other stressful factors are layered on top of the TMJ imbalance, the intensity of the pathologic neural impulses from the TMJ dysfunction may increase substantially. Thereafter, the antagonizing symptoms of the syndrome, seen as the clinical manifestation of TMJ–PDS, begin and progress. If the disturbance persists, the symptoms will increase in magnitude until the patient experiences severe pain. Additionally, psychological distress and in the chronic case, depression, have been noted in these patients (Ieremia *et al.*, 1990; Tversky *et al.*, 1991).

Evidence supporting the psychophysiological theory includes:

- *A higher incidence of bruxism in TMJ–PDS patients.*
- *Nocturnal electromyographic (EMG) activity reveals increased grinding activity especially during stressful periods of life.*
- *TMJ–PDS patients are strong placebo responders: 44 per cent get relief with a placebo; 40 per cent find relief with a sham appliance; 64 per cent get relief with mock equilibration. (Muller, 1989; Paradiso and Scott, 1989)*

3 OCCLUSAL MECHANICAL DYSFUNCTION

Premature occlusal contacts cause muscle disharmony which then become painful. Mandibular dysfunction produced from dental disease, trauma, premature extractions or joint disease can produce secondary stresses (fascial or mechanical) (Curl, 1989)

Dental factors to consider include premature extraction of molars and subsequent drift of adjacent molars, therefore changing the angle of the teeth and losing occlusal contact. This prevents proper spacing of the teeth that erupt later. Dental caries, periodontal and other dental disease, application of excessive force during dental extractions and prolonged dental procedures can have equally damaging effects. The result is suggested to be malocclusion which allows deviation of the sliding action of the mandible from its normal and asymptomatic path (Rocabado, 1983).

Inflammatory diseases of the TMJ, including infectious arthritis, degenerative arthritis, rheumatoid arthritis, as well as mandibular or facial fractures, and recurrent dislocation

of the mandible will influence both occlusion and myofascial aspects (Curl, 1989).

For clinical application it should be noted that incidence of TMJ syndrome occurs maximally with loss of three to five teeth. Extraoral hyperfunction such as sucking or chewing on a pen, nails, tongue, cheek or lip, as well as hyperactivity without dental contact (e.g. biting lips) permit mandibular movements to increase causing greater shear and irritation to the joint (Curl, 1989).

Evidence to support an occlusal theory includes:

- *Fifty per cent of patients with splints show normal EMG activity.*
- *Condylar displacement posteriorly (retrusion) that can be seen on X-ray and can be clinically palpated is associated with TMJ–PDS.*
- *Disc displacement, as seen on arthrography, illustrates the origin of the blockage in movement. (Curl, 1989 and Rocabado, 1983).*

From these discussions a triad of components appear to be necessary for the development of TMJ–PDS:

1 *Tissue alterations including dental attrition, loss of posterior occlusion, iatrogenic causes, local pathology, arthritis and systemic diseases.*
2 *Predisposing factors, including intrinsic (genetic) and extrinsic (trauma, deleterious habits and nutritional changes).*
3 *Psychological factors which may predispose a patient to TMJ–PDS.*

Therefore, we have shown that the condition of TMJ–PDS is multifactorial and requires a multidisciplinary approach. Research into management demonstrates that no one professional discipline can resolve this condition alone. A team approach has been shown to be the most effective. (Chase *et al.*, 1988; Dolwick *et al.*, 1984)

PHYSICAL EXAMINATION, JOINT PLAY AND JOINT ASSESSMENT FOR THE TMJ

Following the introduction of increasing sophistication in TMJ assessment with electronic mandibular gait tracking devices and 'high tech' auscultation, the question of when to initiate treatment arises. While more enhanced equipment may have greater sensitivity in detecting an early or preclinical TMJ problem, earlier intervention provides little or no benefit to the patient (Black and Welch, 1993). In fact studies show that only 3–5 per cent of patients exhibiting signs and symptoms of TMJ dysfunction need treatment (Solberg and Clark, 1980). Logic suggests that it is safer and more effective to begin TMJ treatment when functional impairment can be demonstrated by traditional signs and symptoms (Curl, 1995).

Some clinics have taken to using questionnaires to identify and diagnose TMJ patients. Questionnaires used to define and classify TMJ patients are of questionable clinical value. They are difficult to design and utilize and in use they are either complete or accurate but they cannot be both (Curl, 1995).

A thorough history is the cornerstone of the examination. More information is derived historically than from any instrument. Typically only half of the TMJ patients will be aware of the findings subsequently elicited in the examination.

The questions asked in the history should be used to evaluate the behaviour, social, emotional and cognitive factors of the patient. The common history presented describes the onset of pain as usually insidious. There may be a history of previous clicking. The pain is located unilaterally in the pre-auricular area although it may be within the muscles of mastication. The pain character is steady but may be sharp or dull; sharp pain may be a greater indicator of joint pathology while dull pain indicates muscle dysfunction. The pain may radiate to the temple, jaw, teeth, neck, eye and possibly anywhere within the distribution of the cranial nerves. Aggravating factors include physical or emotional stress, fatigue and mandibular movement while relief is found with rest and immobilization. If the syndrome is of muscular origin moist heat, ice, tranquillizers, muscle relaxants and teeth spacers may be beneficial (Curl, 1995).

An outline for the physical examination is included as Appendix A to this chapter. The specifics include inspection for facial abnormalities, asymmetry, muscle hypertrophy, rheumatoid arthritis in the hands and signs of abusive oral behaviour (bruxing, biting of lips, nails or pens etc.). Signs of trauma such as small cuts, insect bites, furunculosis, abrasions or evidence of impact trauma should be noted. The overlying skin surface of the TMJ must be inspected for signs of inflammation or infection (i.e. redness, warmth, swelling or exudate). Significant swelling is usually seen with acute infection or systemic inflammatory disease. The entire posture should be reviewed, especially that of the neck and mandible. A standard examination for scoliosis, kyphosis and vertebral fixations, particularly in the upper three cervical segments, should also be included (Curl, 1989).

Palpation of the lateral joint and surrounding area follows visual inspection. In cases of suspected joint injury, the surrounding musculature should be evaluated for commonly seen reflex muscle splinting. A three-point grading system can be used when palpating the TMJ and surrounding area.

- *Grade I: patient feels slight tenderness; no obvious pain reaction.*
- *Grade II: pain gives rise to a palpebral reflex.*
- *Grade III: pain gives rise to a protective reflex (Faye and Shafer, 1989).*

Capsulitis and synovitis of clinical significance elicit a grade II or III reaction to palpation that is restricted to the area immediately surrounding the TMJ. Muscle palpation is used to detect pathology, muscle tone, trigger points and swelling. Palpation of the posterior joint is usually performed by placing the distal pad of the smallest finger in the external auditory meatus (EAM) as the patient opens and closes the mouth. This may detect inflammation of the posterior attachment and is used empirically to detect posterior displacement of the condyle, reciprocal clicking or crepitus (Curl, 1989).

Percussion in the TMJ involves two tests; one is general and the other is specific. General percussion is performed as the patient simply closes the teeth sharply. Improper striking sounds or pain suggest acute malocclusion, tooth abscess, periodontal disease etc., and warrant a dental referral. Specific percussion involves tapping each tooth with a tongue depressor to localize the problem to a certain tooth (Curl, 1995).

Auscultation with the bell of a stethoscope may be useful for detecting sounds in the TMJ. However, the clinical significance of being able to detect these sounds with the stethoscope is unknown. It may be no better than detecting sounds with a discriminating sense of touch (Curl, 1995).

A good set of callipers are useful for measurement of mandibular gait or the active range of motion. Normal opening is between 40 and 55 mm. The mandible should move equally and symmetrically without deviation or protrusion. Hypermobility is seen with opening movement greater than 55 mm and indicates the joint may be unstable or may dislocate if excessive force is applied thereby damaging an already lax joint capsule.

JOINT PLAY ASSESSMENT

Joint play measures at the end range of motion are important indicators of the type of pathology. Soft tissue pathologies like muscle or extracapsular structures have limited opening (25–35 mm) and a soft end-feel, while capsular limitations show a springy end-feel. A firm end-feel and limited opening (less than 20 mm) suggests disc derangement (Curl, 1995). Passive range of motion evaluates the ligamentous integrity of the joint and involves medial glide, open end-feel and distractive joint play. Medial glide is performed by contacting the lateral poles of the TMJ and alternately pressing medially. Limitations suggest the presence of intracapsular adhesions (Fig. 7.8).

Open end-feel is performed by using an intraoral contact on the mandibular incisors with a gloved and padded thumb in an inferior and slightly posterior direction at the end range of mandibular opening. A capsular or ligamentous end-feel is expected (Fig. 7.9).

Finally, distractive joint play also uses an intraoral contact with a gloved and protected hand; in this case, the clinician presses on the mandibular molars *inferiorly and laterally* at about 15–20 degrees. A capsular end-feel with little gapping is normal (Fig. 7.10) (Curl, 1993; Faye and Shafer, 1989).

PROVOCATIVE TESTS

Provocative tests for the TMJ include resisted muscle tests, a counter-irritant test, swallowing, jaw clenching, joint

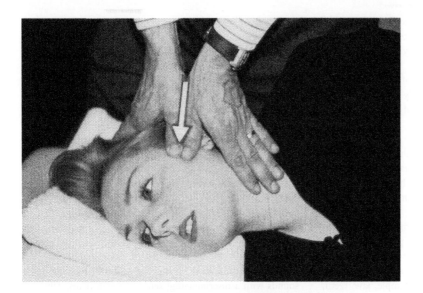

Fig. 7.8

Medial glide joint play assessment to detect intracapsular adhesions

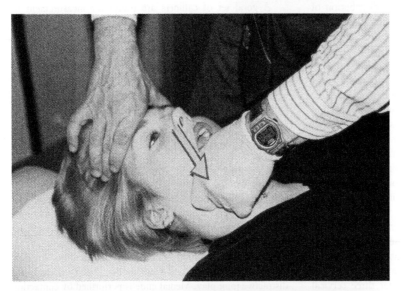

Fig. 7.9

Intraoral contact for open end-feel with posteroinferior distraction to detect capsular or ligamentous pathology

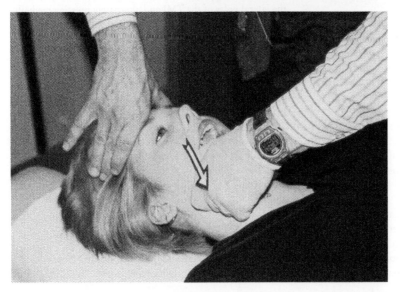

Fig. 7.10

Intraoral contact with distraction inferiorly and laterally to detect capsular involvement

compression-distraction and disc compression-distraction tests. The resisted muscle tests have been listed previously in Table 7.1.

A counter-irritant test looks for a change in the distractibility of the joint following application of ice or fluoromethane across the involved joint. An increase in mandibular opening indicates the problem is an external derangement, most likely muscle (Curl, 1995).

Aberrant swallowing or tongue thrusting is a significant stressor of the throat muscles and neck, and may be an aetiological factor in the patient's TMJ–PDS. A swallowing test has the patient take a sip of water with the lips slightly apart while the clinician observes. If the tongue is seen to thrust between the teeth a dental or speech therapist consultation is advised. Furthermore, involvement of neck and throat muscles in a TMJ condition can be discerned by having the patient attempt to swallow while the tip of the tongue is pressed lightly against the roof of the hard palate. Swan-like movements of the neck are signs of a positive test (Solberg and Clark, 1980; Curl, 1995).

During jaw clenching the clinician should have the patient clench the teeth with and without a tongue depressor between the molars. If pain is present in both cases, the problem is likely to be muscular since the muscles were active in the two situations. However, if biting on the tongue blade causes no pain while biting without a tongue blade reproduces the pain, the problem is a synovitis. This happens because the tongue blade is thick enough to disengage the condyle from the RDT and decrease the impact loading in the area (Curl, 1995; Solberg and Clark, 1980).

The joint compression–distraction test identifies internal joint involvement. In this case the mandible is first pressed posteriorly and superiorly (Fig. 7.11). Pain in this direction indicates retrodiscal tissue involvement. Conversely, pain provoked by distraction of the mandible (Fig. 7.12) indicates capsular or ligamentous involvement (Curl, 1993).

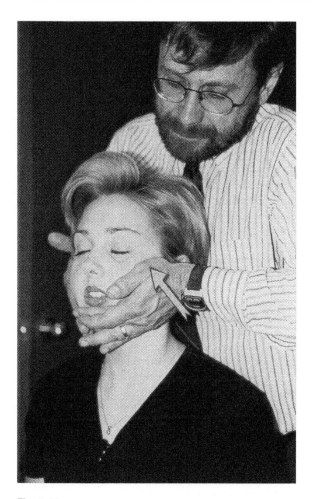

Fig. 7.11

Compression of the condyle (arrow) into the posterior attachment will recreate the pain if the RDT is inflamed

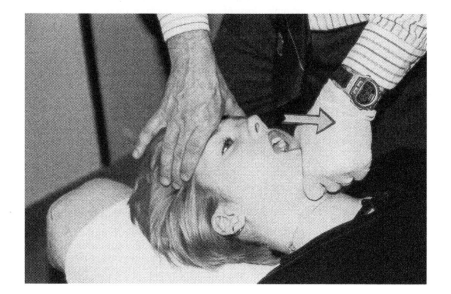

Fig. 7.12

Long-axis distraction (arrow) of the TMJ stressing the fibrous capsule to detect capsulitis

Finally, a disc compression–distraction test is used when clicking is found on mandibular opening. The clinician must first identify the point in millimetres where the click occurs during the opening cycle. Then, with pressure applied to the mandible in an anterior and superior direction to enhance contact of the condyle against the anterior articular eminence (Fig. 7.11), the mandible is moved from a closed to an open position. The opening gait measurement to the point of the click is re-taken. The procedure is repeated to verify the position of the click. A consistent click and measurement indicates an immobile, malpositioned disc with adhesions. An inconsistent measurement suggests a mobile anteriorly displaced disc (Curl, 1995).

The final two aspects of the examination for the chiropractor are: (a) a cursory look at the dentition to assess the state, presence and absence of teeth, and (b), most importantly, a neurological examination.

In general, the first goal in TMJ management should be to exclude conditions not amenable to chiropractic treatment. From the group of conditions remaining, specifically diagnose the exact pathology using the tests outlined. By doing this the clinician will greatly improve the success of any treatment. In summary, if the pain is historically and presently localized to the area of the TMJ and physical as well as laboratory findings do not indicate systemic, tumorous or infectious involvement, local causes should be considered.

DIAGNOSIS AND DIFFERENTIAL DIAGNOSIS

It has been shown thus far that the term TMJ–PDS is not an adequate or appropriate diagnosis. Since the illness is a multifactorial problem, a number of combinations and permutations in presentation are possible. It is essential that the diagnosis rendered be specific and relevant to the examination findings encountered. In addition the treatment must reflect the distinctive findings of the case at hand.

In establishing a diagnosis it is suggested first to exclude the 'worst' conditions and those not amenable to chiropractic treatment. Systemic diseases such as cardiovascular, renal disease, arthritis and hypothyroidism (as a cause of generalized muscle symptoms) must be ruled out. Local pathology in the ears, nose, throat or cervical spine, including trigeminal or glossopharyngeal neuralgia, vascular headaches, temporal arteritis and styloid process fracture, must also be excluded (Curl, 1989; Rocabado, 1983).

Growth disorders such as condylar hypoplasia are rare and seldom painful. Neoplasms are also rare but must be considered. The most typical types are:

1 *Benign: osteoma, haemangioma, chondroma, osteochondroma.*
2 *Malignant: osteosarcoma, chondrosarcoma, multiple myeloma.*
3 *Metastases: adenosarcoma, bronchogenic carcinoma.* *(Guralnick et al., 1978)*

Among the arthritides, infectious arthritis occurs most often in the second to fourth decades. It is spread haematogenously, most commonly from staphylococcal or streptococcal pneumococci. The patient will present with fever and joint pain on active and passive motion.

Gout occurs very rarely in the TMJ, as does osteochondritis. Acute necrosis of the mandibular condyle of unknown aetiology is most common in females from age 14 to 17.

The TMJ is usually one of the last joints affected by rheumatoid arthritis. The condition often presents as ear pain, or a dull, aching pain that is worse in the morning and better through the day. In patients with rheumatoid arthritis, review of their disease status and its involvement in the TMJ is warranted every 3–6 months because of the potential for rapid, destructive progression. In rheumatoid arthritis, the gradual destruction of the joint leads to a fibrous ankylosis. This in turn leads to non-functional mouth opening (approaching zero mm). Gentle assisted mobilization techniques and exercises have been used successfully if the procedures are started early in the course of the disease. When destruction is visible on X-ray there is great risk in damaging remaining joint structures (for example, rupturing the capsule) and, therefore, intervention is contraindicated.

Osteoarthritis has a reported incidence of between 8 and 40 per cent. It occurs in the fourth to fifth decades. Maximal opening is difficult and there is pain noted on condylar translation. Patients are usually asymptomatic for 9–12 months. Degenerative arthrosis usually affects only one side of the TMJ at a time. It is signalled by a loss of movement of the condyle. Patients can open approximately 20 mm in the rotational aspect of motion but not beyond that since the condylar translation is too painful.

There is a risk of damaging the capsule in a degenerated joint. If degenerative changes are seen on X-ray, mobilizing and/or manipulating techniques are not indicated for that joint.

One must also consider other mechanical causes and effects of TMJ–PDS as it relates to the patient's pain. For example, loss of posterior teeth permits a leverage and concentration of forces between the condyle and the fossa or articular eminence. The opposite joint may be relatively hypermobile which may also cause pain. Treatment in such a case will consist of mobilizing the hypomobile joint and using pain relieving treatment (ultrasound, interferential current or microcurrent), as well as non-painful exercise to the hypermobile side.

Imaging techniques are infrequently used and generally not required for the diagnosis of TMJ–PDS (Guralnick et al., 1978). However, if short-term efforts to reduce the problem fail, then investigatory radiographs are needed (Curl, 1989; Rocabado, 1983).

Every chiropractor must screen and consider whether or not to treat a patient with a TMJ disorder. Reviewing patients for evidence of a pre-existing condition or predisposing factor is paramount since very few TMJ disorders are caused by a single traumatic event (Curl, 1995). A poor treatment outcome is almost assured when there is

Table 7.3

Signs and symptoms commonly observed in TMJ conditions

Painful or painless noises arising from the TMJ
Pain initiated or provoked by jaw activity
Deviations or limitations in jaw movement
Locking of the jaw
Pain arising from the TMJ
Sudden changes in the bite
Swelling arising from the TMJ
Pain of the chief complaint worsened by palpation
Pain of the chief complaint worsened by provocative tests
Abnormal changes as seen in imaging studies
Early fatigue of the jaw muscles with normal activity

---

failure to properly interview and scrutinize each case. Once the diagnosis is made and felt to be within the acceptable inclusion conditions, it is important to choose the appropriate and most successful course of treatment.

COMMON CONDITIONS

Fortunately, the most common TMJ conditions are those routinely seen in clinical practice and are easily identified by standard history and examination efforts. Curl (1995) offers a list of symptoms which provide immediate hints that the patient has a TMJ disorder (Table 7.3).

The cardinal signs in TMJ conditions include:

1   *Preauricular pain.*
2   *Joint sounds such as clicking with or without pain progressing to locking and crepitus.*
3   *Dysfunction, limitation in mandibular movement, and/or abnormal jaw movements.*
4   *Tenderness of muscles of mastication (Curl, 1989; Solberg and Clark, 1980).*

There are six common conditions affecting the TMJ and these can be divided into three groups:

1   *Disorders affecting the TMJ –*
    (a)   synovitis
    (b)   capsulitis
    (c)   osteoarthritis.
2   *Disorders of the muscles of mastication –*
    (a)   myofascial pain syndrome.
3   *Disorders of mandibular mobility –*
    (a)   acute disc dislocation or acute closed lock
    (b)   disc adhesion (Curl, 1995).

Disorders affecting the TMJ refer to intra-articular conditions. It is believed that there are various factors that alter joint dynamics and contribute to the formation of capsulitis and synovitis. For example, changes in occlusion, occlusal interference, loss of posterior support, iatrogenic malocclusion, abusive oral habits, occupational conditions (e.g. holding a telephone receiver in the angle of the neck),

bruxism, microtrauma and conditions of muscular imbalance, all increase the load on the TMJ (Saghafi and Curl, 1995).

SYNOVITIS

Synovitis (also known as retrodiscitis or pre-arthritis) involves inflammation of the retrodiscal tissue (RDT). The most frequent cause is an 'excessively posteriorly positioned condyle' which impacts into the fossa, traumatizes the synovial membrane and encroaches on the highly vascularized retrodiscal tissue. The extrinsic trauma may originate from a jaw impact (e.g. motor vehicle accident) or abusive use such as repetitive behaviours (e.g. bruxism, gum chewing, atypical chewing habits). The condition follows a typical course: the posterior attachment becomes oedematous; the intracapsular pressure increases; the condyle displaces anteriorly causing a midline shift and ipsilateral disocclusion; joint pain develops and is aggravated as the patient attempts to occlude the ipsilateral teeth thereby forcing the condyle back against the inflamed posterior attachment (Solberg and Clark, 1980; Curl, 1993).

Characteristics seen in synovitis are local discitis with pain on digital palpation, pain on clenching the teeth, facial grimacing, pain increased with compression but usually relieved with distraction, and swelling on the involved side often disengaging contact between the ipsilateral teeth.

Treatment is often simple: the immediate goals are to decrease the pain and inflammation. Therefore, use of ice, anti-inflammatory medication and adjunctive physiotherapy using ultrasound or electric stimulation with TENS or interferential current are advised. The patient is advised to avoid abusive habits, rest the jaw, avoid belly sleeping and change to a soft food diet. Consultation with a dentist is suggested for a stabilization appliance (i.e. night guard or bite plate). This may be useful since it will disengage the condyle from the inflamed posterior attachment. Mobilization should use only low force techniques to prevent reaggravation of the area but is useful to stimulate flow of the synovial fluid, enhance nutrition to the area, prevent associate muscle guarding and adhesion formation. As the acute phase resolves mobilization and manipulation are useful to accelerate tissue repair in the final stages of healing. The prognosis is good to excellent within 2–4 weeks (Curl, 1995 and 1993).

CAPSULITIS

Capsulitis refers to inflammation of the structures comprising the joint capsule, namely the fibrous capsule itself and its inner synovial lining. This creates the clinical difficulty of trying to distinguish between inflammation of each component. Historically, the term capsulitis was used interchangeably with synovitis. A better understanding of the region's anatomy allows us to differentiate the two terms. Capsular pain is provoked when the inflamed capsule is stretched as in translatory motion and further exacerbated by protrusion or lateral excursion of the mandible, contralateral chewing and wide mouth opening. Capsulitis is further characterized by palpable tenderness or pain directly over the condyle and minor swelling detected over the joint.

Clinical characteristics that differentiate capsulitis from synovitis and other conditions are a lack of pain on clenching and pain on stretching as in yawning or making large bites. The patient may complain of malocclusion or perception that the contralateral side strikes first. Distraction tests increase the pain while compression relieves it.

Treatment of capsulitis is similar to that of synovitis. The first goal is to decrease the pain and inflammation therefore rest, soft diet, ice, anti-inflammatories and adjunctive physiotherapy are similarly warranted. Early mobilization and manipulation are delayed until the acute inflammatory phase resolves (at least 3–5 days). Thereafter, mobilization and manipulation can be used as tolerated by the patient to facilitate tissue repair in the final stage of healing and to prevent adhesion formation.

Complications include adhesion formation, joint inflammation and haemarthrosis. These occur owing to either the initial trauma or manual treatment performed too early or too aggressively. With a conservative but appropriate programme the prognosis is good to excellent within 2–4 weeks (Curl, 1993).

OSTEOARTHRITIS

Degenerative changes within the TMJ are an unwelcome consequence of long-term impact loading within the joint but one that must be considered at the beginning of any treatment protocol. Osteoarthritis is of gradual onset (compared to the other common conditions) and probably has a history of joint noises and crepitus. The condition also involves local pain and difficulty in opening. The patient usually cannot open more than 25 mm in translation without pain. The pain is often unilateral with pain on distraction and compression.

Management of osteoarthritis should begin with an X-ray as indicated by the history and clinical findings. Recall from earlier discussions that 8 per cent of TMJ–PDS patients have degenerative findings on radiographs but 40 per cent of cadavers over age 40 have TMJ degeneration without previous history of TMJ symptoms. As well, approximately 30 per cent bony changes are needed for arthritis to be apparent on plain radiographs. Patients without visible degenerative changes can be given a course of light to moderate force mobilization and manipulation to their tolerance. The purpose of this treatment would be to break down adhesions and provide some degree of improved joint play motion to bathe the joint with synovial fluid. Adjunctive physiotherapy, including heat, ultrasound and electrotherapy is beneficial, as are anti-inflammatories, a soft diet, remedial home exercises, limitation of large yawning and avoidance of belly sleeping. Consultation with a dentist is suggested for a stabilization appliance.

MYOFASCIAL PAIN SYNDROME

Most common amongst TMJ conditions, muscle pain is usually the result of macrotrauma (e.g. blunt injury), microtrauma (e.g. bruxing) or myofascial dysfunction. This condition involves moderate to severe local and referred pain. It too benefits from a multidisciplinary team approach for appropriate management.

The myofascial pain is characteristically a dull depressing pain. There is local tenderness with a typical referral as defined by Travell and Simons (1983). The pain is related to functional demands while rest provides relief. Mouth opening is limited by pain to 25–30 mm. Distraction increases the pain while passive compression shortens the muscle and relieves the discomfort. There is pain on resisted muscle testing (see Table 7.1) which delineates the muscle involved. A counter-irritant test should be used to discriminate muscle involvement from other extracapsular soft tissue conditions. An increase in the range of motion after application of ice or fluoromethane is a positive test and confirms myofascial involvement.

Successful treatment includes trigger point therapy, soft tissue therapy or light massage, ice, ultrasound, electrotherapy and muscle relaxants. The patient must rest from the aetiological abusive factors, use a soft diet and consider dental consultation for a splint to lightly stretch and relax the hypertonic muscle(s). Home care includes stretching, range of motion and proprioceptive neuromuscular facilitation exercises. Manipulation is an effective measure to restore normal mechanics and prevent contracture. The prognosis is good to excellent within 2–3 weeks. If the problem fails to promptly respond to therapy infectious causes must be considered (Curl, 1989 and 1995; Diakow, 1988).

ACUTE ANTERIOR DISC DISLOCATION OR ACUTE CLOSED LOCK

This condition involves an acute onset of intense local pain. It usually results from laxity of the TMJ ligaments or from trauma. The patient will often describe a history of trauma or multiple episodes of joint locking which previously he/she was able to reduce. The disc dislocates anteromedially owing to traction of the superior lateral pterygoid and failure of the ligaments to stabilize the disc and prevent movement.

Characteristics of acute disc dislocation include an acute, sudden onset of pain, absence of joint sounds such as clicking and an inability to open more than 15–20 mm. This is a closed lock (see Fig. 7.6). There will be ipsilateral malocclusion and premature dental contact. The patient may also have suboccipital pain, dysphagia and tinnitus. Soft over-pressure may elicit guarding or an apprehension sign. Clenching or compression cause pain while distraction in a direction perpendicular to the slope of the eminence relieves the pain. A counter-irritant test with ice or fluoromethane is negative.

Mobilization and especially manipulation are successful when performed promptly and correctly. The goal is to increase mobility, decrease pain and reposition or recapture the disc to an anatomically normal position. Segami et al. (1988) demonstrated a 72 per cent success rate using manual manipulation. Manipulation is an effective means for restoring normal mechanics and preventing adhesion formation. Ice, anti-inflammatories and adjunctive physiotherapy are also useful. A dental splint is used to hold the jaw in correct position while the ligaments heal after the disc has been recaptured. At home the patient should use ice, rest, a soft diet, minimize mouth opening and perform small movement range of motion exercises (Curl, 1991).

The prognosis is good to excellent within days if the condition is dealt with while acute. If treatment is delayed by weeks, adhesion formation may be enough to prevent reduction by either manual or surgical manipulation. Similarly a history of laxity affects the prognosis since the lateral collateral discal ligaments may be so lax as to be unable to secure the disc in position over the condyle. Complications from inappropriate management include adhesion formation, joint inflammation and haemarthrosis (Saghafi and Curl, 1995; Curl, 1991 and 1995; Evan, 1990).

DISC ADHESION

As in all synovial joints, the TMJ is susceptible to formation of adhesions during the course of the inflammatory episode and healing. Disc adhesions in the TMJ can be a consequence of traumatic haemarthrosis, disc derangements, coexistent inflammatory conditions or prolonged persistent static loading of the joint, as in bruxing and prolonged mouth opening with difficult dental or orthodontic procedures. Adhesions impair the normal biomechanics and disc nutrition thus accelerating the degenerative process. Adhesions may occur in either TMJ space but they are more likely to occur in the superior compartment, or upper joint space, cementing the disc to the anterior articular eminence. Patients are observed to lose condylar translation, resulting in painful limited mouth opening. Permanent adhesions or fibrous ankylosis occurs if the temporary adhesions are allowed to remain.

Characteristics of disc adhesions are mild to moderate pain with a history of joint noise, especially a 'click or pop' at a specific reproducible amount of mouth opening (see Fig. 7.7). There is limited mandibular opening with slight to moderate deviation to the affected side and laterotrusion of the contralateral aspect. Soft tissue imaging (if available) reveals a stationary disc during condylar translation. Provocation tests for adhesions are positive; if the mandible is lifted in an anterosuperior direction as the patient opens the mouth there will be a loss of motion limited by pain and the adhesion will reproduce the click (see Fig. 7.24). This happens because the condyle has been lifted to trap the disc against the anterior articular eminence. The clinician should take note if the click reoccurs at the same amount of mouth opening on retesting. A disc that 'pops' at different positions is less stable and has a poorer prognosis.

Treatment for disc adhesions includes mobilization and manipulation, a soft diet, use of a splint to prevent bruxing and home care mobilization exercises. The prognosis is best with earlier intervention. Adhesions that have been present for several weeks to months may not resolve (Curl, 1995).

TREATMENT

Treatment of the TMJ is directed to decrease pain, tenderness and adverse loading within the joint. This will improve synovial fluid flow and nutrition to the joint and disc. In addition it will decrease the rate of disc degeneration. Mobilization, manipulation and exercise will restore normal joint mechanics and return the patient to painless activities of daily living. At home the patient can modify diet, work environment and sleeping postures to decrease many of the aetiological factors that initiated the condition.

Of greatest interest to the chiropractor is the ability to decrease pain, improve the health of the joint, enhance healing, improve the biomechanics and prevent deleterious consequences of chronic joint inflammation or adhesion formation. This all can be accomplished with mobilization and manipulation techniques in conjunction with the comprehensive approach previously outlined.

The crucial consideration for the clinician is the timing of the mobilization and manipulation interventions as well as the degree of effort applied.

The acute inflammatory phase usually lasts for 3–5 days. Aggressive intervention is contraindicated at this time. During this phase the preferred therapy is rest and minimal movement. Immobilization will limit pain, provide support or protection to the injured tissues and provide a suitable healing environment. The physiological rationale for rest and immobilization is to prevent: (a) exacerbation of the condition; (b) prolonged inflammation and (c) disruption of new blood vessels and collagen while promoting ground substance synthesis. Modalities used include rest, ice, anti-inflammatories, stabilization devices for support as well as any means of decreasing tension and strain across the injured joint.

Immobilization, while important initially, does have its limits. Morbidity due to excessive immobilization is caused by:

1 *Muscle inhibition and atrophy.*
2 *Joint hypomobility.*
3 *Adaptive shortening of capsules and other connective tissues leading to a lack of support.*
4 *Loss of joint lubrication due to immobility and lack of alternating compression and distraction. This deprives the cartilage of nourishment and hastens degeneration of the cartilage matrix.*
5 *Loss of important stresses to ligament and tendon fibres causing collagen to weaken and stability to diminish.*

Between the fifth and twenty-first day after an injury, the joint undergoes repair and regeneration. Repair is the process of fibroblastic proliferation. The scar tissue formed is necessary but excessive. It must be limited to as great a degree as possible to prevent weakness and adhesions. In this phase light mobilization and manipulation should begin. The therapeutic goals of mobilization and manipulation are to:

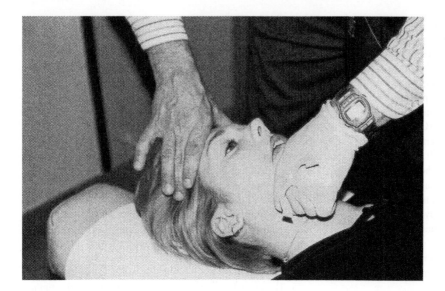

Fig. 7.13

Distraction mobilization or manipulation

1 *Restore the intrinsic range of motion through joint play.*
2 *Gradually reintroduce stress across the tissues to build strength and stability.*
3 *Prevent muscle and joint atrophy.*

Using mobilization within the passive range of motion and to the patient's tolerance improves collagen cross-linking and stability. Fibril size and alignment in the direction of tensile strength also is enhanced. In addition, mobilization breaks down inappropriate fibrosis and excessive adhesions.

The final phase of remodelling, regeneration and maturation occurs after 20 days. In this phase progressive stress through mobilization, manipulation and graduated exercise is used to improve:

1 *Load tolerance.*
2 *Tensile strength and fibre orientation.*

3 *Speed of movement followed by magnitude of motion.*
4 *Cross-linking of ligaments and tendons.*
5 *Proprioception (Zachazewski et al., 1996).*

Management, therefore, is not just a single process. It is the immediate and accurate initial diagnosis of the nature and severity of the injury. It is initiation of appropriate treatment directed at moderating the secondary effects of the inflammatory reaction and enhancing repair by mobilizing, manipulating and strengthening during the remodelling and maturation phases. In addition, it is the ordered sequence of rehabilitation including progressive exercises to enhance the healing of the tissues involved. Management also integrates functional activities to assist in coordinated movement patterns and proprioception. Lastly, management is the successful return to activities of daily living with confidence and bodily control, while being mindful of aetiological factors to prevent recurrence.

Table 7.4
Grades of effort and force in mobilization and manipulation

Grade	Procedure Type	Amplitude	Site of Action	Purpose
I	mobilization	small	performed at the beginning of the functional or AROM	Doctor confidence, patient relaxation, reduce joint pain
II	mobilization	large	performed within the ROM but not reaching the limit of the range or the elastic barrier, i.e. physiologic PROM	reduce joint pain, joint stiffness or both
III	mobilization/ manipulation	large	performed to the limit of the physiologic range	increase joint play (increase ROM), decrease pain after grade IV treatment
IV	manipulation	small	performed at the limit of the range or at the elastic barrier; accessory motion or joint play	increase joint play, increase ROM, decrease adhesions and muscle spasm

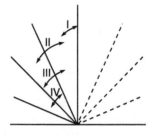

MOBILIZATION AND MANIPULATION

Mobilization is an important but often overlooked stage in the treatment paradigm. The TMJ injury requires patience for the resolution of the inflammatory and repair phases prior to performing more aggressive interventions. Mobilization provides a low force precursor to manipulation. Both are of therapeutic benefit and are similar except for degree (Table 7.4).

The review of the anatomy of this region identified certain areas of weakness as well as areas more susceptible to injury. A graded application of force ranging from mobilization to manipulation is therefore required, especially in the TMJ. The amount of force, the procedure, its amplitude, site of action and purpose are outlined in Table 7.4 (Maitland, 1979; Sandoz, 1976). Use of grades of therapeutic force is based on the clinician's assessment of the patient's pain tolerance and the estimated phase of healing. The specific direction of mobilization and/or manipulation is dictated by joint play assessment and provocative tests outlined previously. An example of mobilization to improve opening of the mouth is demonstrated in Figure 7.13. Using a gloved hand the chiropractor mobilizes the jaw in the direction of joint play restriction. The technique in Fig. 7.13 uses motion oscillating between anterior–inferior and posterior–inferior directions.

TECHNIQUES FOR THE TMJ

Each of the following six technique procedures are adjustments for the TMJ.

TECHNIQUE: TRANSLATION

Indications
Synovitis, positive joint compression–distraction test, loss of anteroinferior joint play, limited opening (e.g. 25–35 mm), myofascial pain syndrome, capsulitis, disc adhesions limiting translation, crepitus suggesting osteoarthritis without radiographic signs.

Position of patient
Supine with mouth open ⅓ or to the point of restriction with involved side exposed.

Position of chiropractor
Standing at the head of the table facing the patient.

Primary contact
Pisiform contact slightly distal to the condyle but superior to the angle of the mandible.

Indifferent hand
Supporting the patient's head.

Line of drive
Anteroinferior along the jaw through the mental protuberance parallel to the slope of the anterior articular eminence.(see Figs. 7.14, 7.15, 7.16).

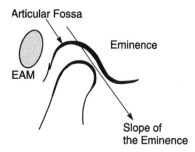

Fig. 7.14

Translation mobilization or manipulation illustrating line of drive parallel to the slope of the anterior articular eminence (adapted from Saghafi and Curl, 1994)

Fig. 7.15

Distraction mobilization or manipulation

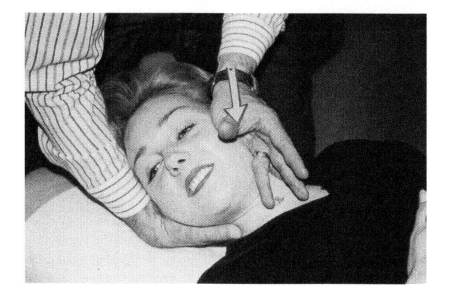

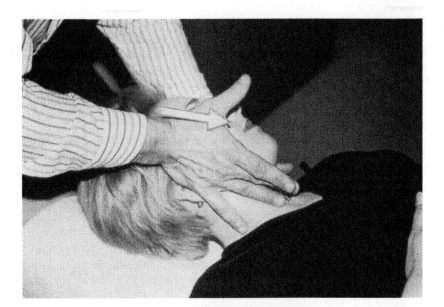

Fig. 7.16

Translation mobilization or manipulation

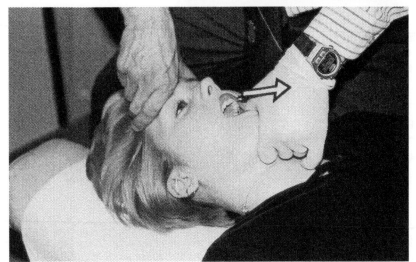

Fig. 7.17

Intraoral translation mobilization or manipulation to draw the condyle out of the fossa or to break adhesions

Technique: Intraoral distraction

Indications
Synovitis, positive joint compression–distraction test, loss of anteroinferior joint play, limited opening (e.g. 25–35 mm), myofascial pain syndrome, capsulitis, disc adhesions limiting translation, decreased protrusion more than retrusion, crepitus suggesting osteoarthritis without radiographic signs.

Position of patient
Supine with the head in a midline position and the mouth open to the point of restriction.

Position of chiropractor
Standing on the non-involved side.

Primary contact
Using a gloved and padded caudal hand, the thumb contacts the mandibular molars.

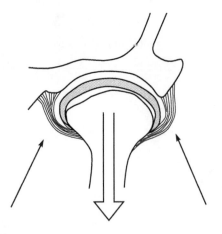

Fig. 7.18

Intraoral distraction mobilization or manipulation anterior view

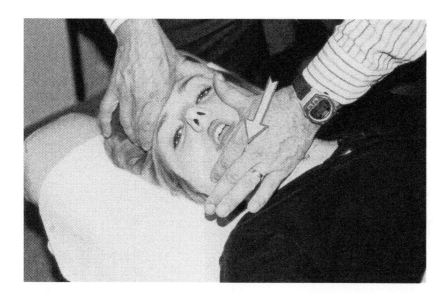

Fig. 7.19

Lateral mobilization or manipulation

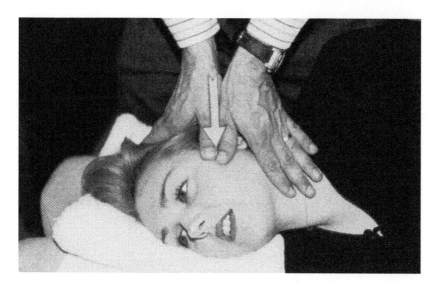

Fig. 7.20

Optional position for lateral mobilization or manipulation

Indifferent hand
Stabilizing the patient's forehead.

Line of drive
Anteroinferior along the jaw through the mental protuberance parallel to the slope of the anterior articular eminence (see Figs. 7.14, 7.17, 7.18).

Option
Patient seated.

TECHNIQUE: LATERAL MANDIBLE

Indications
Loss of lateral to medial joint play, limited opening (e.g. 25–35 mm), myofascial pain syndrome, (synovitis, capsulitis, disc adhesions limiting translation, crepitus suggesting osteoarthritis without radiographic signs limiting lateral movement).

Position of patient
Supine with mouth open ⅓ or to the point of restriction with involved side slightly exposed.

Position of chiropractor
Standing at the head of the table facing the patient.

Primary contact
Thenar contact between the angle of the jaw and the mental protuberance.

Indifferent hand
Stabilizing the patient's forehead on the uninvolved side.

Line of drive
Lateral to medial along the line of diminished joint play (see Fig. 7.19).

Option
Double thumb contact on the involved side (see Fig. 7.20).

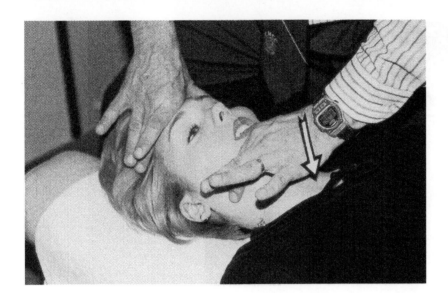

Fig. 7.21

Retrusion mobilization or manipulation

TECHNIQUE: RETRUSION

Indications
Loss of protrusion and retrusion joint play, limited opening (e.g. 25–35 mm), myofascial pain syndrome, joint adhesions, decreased retrusion more than protrusion.

Position of patient
Supine with the head in a midline position and the mouth open to the point of restriction.

Position of chiropractor
Standing on the non-involved side.

Primary contact
Web contact on the chin.

Indifferent hand
Stabilizing the patient's forehead.

Line of drive
Posterior (see Fig. 7.21).

TECHNIQUE: REDUCTION OF ACUTE DISCAL LOCK

Indications
Decreased rotation during opening, opening less than 15–20 mm, positive compression, pain on clenching, jaw deviation, absence of clicking, apprehension sign.

Position of patient
Supine with mouth open ⅓ or less than the point of restriction.

Position of chiropractor
Standing on the non-involved side.

Primary contact
Using a gloved and padded caudal hand, the thumb contacts the mandibular molars.

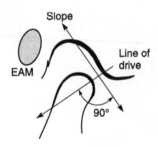

Fig. 7.22

Line of drive for acute discal lock (joint gapping) mobilization or manipulation (adapted from Curl, 1991)

Indifferent hand
Stabilizing the patient's forehead from the un-involved side.

Line of drive
Posteroinferior direction perpendicular to the slope of the articular eminence. (see Figs. 7.22, 7.23).

TECHNIQUE: ANTERIOR DISC DISLOCATION WITH ADHESIONS

Indications
Opening click, decreased distraction joint play, positive disc compression–distraction test, limited opening (e.g. 20–35 mm).

Position of patient
Seated with the head in a midline and the jaw open just past the point where the click is felt.

Position of chiropractor
Standing behind the patient.

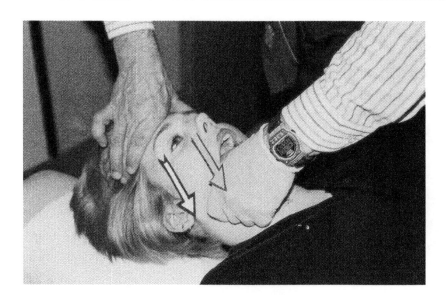

Fig. 7.23

Acute discal lock (joint gapping) mobilization or manipulation

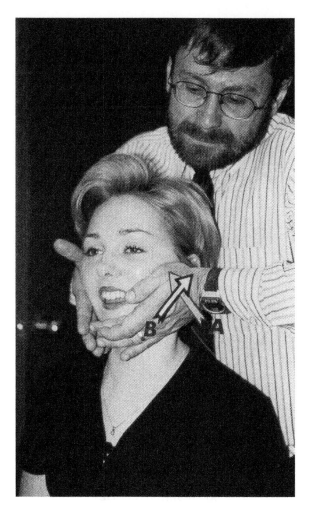

Fig. 7.24

Mobilization or manipulation for anterior disc dislocation with adhesions.

Primary contact
Soft pisiform contact on the patient's mandible with the doctor's ipsilateral hand.

Indifferent hand
Stabilizing the patient's contralateral side.

Line of drive
With the contact hand pressing superoanterior to approximate the condyle and the adherent disc (see 'A' in Fig. 7.24), a series of superoposterior thrusts are applied parallel to the slope of the eminence (see 'B' in Fig. 7.24 and Fig. 25).

Option
Patient supine (see 'A' and 'B' in Fig. 7.26).

Contraindications for TMJ mobilization and manipulation are presented earlier in the differential diagnosis discussion.

Complications from delayed treatment are primarily the formation of adhesions. Prolonged impact loading, an

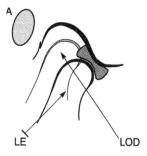

Fig. 7.25

Loading force that holds the disc in position for the manoeuvre (A) and the line of drive (B) for the mobilization or manipulation in cases of anterior disc dislocations or adhesions (adapted from Saghafi and Curl, 1994)

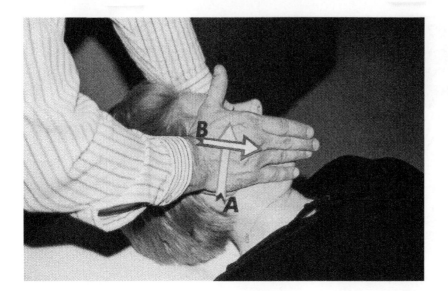

Fig. 7.26

Optional supine patient position for mobilization or manipulation for anterior disc dislocation with adhesions

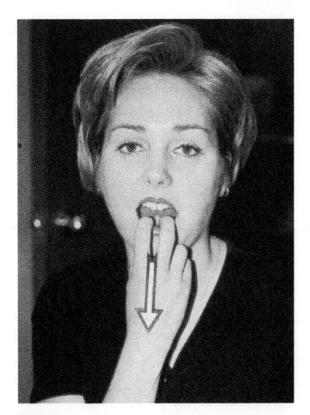

Fig. 7.27

Remedial exercises: passive stretching to restore range of motion

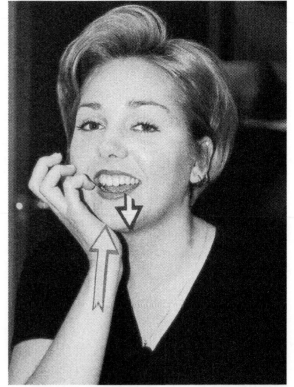

Fig. 7.28

Remedial exercises: proprioceptive neuromuscular facilitation

unresolved inflammatory phase or sustained immobilization affect the health of the joint and permit the proliferation of adhesions which in themselves have detrimental effects. Furthermore, perseverant joint compression leads to early degeneration of the disc and joint surfaces.

REMEDIAL EXERCISES

A course of treatment would be incomplete without exercise. Studies that have reviewed the success of TMJ treatment have found overwhelmingly that active patient participation is

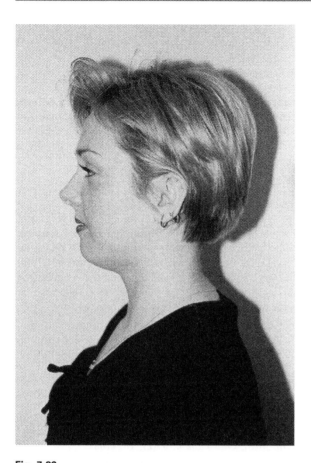

Fig. 7.29

Postural exercises

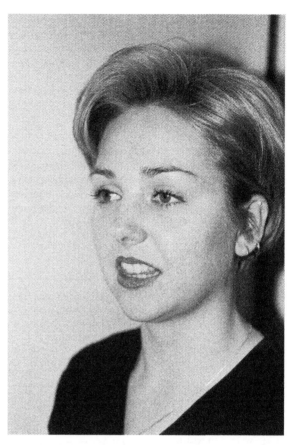

Fig. 7.30

Mandibular postural resting position (MPRP).

mandatory (Reisine and Weber, 1989). The patient should be given a course of passive range of motion exercises (see Fig. 7.27) followed by isometrics and then proprioceptive neuromuscular facilitation (see Fig. 7.28). The latter two forms of exercise should never force the patient through pain or the 'click'.

Posture has been shown to be an important aetiological factor in this condition. The programme should incorporate this aspect. Exercises for general spinal posture, cervical posture and head carriage in particular (Fig. 7.29), as well as exercise to maintain the mandibular postural resting position (MPRP) discussed in the biomechanics section (Fig. 7.30) complete the programme.

In cases of joint hypermobility, Berkman (1985) prescribes a series of active retrusion exercises over the course of 4–12 weeks to correct this problem.

PROGNOSIS

Chiropractic treatment of TMJ–PDS has been shown in the literature to have empirical and statistical value. Studies by Curl and Saghafi (Saghafi and Curl, 1995; Curl and Saghafi, 1995) have shown the clinical efficacy of manipulative treatment for acute discal lock and discal displacement with adhesions. This is corroborated by Rocabado (1983) and Solberg and Clark (1980). Manipulation decreased adhesion formation, capsular fibrosis, capsular contracture and muscle shortening. Vernon and Ehrenfeld (1982) demonstrated the successful management of a TMJ case with cervical rather than TMJ manipulation.

In 75 per cent of cases, patients experience an improvement in their condition within 2–4 weeks of chiropractic manual treatment (Ricken and Siebert, 1989). This improvement includes a decrease in pain, clicking and muscle dysfunction, as well as an improved range of motion. Fifteen per cent of the remaining cases usually require more extensive treatment, often in conjunction with other disciplines (i.e., dentistry, oral surgery, rheumatology, psychology, etc.). From the final 10 per cent of cases, 5 per cent may go on to surgery and 5 per cent will not respond to any treatment and are termed clinical failures (Ricken and Siebert, 1989 and Wilkinson, 1987).

As well as diagnosis and treatment, the chiropractor may be called upon to assess the degree of impairment and disability in a TMJ patient. 'Impairment is a medical condition involving a loss of function. Its degree of severity is determined by the treating chiropractor only after the maximal response to treatment is achieved.' The chiropractor should bear in mind that TMJ injuries are not known to result in permanent disability that would prohibit the patient from engaging in gainful employment (Curl, 1995).

Success in chiropractic TMJ management will always depend on the skill of the clinician, nature of the pathology, duration of the condition, status of the mandible and dentition as well as the participation of the patient.

The best success in these cases is furthermore derived from a multidisciplinary approach. In most of the common conditions presented a dental consultation to review the health of the teeth or to construct a stabilizing appliance is suggested. Research supports this; the success rate for patients with combined chiropractic and dental management is over 80 per cent (Ricken and Siebert, 1989).

CONCLUSION

Chiropractic management of the temporomandibular joint conditions is very successful when the examination is thorough, the differential diagnosis is comprehensive and the treatment is timely and appropriate for the diagnosis.

The purpose of this chapter has been to illustrate the most common conditions affecting this joint, the types of tissues injured and the mechanisms of injury. The simple, inexpensive but sensitive tests provided will enable the clinician to specifically diagnose the subcategories of TMJ–PDS. Treatment for each condition has been reviewed, with demonstration of chiropractic procedures, and a comprehensive treatment programme outlined.

ACKNOWLEDGEMENTS

I would like to acknowledge the support and encouragement of my office personnel and especially my family during the preparation of this chapter, as well as the efforts of Dr Ray Broome who provided me with the time needed to complete the topic properly. Lastly, I would like to acknowledge the work and support of my colleague, friend and mentor Dr Darryl Curl.

REFERENCES

Berkman, E. (1985) TMJ and chiropractic. *American Chiropractor*, **Nov.**

Black, W.C. and Welsh, H.G. (1993) Advances in diagnostic imaging and overestimation of disease prevalence and benefits of therapy. *N. Engl. J. Med*, **326**, 1237–1243.

Brand, R.W. and Isselhard, D.E. (1986) *Anatomy of Orofacial Structures*, 3rd edn. Toronto, Mosby.

Chase, D.C., Hendler, B.H. and Kraus, S.L. (1988) A commonsense approach to TMJ pain. *Patient Care.*

Curl, D.D. (1989) *The Chiropractic Approach to Temporomandibular Disorders, Seminars in Chiropractic*. Baltimore, MD: Williams and Wilkins.

Curl, D.D. (1991) Acute closed lock of the temporomandibular joint: manipulation paradigm and protocol. *Chiro. Technique*, **3**(1), 13–18.

Curl, D.D. (1993) Chiropractic management of capsulitis and synovitis of the temporomandibular joint. *J. of Orofacial Pain* **7**(3), 283–293.

Curl, D.D. (1995) The temporomandibular joint. *Advances in Chiropractic*, Vol. 2. Toronto: Mosby.

Curl, D.D. and Saghafi, D. (1995) Manual reduction of adhesion in the temporomandibular joint. *Chiro. Technique*, **7**(1), 22–29.

Diakow, P. (1988) Pseudo-temporomandibular joint pain-dysfunction syndrome. *JCCA*, **32**(3).

Dolwick, M.F., Hendler, B.H. and Kraus, S.L. (1984) Commonsense management for TMJ trouble. *Patient Care.*

Evan, P. (1990) A three-year follow-up of patients with reciprocal temporomandibular joint clicking. *Oral Surg., Oral Med., Oral Pathol.*, **69**(2), 167–168.

Faye, L. and Shafer, R.C. (1989) *Motion Palpation and Chiropractic Technic*. Huntington Beach, CA, Motion Palpation Institute.

Guralnick, W., Kaban, L.B. and Merrill, R.G. (1978) Temporomandibular-joint afflictions. *New Engl. J. Med.*

Helland M.M. (1986) Anatomy and function of the TMJ. In: *Modern Manual Therapy* (G.P. Grieve, ed.). Edinburgh: Churchill Livingstone.

Ieremia, L., Podoleanu, G., Balas-Chirila, M. and Kovacs, D. (1990) Estimating some perspective of certain epidemiological, clinical and paraclinical investigations aiming at discovering the etiopathogenesis of the painful dysfunctional meniscus-condyle syndrome of temporomandibular joint for prophylaxis and individualized treatment. *Stomatologie*, **37**, 149–159.

Kelsey, J.L. (1982) *Epidemiology of Musculoskeletal Disorders*. Oxford: Oxford University Press.

Maitland, G.D. (1979) *Peripheral Manipulation*, 2nd edn. Oxford: Butterworth-Heinemann, pp. 28–31.

Marbach, J.J., Lennon, M.C. and Dohrenwend, B.P. (1988) Candidate risk factors for temporomandibular pain and dysfunction syndrome: psychosocial, health behaviour, physical illness and injury. *Pain*, **34**, 139–151.

Marotta, J.T. (1983) Chronic facial pain: a clinic approach. *Can. Fam. Physician*, **29**.

Muller, F. (1989) Biofeedback as a part of the treatment of mandibular dysfunctions. *Deutsche Zahnarztliche Zeitschrift*, 44, 938–941.

Paradiso, M. and Scott, R. (1989) Evaluation of the clinical effectiveness of biofeedback EMG on muscular relaxation and painful symptomatology. *Minerva Stomatologia*, 38, 19–22.

Reik, L. and Hale, M. (1981) The temporomandibular joint pain–dysfunction syndrome: A Frequent Cause of Headache. *Headache* **Jul 21**(4), 151–156.

Reisine, S. and Weber, J. (1989) Motivations for treatment and outcomes of care. The relationship between motivation for seeking dental treatment and the evaluation of outcomes of care. *J. Am. Coll. Dentists*, 56(2), 19–25.

Ricken, C. and Siebert, G. (1989) Comparative post-treatment evaluation of patients with pain–dysfunction syndrome. *Deutsche Zahnarztliche Zeitschrift*, 44(11), 20–22.

Rocabado, M. (1983) Arthrokinematics of the Temporomandibular Joint. In *Temporomandibular Joint Dysfunction and Treatment. The Dental Clinics of North America* (H. Gelb, ed.), pp. 573–594.

Royder, J.O. (1981) Structural influences in temporomandibular joint pain and dysfunction. *JAOA*, 80(7).

Saghafi, D. and Curl, D.D. (1995) Chiropractic management of anteriorly displaced temporomandibular disc with adhesion. *JMPT*, 18(2), 98–104.

Sandoz, R. (1976) Some physical mechanisms and effects of spinal adjustments. *Swiss Annals VI* (Swiss Chiropractors' Association), Grounauer, pp. 91–141.

Schnurr, R.F., Brooke, R.I. and Rollman, G.B. (1990) Psychosocial correlates of temporomandibular joint pain and dysfunction. *Pain*, 42(2), 153–165.

Segami, N., Murakami, K., Matsuki, M. (1988) Clinical assessment for treatment of patients with TMJ closed-lock by means of manipulation and pumping technique. *Jpn. J. Oral Maxillofac. Surg.*, 34, 1123–1131.

Solberg, W.K. and Clark, G.T. (1980) *Temporomandibular Joint Problems; Biologic Diagnosis and Treatment.* Chicago, IL: Quintessence Publishing Company.

Toller, P.A. (1974) Temporomandibular Capsular Rearrangement. *Br. J. Oral Surg.*, 70, 461–463.

Travell, J.G. and Simons, D.G. (1983) *Myofascial Pain and Dysfunction: The Trigger Point Manual.* Baltimore, MD: Williams and Wilkins.

Tversky, J., Reade, P.C., Gerschamn, J.A., Holwill, B.J. and Wright, J. (1991) Role of depressive illness in the outcome of treatment of temporomandibular joint pain–dysfunction syndrome. *Oral Surg., Oral Med., Oral Pathol.*, 71, 696–699.

Vernon, L.F. and Ehrenfeld, D.C. (1982) Treatment of temporomandibular joint syndrome for relief of cervical spine pain: case report. *JMPT*, 5(2).

White, A.A. and Gordon, S.L. (1982) *American Academy of Orthopedic Surgeons Symposium on Idiopathic Low Back Pain.* Toronto: Mosby.

Wilkinson, T.M. (1987) A multi-disciplinary approach to the treatment of craniomandibular disorders. *Aust. Prosthodontic J.*, 1, 19–24.

Zachazewski, J.E., Magee, D.J. and Quillen, W.S. (1986) *Athletic Injuries and Rehabilitation.* Toronto: Saunders.

APPENDIX A: TMJ PHYSICAL EXAMINATION SUMMARY

- *History*

- *Inspection*
  - *facial asymmetry: mastoid, lips, cheeks*
  - *hypertrophy/hypertonicity of muscles of mastication, posterior cervical muscles, accessory muscles of respiration*
  - *hands: evidence of rheumatoid arthritis*
  - *assess speech*
  - *auditory acuity*
  - *swallowing*

  posture
  - *head carriage, head position, head tilt, head movement*
  - *resting position of the jaw*
  - *musculature of the head, neck, back, chest and leg*
  - *any tenderness to touch, trigger points or spasm?*

ROM: active, passive and resited for
- *cervical spine*
- *shoulder*
- *thoracic spine*
- *lumbar spine*
note: unlevelling, scoliosis, kyphosis, leg-length inequality

- *mandibular gait*
  opening 40–60 mm, three knuckle test
  closing: pain or double contact
  repeat with tongue depressors to delineate muscle from joint pain
  lateral deviation 5–10 mm
  ratios of opening: lateral deviation
      1:4 normal, 1:3 extracapsular, 1:6 intracapsular
  protrusion 5 mm
  retrusion 3–4 mm

- *Palpation*
  - *joint tenderness to touch*
  - *crepitus, cracking, clicking*
  - *bruxomania*
  - *trigger points: lateral pterygoid, medial pterygoid, masseter, temporalis, SCM, digastric*
  - *joint play and end-feel: soft (muscle), hard (capsule/disc)*
  1 *distraction, inferolateral at 20 degrees*
     (i) at rest ⎫ *(a) extraoral*
     (ii) open ⎭ *(b) intraoral*
  2 *lateral deviation*
  3 *posterosuperior (disc, RDT)*

- *Resisted muscle tests*
  Opening (O), Closing (C), Protrusion (P), Retrusion (R), Lateral Deviation (LD)

Muscle	O*	C	P	R	LD
Masseter		+	+		
Temporalis		+		+	+
Medial pterygoid		+	+		+
Inferior lateral pterygoid	+		+		+
Digastric	+			+	
Superior lateral pterygoid		+			+

*Repeat resisted opening: if there is a fixed click on opening then the patient has a fixed disc, if the click occurs at a different point then the patient has a mobile disc.

- *Percussion*
  - *general: sharply close teeth – pain?*
    → periodontal disease
  - *specific: tap tooth with a blunt instrument*

- *Counter-irritant spray test*

- *Cervical spine exam*

- *Neurologic exam*

8

The evaluation of joint play and adjustive procedures for the peripheral joints

Raymond T. Broome

ADJUSTIVE PROCEDURES

The techniques presented in the following chapter aim to treat abnormal biomechanics to restore normal function, using as gentle, specific and efficient methods as possible. They are arranged in two major sections, the upper and lower extremities. Each section starts with descriptions of techniques on the joints closest to the trunk, working distally towards the joints of the extremities.

In the regions such as the wrist and hand or in the foot and ankle, where anatomical parts are relatively small, as much use as possible has been made of line drawings to accompany the photographs. These are to better illustrate and clarify the hand positions, contacts and the directions of adjustive thrusts used.

For the sake of uniformity, all techniques are demonstrated on the **right side** of the body. Obviously the practitioner and student must be just as proficient with the application of the techniques on both sides of the body and this also necessitates practice. To address the left limbs, the descriptions given in the text, photographs and line drawings are simply reversed by the reader.

As aids to proficiency, there are no substitutes for anatomical models of the wrist and hand and foot and ankle, which are invaluable for familiarizing student practitioners with the exact location of contact points, anatomical landmarks, the complexity of the joint angles, and for giving assistance in technique practice set-ups and diagnosis (Logan, 1995). Every student of peripheral joint technique is strongly advised to use them.

NOMENCLATURE

Although the author is aware of the emotive and connotative implications, the terms 'adjustment' and 'manipulation' are deemed in this text to be interchangeable. The term 'mobilization' also means different things in different countries. In the following chapter, mobilization is deemed to mean the partial or full passive movement of a joint without the explicit intention to produce a cavitation.

CHOICE OF TECHNIQUE

If a peripheral joint dysfunction is chronic and/or the patient is elderly, or if the joint is stiff due to its being a healed fracture site, the treatment should be commenced by selecting mobilization methods and carrying out appropriate soft tissue work first before attempting more vigorous methods.

The techniques described follow the typical thrust directions of superior to inferior, anterior to posterior and so forth, but these are intended simply as practical guidelines. In practice the thrust directions must follow directly and precisely along the plane lines of the articulations involved. These variations must be accommodated when performing the techniques.

THE EVALUATION OF JOINT PLAY

The method used in this book for examination purposes is motion palpation (Gillet, 1964, 1981; Schafer and Faye, 1990; Gillet, 1996), but taken beyond the range of voluntary movement into the remaining passive movement still normally available in the joint before the elastic barrier is reached (Sandoz, 1976). Joint dysfunction in this passive area is described as a loss of mechanical play in the synovial joint (Mennell, 1964; Gale, 1991). Loss of this joint play causes pain and joint disability. Exercise, either active or passive, does not produce or restore it (Schafer and Faye, 1990). Mechanoreceptors when activated under extreme conditions inhibit adjacent muscles (Hearon, 1991). Impaired muscle function leads to impaired joint function and impaired joint function leads to the impairment of muscle function (Schafer and Faye, 1990).

The successful outcome of chiropractic examinations and treatment methods depends on a number of factors. The main ones are the exclusion of non-skeletal sources of disability, the careful testing of the presence and direction of the loss of joint play function, thorough knowledge of the plane lines of the joints involved and a very high level of proficiency in the delivery of the adjustment.

Faye states that it is not unusual for joint play to be restricted in a joint in some planes but not others (Schafer and Faye, 1990). It has also been observed clinically that mobilizing a joint in one direction does not always restore the joint play in all other directions in which that joint can function normally. The consequence of this is that occasions may arise where the restoration of joint play in all planes may require separate adjustive thrusts in several directions, administered to tolerance, during the same or subsequent patient visits.

Insufficient studies have been made so far on the inter- and intra-examiner reliability of motion palpation of the spine and pelvis and even fewer on the motion palpation studies of the peripheral joints. Shaw and Perth (1987) showed in their study of the motion palpation of the tarsals in the non-weight-bearing position a high average – 88.09% – inter-examiner reliability and an even higher – 90% and 93% – intra-examiner reliability. No comparisons for these figures can yet be made.

APPLICATION OF JOINT PLAY EVALUATION

Motion palpation of the peripheral joints for joint play differs from passive osteokinematic motion palpation (POMP) (see Chapter 4) in that joint play examination is concerned only with that motion at the end of travel in the directions permitted by the plane lines of the joints and not with the quality in the voluntary or mid-range of motion.

1   *The joint to be examined is isolated as efficiently as possible by blocking the movement of the neighbouring joint(s) with one hand, leaving the other hand free to check the mobility of the joint in question.*
2   *The joint is then moved passively through its range of movement as in POMP, and from this point onwards the technique differs.*
3   *The joint movement is continued until resistance is felt by the palpating thumb or fingers against the ligamentous tightness at the end of the range of travel. Without releasing the pressure, a further firm compressive force is then applied.*
4   *Normal peripheral joint movement at this end range of motion is perceived as an elastic sensation, similar in feeling to compressing a pencil eraser or a hard rubber ball. This perception of elasticity has been termed end-play (Schafer and Faye, 1990). The patient perceives this solely as a passive sensation.*
5   *Absence of end-play is perceived by the doctor as a sensation of hardness similar to pressing against a block of wood and is accompanied by a local pain and tenderness experienced by the patient.*
6   *Loss of end-play may be present in one or more directions so examination of the joint is made in all the directions which the joint planes permit.*
7   *Adjustive corrections are made in the direction or directions in which end-play is lost.*

With this information, the practitioner is in a position to select a technique to specifically correct the motion loss.

For ease of use in this text, detailed descriptions of joint play evaluation methods are included at the beginning of each section and throughout. **All techniques are described for the right extremity.** For application on the left extremity, the opposite hands are used for the contact and support, the stance is reversed etc.

If the chiropractor has a clear perception of what needs to be achieved biomechanically, then techniques do not need to be memorized. Instead they become a logical progression from the joint examination findings. Since the joint must be released in the direction that motion is lost, Henri Gillet's rhetorical question comes to mind: 'At what point does examination end and treatment begin?' (Lecture given to the European Chiropractors Union, Switzerland, 1969).

Diligent practice ultimately provides expertise. With expertise, manual joint evaluation using joint play analysis followed by efficient technique application is performed thoroughly and rapidly as required in a clinical practice setting. This allows peripheral joint correction to be routinely incorporated into existing practice procedures. It is a powerful ally for the chiropractor to use in the delivery of an efficient means of improving the patient's neuro-biomechanical integrity.

GUIDELINES FOR ADJUSTING THE PERIPHERAL JOINTS

1   *Work methodically, especially when evaluating a complex of joints.*
2   *Evaluate, adjust, re-evaluate. Repeat this sequence if necessary.*
3   *When selecting a technique, consideration should be given to the physical size of the patient compared to the size of the chiropractor.*
4   *If there is evidence of chronicity or arthrotic changes, consider using mobilization techniques first, before more aggressive methods are chosen.*
5   *Always work within the patient's tolerance.*
6   *The direction of the thrust must conform to the plane line of the joint.*
7   *Consider adjusting and treating the proximal joint problem before the distal one.*
8   *If the peripheral joint problem is chronic, consider the use of supports or taping following the manual treatment.*
9   *If the peripheral joint problem is acute, use cryotherapy first to control effusion before manual techniques are employed.*

REFERENCES

Gale, P. (1991) Joint mobilization. In *Functional Soft Tissue and Treatment by Manual Methods*. (W.I. Hammer, ed.) pp. 10–197, Gaithersburg, MD, Aspen Publishers.

Gillet, H. (1964) *Belgian Chiropractic Research Notes*, 5th edn. 5 Rue de la Limite, Brussels, Belgium.

Gillet, H. (1981) *Belgian Chiropractic Research Notes*, 11th edn. Huntington Beach, CA, Motion Palpation Institute.

Gillet, J. (1996) New light on the history of motion palpation. *J. Manip. Physiol. Ther.* **19**(1).

Hearon, K.G. (1991) *What You Should Know About Extremity Adjusting*, 7th edn. Sequim, WA, Vanity Press.

Logan, A.L. (1995) *The Foot and the Ankle: Clinical Applications*. Gaithersburg, MD, Aspen Publishers.

Mennell, J.Mc.M. (1964) *Joint Pain Diagnosis and Treatment Using Manipulative Techniques*. London, Little Brown and Company.

Sandoz, R. (1976) Some physical mechanisms and effects of spinal adjustments. *Ann. Swiss Chiro. Assoc.* **VI**.

Schafer, R.C. and Faye, L.J. (1990) *Motion Palpation and Chiropractic Technique – Principles of Dynamic Chiropractic*. 2nd edn. Huntington Beach, CA, Motion Palpation Institute.

Shaw, A.J. and Perth, F.R.J. (1987) *An Inter- and Intra-Examiner Reliability Study of Motion Palpation of the Tarsals in the Non-weight-bearing Position*. D.C. Thesis, Anglo-European College of Chiropractic.

REFERENCES

Section

1

The Upper Extremity

8.1

The sterno-clavicular joint

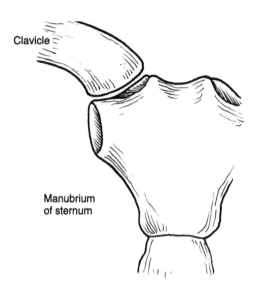

Clavicle

Manubrium
of sternum

8.1.A   Joint play evaluation of the sterno-clavicular joint medial to lateral, lateral to medial and anterior to posterior glide

8.1.B   Joint play evaluation of the sterno-clavicular joint superior to inferior and inferior to superior glide

8.1.1   Supine sterno-clavicular joint superior to inferior thrust technique

8.1.2   Sitting sterno-clavicular joint superior to inferior thrust technique

8.1.3   Supine sterno-clavicular joint inferior to superior thrust technique

8.1.4   Sitting sterno-clavicular joint medial to lateral thrust technique

8.1.5   Sitting sterno-clavicular joint anterior to posterior unilateral or bilateral pull technique

8.1.6   Supine sterno-clavicular joint anterior to posterior crossed arms mobilization technique

8.1.7   Supine sterno-clavicular joint recoil technique

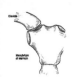

8.1.A Joint play evaluation of the sterno-clavicular joint medial to lateral, lateral to medial and anterior to posterior glide

Procedure

The patient is placed supine and the chiropractor places a heel of hand (see Glossary of Terms, p. 285) contact on the anterior medial end of the clavicle. On occasions, it may be found helpful to detect for the presence or absence of joint play if the shoulder is first abducted and held at an angle of more than 90° before the sterno-clavicular joint is tested for joint play glide.

1) Medial to lateral glide

The chiropractor's hand is first pressed downwards from anterior to posterior to compress the patient's rib cage before exerting short, firm pressures into joint play from medial to lateral. Elasticity should be felt if joint play is normal.

2) Lateral to medial glide

The chiropractor's hands are reversed and again pressed first downwards to compress the patient's rib cage before short, firm pressures from lateral to medial are exerted. Elasticity should be felt if joint play is normal.

3) Anterior to posterior glide

Anterior to posterior pressure is exerted until the rib cage is compressed. Further pressure is then exerted, taking the joint into joint play. Elasticity should be felt if joint play is normal.

8.1.B Joint play evaluation of the sterno-clavicular joint superior to inferior and inferior to superior glide

Procedure

The patient is placed supine and the chiropractor places a heel of hand (see Glossary of Terms, p. 285) contact on the anterior medial end of the clavicle.

1) Superior to inferior glide

The Chiropractor stands at the head end of the treatment table facing caudad. The **right hand** is used for the contact. The **left hand** may be used to stabilize the other shoulder girdle by placing it over the distal end of the opposite clavicle.

The patient's clavicle is first pressed downwards from anterior to posterior to compress the rib cage then pressed firmly with short pressures from superior to inferior into joint play. Elasticity should be felt if joint play is normal.

2) Inferior to superior glide

The chiropractor stands on the homolateral side, close in to the patient, so that the fingers point cephalad. The patient's clavicle is again pressed downwards from anterior to posterior to eliminate as much rib cage movement as possible. Pressure into joint play is then applied from inferior to superior. Normal joint play is felt as an elastic sensation at the end of the travel.

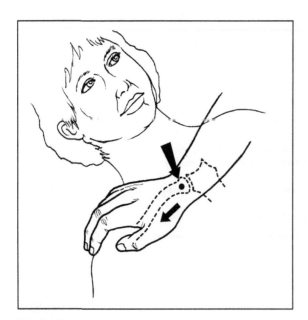

Fig. 8.1.A

Joint play evaluation of the sterno-clavicular joint from medial to lateral and anterior to posterior glide

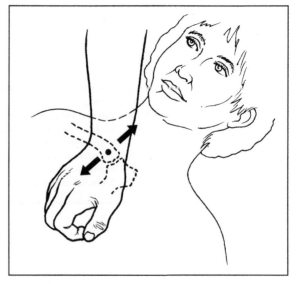

Fig. 8.1.B

Joint play evaluation of the sterno-clavicular joint from superior to inferior and inferior to superior glide

8.1.1 Supine sterno-clavicular joint superior to inferior thrust technique

Application
Joint play glide loss from superior to inferior of the clavicle on the sternum.

Patient's position
The patient is placed supine on the affected side with the arm fully extended and the shoulder hyper-abducted.

Chiropractor's stance
The chiropractor stands at the head end of the table facing caudad and favouring the side of involvement.

Contact
(a) The left hand is placed over the superior aspect of the medial end of the clavicle using a pisiform or heel of hand contact.
(b) The right hand holds the patient's forearm just proximal to the wrist.

Procedure
Joint pre-load tension is achieved by tractioning the patient's right arm in long axis with the right hand, and by gently pressing against the clavicle with the left hand. Without releasing the tension, an impulse is made from superior to inferior on the clavicle with the left hand.

8.1.2 Sitting sterno-clavicular joint superior to inferior thrust technique.

Application
Joint play glide loss from superior to inferior of the clavicle on the sternum.

Patient's position
The patient is placed sitting on a chair with a back rest, with the shoulder on the affected side abducted and the elbow flexed. The patient's head is flexed slightly forwards.

Chiropractor's stance
The chiropractor stands behind the patient favouring the side of involvement, so that the left shoulder is above the clavicular contact.

Contact
a) The left hand is placed over the patient's shoulder with a pisiform contact on the medial end of the right clavicle, with the fingers pointing downwards. If the direct pisiform contact is uncomfortable for the patient, the contact may be cushioned with the use of a pad or folded hand towel.
b) The right hand is placed palm upwards against the inferior aspect of the patient's distal humerus holding the shoulder in abduction.

Procedure
Joint pre-load tension is achieved by pressing the clavicle downwards with the left hand and simultaneously elevating the patient's shoulder with the right hand. Without slackening the contact, the impulse is applied from superior to inferior with minimal depth of thrust.

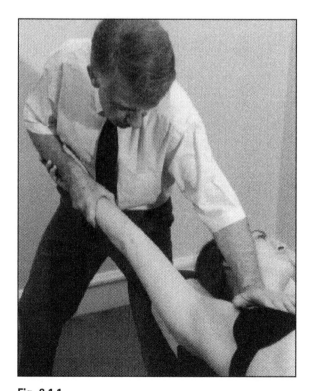

Fig. 8.1.1

The patient's arm is tractioned in long axis and a steady pressure applied to the clavicle before an impulse is made

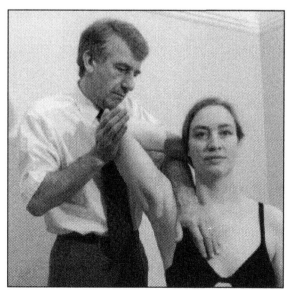

Fig. 8.1.2

The patient's arm is elevated simultaneously with the downward thrust on the clavicle

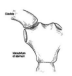

8.1.3 Supine sterno-clavicular joint inferior to superior thrust technique

Application
Joint play glide loss from inferior to superior of the clavicle on the sternum.

Patient's position
The patient is placed supine with the shoulder on the affected side flexed.

Chiropractor's stance
The chiropractor stands on the contralateral side facing the patient, flexing the trunk forwards so that the right shoulder is almost above the patient's sterno-clavicular joint.

Contact
a) The left hand holds the patient's right forearm just proximal to the wrist.
b) The right hand is placed over the anterior aspect of the medial end of the clavicle with a pisiform, low arch (see Glossary of Terms, p. 285) contact. If the contact is uncomfortable for the patient, a pad to cushion the pressure may be used.

Procedure
Joint pre-load tension is achieved by long axis traction of the patient's right arm until the shoulder girdle begins to rise from the treatment table. At the same time, gentle pressure is exerted on the clavicular contact with the right hand. Without releasing the tension, an impulse is applied with an inferior to superior vector.

8.1.4 Sitting sterno-clavicular joint medial to lateral thrust technique

Application
Joint play glide loss from medial to lateral of the clavicle on the sternum.

Patient's position
The patient is placed sitting on a chair with a back rest and with the arm on the affected side abducted and the elbow flexed.

Chiropractor's stance
The chiropractor stands directly behind the patient.

Contact
a) The left hand reaches around to the anterior of the patient on the left of the patient's neck, to contact the medial end of the right clavicle with the thenar eminence. The fingers point obliquely downwards.
b) The right hand reaches across behind the patient and holds under the distal end of the humerus to abduct and extend the shoulder.

Procedure
The joint is stabilized by lightly pressing the patient back against the chair with the left hand and by slightly extending the patient's right shoulder with the right hand. Joint pre-load tension is achieved by further elevating the patient's right arm and without slackening the tension, an impulse is delivered from medial to lateral with the left arm.

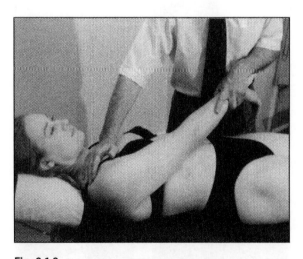

Fig. 8.1.3

Before the impulse is made, the patient's arm is tractioned in long axis until the shoulder girdle is just lifted off the treatment table

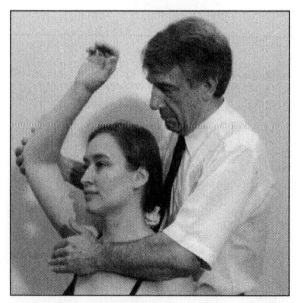

Fig. 8.1.4

Joint tension is achieved by gently pressing the patient against the chair and by abducting and extending the right shoulder

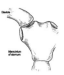

8.1.5 Sitting sterno-clavicular joint anterior to posterior unilateral or bilateral pull technique

Application
Joint play glide loss from anterior to posterior of the clavicle on the sternum.

Patient's position
The patient is seated on a chair without a back rest.

Chiropractor's stance
The chiropractor either sits or stands behind the patient, depending on the relative sizes of patient and chiropractor, and stabilizes the patient by pressing the chest against the patient's scapulae.

Contact
Both arms are wrapped around the patient's shoulders. Both wrists are held in extension and the anterior bases of the metacarpals placed over the sterno-clavicular joints. The fingers may be laced together.

Procedure
Joint pre-load tension is achieved by gently tractioning laterally with the arms. Without releasing the tension, an impulse is made from anterior to posterior on patient exhalation.

If the joint play glide loss is bilateral then the impulse is made equally with both arms. If the joint play glide loss is unilateral then the thrust is also unilateral, with the inactive arm acting as a stabilizer.

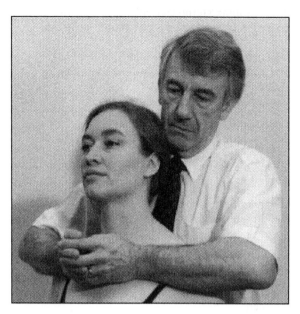

Fig. 8.1.5(a)

The chiropractor's wrists are both held in extension to assist in making firm contact with the sternum

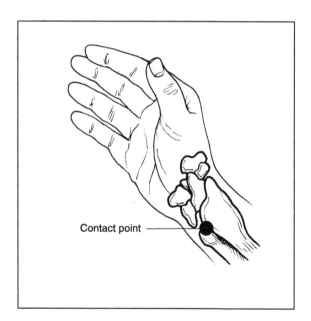

Fig. 8.1.5(b)

The contact point is the anterior distal aspect of the radius

8.1.6 Supine sterno-clavicular joint anterior to posterior crossed arms mobilization technique

Application
The technique is adaptable for general joint stiffness, anterior to posterior or medial to lateral joint play glide loss of the clavicle on the sternum.

Patient's position
The patient is placed supine with a rolled hand towel or a small cylindrical-shaped cushion inserted lengthways between the scapulae. The arms remain down at the patient's sides throughout the procedure.

Chiropractor's stance
The chiropractor stands facing cephalad on either the left or right side of the patient.

Contact
The chiropractor crosses the arms and places the heels of the hands midway along the clavicles.

Procedure
The mobilization may be applied unilaterally or bilaterally as required. Using the hand towel or cushion as a fulcrum between the scapulae, a downward stretching pressure is applied. The pressure is evenly applied with both arms when both clavicles are to be mobilized. If the application is unilateral, then the inactive arm acts as a stabilizer against the clavicle while the impulse is given with the other arm. The pressure is repeated as often as necessary.

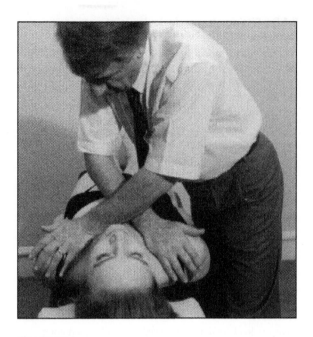

Fig. 8.1.6(a)

The contacts are midway along the anterior border of the clavicles and rhythmic stretching thrusts are used

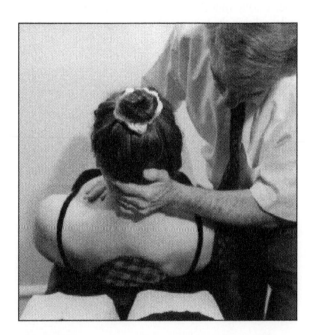

Fig. 8.1.6(b)

To act as a fulcrum, a cushion or rolled towel is placed between the scapulae

8.1.7 Supine sterno-clavicular joint recoil technique

Application
Joint play glide loss from anterior to posterior, superior to inferior, inferior to superior, lateral to medial or medial to lateral, as found by examination, of the clavicle on the sternum.

Patient's position
The patient is placed supine with the arms to the sides.

Chiropractor's stance
a) On the **contralateral side** facing the patient for joint play glide loss from medial to lateral or anterior to posterior.
b) At the **head end** of the treatment table facing caudad favouring the side of involvement for joint play glide loss from superior to inferior or lateral to medial.

Contact
a) The left hand is placed over the posterior of the right wrist using a high or low arch (see Glossary of Terms, p. 285).
b) The right hand is placed over the medial end of the clavicle with a pisiform contact.

Procedure
A high velocity shallow pectoralis/triceps/anconius recoil thrust (see Chapter 2) is applied. If the treatment table is equipped with a thoracic section drop mechanism, this can be employed for this technique.

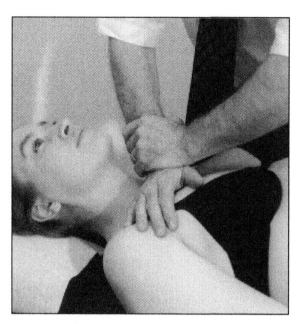

Fig. 8.1.7(a)

Recoil technique showing the stance on the contralateral side

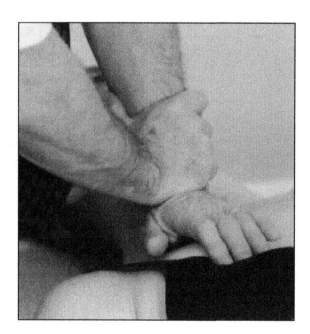

Fig. 8.1.7(b)

Recoil technique showing the stance at the head of the treatment table

8.2

The acromio-clavicular joint

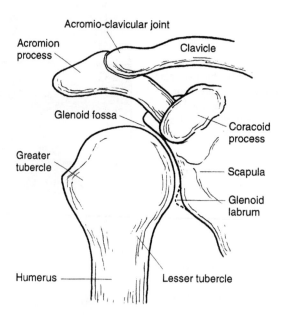

Acromio-clavicular joint

Acromion process

Clavicle

Glenoid fossa

Coracoid process

Greater tubercle

Scapula

Glenoid labrum

Humerus

Lesser tubercle

8.2.A Joint play evaluation of the acromio-clavicular joint superior to inferior and anterior to posterior glide

Procedure

The patient is placed supine and the chiropractor stands at the head end of the treatment table. The heel (see Glossary of Terms, p. 285) of the left hand is placed over the anterior superior border of the distal end of the clavicle. The right hand stabilizes the right upper arm holding around the lower biceps region, abducting and extending the arm a little.

1) Superior to inferior glide

Whilst respecting the oblique plane line of the joint, pressure is exerted from superior to inferior and lateral to medial, taking the joint into joint play. This is felt as an elasticity right at the end of the joint travel.

2) Anterior to posterior glide

The patient is supine and with the hands placed in a similar position as described in (1) above, the left hand presses the joint from anterior to posterior into joint play.

8.2.B Joint play evaluation of the acromio-clavicular joint superior to inferior glide – alternative patient position

Procedure

An alternative position for examining for superior to inferior joint play glide loss is for the chiropractor to stand behind the seated patient. The heel (see Glossary of Terms, p. 285) of the left hand is placed over the anterior superior border of the distal end of the clavicle. The thumb can be used instead of the heel of the hand. The right hand holds the ipsilateral upper arm just proximal to the elbow and abducts and extends the shoulder. As the upper arm rises and the shoulder is extended, the left hand or thumb presses downwards on the acromio-clavicular joint and takes it into joint play. The acromial extremity of the clavicle has a small flattened oval surface facing obliquely downward (Gray, 1959). The downward pressure of the left hand must therefore be directed appropriately at a lateral to medial oblique angle to elicit joint play mobility. It may be necessary to repeat the movement several times to fully assess the presence or absence of joint play in this joint.

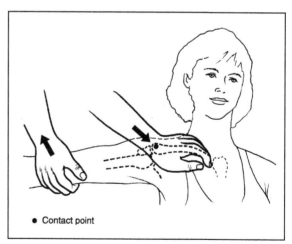

Fig. 8.2.B

An alternative position for examination for superior to inferior joint play glide loss of the acromio-clavicular joint is to have the patient sitting

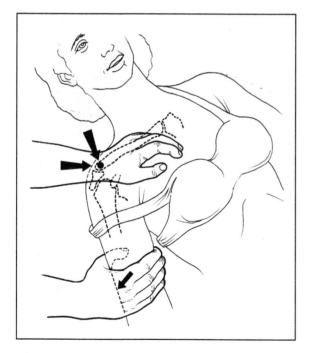

Fig. 8.2.A

Joint play evaluation of the acromio-clavicular joint. The patient is placed supine

8.2.1 Supine acromio-clavicular joint anterior to posterior thrust technique

Application
Joint play glide loss from anterior to posterior of the clavicle on the acromion process.

Patient's position
The patient is placed supine with the arm on the affected side abducted.

Chiropractor's stance
The chiropractor stands on the affected side facing cephalad with the trunk flexed forwards and rotated slightly so that the shoulder is directly above the contact.

Contact
a)   The left hand holds around the patient's right elbow to support the abducted arm.
b)   The right hand is placed over the distal end of the clavicle using a pisiform contact.

Procedure
A variety of methods may be employed for joint correction of this fixation with this contact:

• *Drop technique – see Chapter 2*
• *Body drop technique – see Chapter 2*
• *Slow stretch mobilization technique – see Chapter 2*
• *Recoil technique – see Chapter 2 and Fig. 8.2.1(b)*

A further alternative would be to use an 'Activator' or adjustable spring-loaded centre punch with the right hand, instead of using a direct contact with the pisiform.

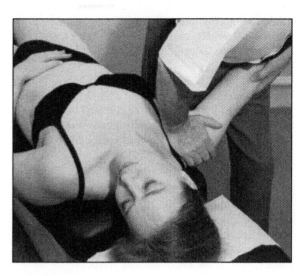

Fig. 8.2.1(a)

The chiropractor's trunk is rotated away from the affected side to bring the shoulder directly above the point of contact

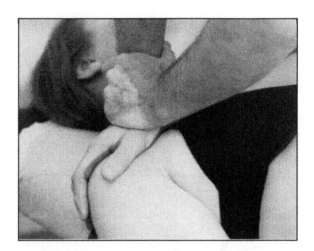

Fig. 8.2.1(b)

As an alternative, the chiropractor stands on the contralateral side using a drop section on the treatment table and recoil high velocity thrust technique

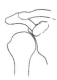

8.2.2 Sitting acromio-clavicular joint superior to inferior thrust technique – Method I

Application
Joint play glide loss from superior to inferior of the clavicle on the acromion process.

Patient's position
The patient sits without a back rest, with the shoulder on the affected side abducted and internally rotated so that the forearm hangs downwards.

Chiropractor's stance
The chiropractor kneels close in to the patient on the affected side with the arm placed over the patient's right shoulder. This procedure places the chiropractor's head conveniently behind the patient's upper trunk.

Contact
Both hands are laced together so that the middle fingers contact the clavicle.
a) The left hand is placed over the distal end of the clavicle from the posterior.
b) The right hand is placed over the distal end of the clavicle from the anterior.

Procedure
Joint pre-load tension is achieved by drawing both arms downwards. Without slackening the tension, a swift downward impulse is applied using minimal depth of thrust.

Note
When utilizing this technique, great care must be taken to reach joint pre-load tension before the impulse is made because in this position the shoulder girdle is anchored by the glenohumeral joint.

8.2.3 Sitting acromio-clavicular joint superior to inferior thrust technique – Method II

Application
Joint play glide loss from superior to inferior of the clavicle on the acromion process.

Patient's position
The patient sits erect with or without a back rest with the arm on the affected side abducted, externally rotated, the elbow flexed and the hand held behind the head.

Chiropractor's stance
The chiropractor stands behind the patient favouring the affected side.

Contact
a) The left hand is placed so that the lateral aspect of the 2nd metacarpo-phalangeal joint is placed over the distal end of the clavicle, fingers pointing downwards over the anterior upper ribs and the thumb pointing down at the posterior to stabilize the scapula.
b) The right hand is placed under the distal end of the humerus.

Procedure
Joint pre-load tension is achieved by holding the clavicle down with the left hand and simultaneously abducting the patient's shoulder with the right hand. The impulse is made downwards with the left arm. Body drop technique (see Chapter 2) is applied by holding the contact arm rigid at the wrist, elbow and shoulder.

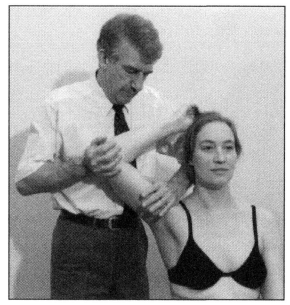

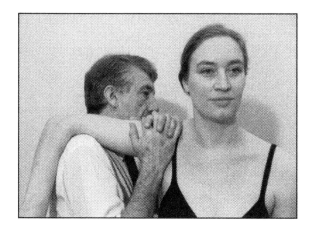

Fig. 8.2.2

To achieve the correct patient/practitioner height ratio, it may be necessary for the chiropractor to kneel on a cushion or to have the patient on a variable height chair

Fig. 8.2.3

To achieve joint pre-load tension, the contact on the clavicle is held down as the arm is further abducted

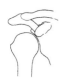

8.2.4 Supine acromio-clavicular joint superior to inferior body drop technique with shoulder hyper-abduction

Application
Joint play glide loss from superior to inferior of the clavicle on the acromion process.

Patient's position
The patient is placed supine with the arm on the affected side hyperabducted.

Chiropractor's stance
The chiropractor stands at the head end of the treatment table favouring the side of involvement, facing caudad.

Contact
a) The thenar eminence of the left hand is placed over the distal end of the clavicle and the wrist is held in extension, the elbow held stiff and slightly flexed.
b) The right hand holds the patient's right mid-forearm from the lateral side and holds the arm in hyperabduction.

Procedure
To produce joint pre-load tension, the patient's right arm is tractioned headwards to stabilize the shoulder girdle. The chiropractor, whilst keeping the left arm rigid, leans towards the contact. The impulse is made by using a gentle body drop technique (see Chapter 2) with a unilateral thrust along the left arm.

8.2.5 Sitting acromio-clavicular joint superior to inferior and posterior to anterior thrust technique

Application
Joint play glide loss from superior to inferior and posterior to anterior of the clavicle on the acromion process.

Patient's position
The patient sits with or without a back rest, with the shoulder on the affected side abducted, internally rotated and slightly extended. The elbow is flexed to approximately 90–100°. The patient's hand falls just behind the trunk and the head is tilted laterally away from the side of contact.

Chiropractor's stance
The chiropractor stands directly behind the patient favouring the side of involvement.

Contact
a) The web of the left hand, with the elbow held high, is placed over the distal end of the clavicle, the fingers anterior and pointing downwards, the thumb to the posterior.
b) The fingers of the right hand are wrapped around the lateral aspect of the patient's forearm, to stabilize and help depress the shoulder girdle.

Procedure
Joint pre-load tension is achieved by both hands depressing the shoulder girdle and a high velocity, low amplitude impulse is applied downwards and towards the anterior.

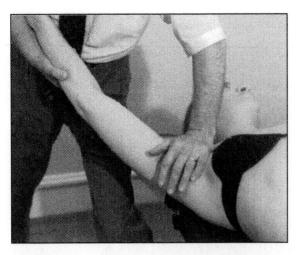

Fig. 8.2.4

A unilateral body drop technique is applied whilst maintaining traction on the hyper-abducted arm

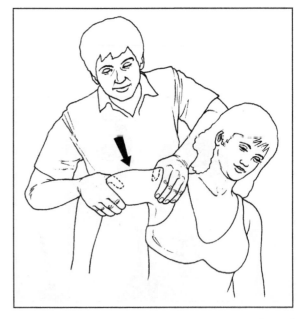

Fig. 8.2.5

The shoulder girdle is depressed to achieve joint pre-load tension before the oblique downward thrust is applied

8.2.6 Supine acromio-clavicular joint circumduction mobilization technique

Application
General mobilization of the acromio-clavicular joint.

Patient's position
The patient is placed supine with the shoulder on the affected side flexed and abducted. The patient's elbow remains extended.

Chiropractor's stance
The chiropractor stands facing cephalad on the affected side, close against the patient. The right knee is flexed and placed close to the patient's axilla allowing the posterior of the upper arm to rest against the chiropractor's anterior lower thigh.

Contact
a) The left hand holds the patient's upper arm and the fingers are wrapped around the posterior of the triceps area. Traction is then applied, elevating the shoulder girdle and pulling the patient's upper arm closer against the chiropractor's thigh.

b) The right hand is placed over the distal end of the clavicle and the fingers are flexed to tightly clasp the superior border. It is advisable to use a towel under the hand to soften the contact. The traction and shoulder girdle elevation applied with the left hand exposes the clavicle, to make a firmer and more accessible contact with the right hand.

Procedure
The chiropractor circumducts the patient's shoulder girdle in as wide a circle as is tolerable for the patient. The anterior thigh contact is maintained close against the patient's axilla throughout the manoeuvre by coming up on the toes, flexing and followed by extension of the hip in order to stabilize the patient's glenohumeral joint. The manoeuvre is repeated several times as required.

Note
This technique does not confine the movement to the acromio-clavicular joint alone but may be considered as a mobilization method for all the joints of the shoulder girdle.

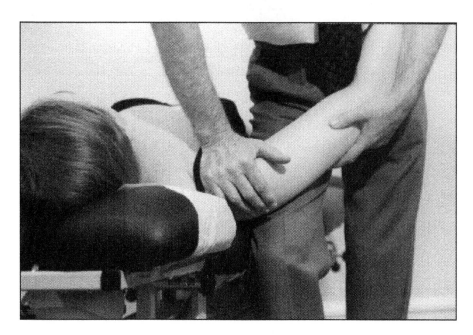

Fig. 8.2.6

The chiropractor's knee is placed at the posterior of the upper humerus. The knee remains in contact throughout

8.2.7 Supine acromio-clavicular joint superior to inferior pull technique – Method I

Application
Joint play glide loss from superior to inferior of the clavicle on the acromion process.

Patient's position
The patient is placed supine with the arm on the affected side elevated to about 45°.

Chiropractor's stance
The chiropractor stands facing cephalad on the homolateral side.

Contact
a) The left hand grasps the upper part of the humerus from the posterior. The patient's elevated forearm is held with the elbow against the chiropractor's side.
b) A towel is placed over the affected clavicle to cushion the contact. The right hand is placed on the towel with all four fingers holding the distal end of the clavicle from the superior. To facilitate this, the patient's shoulder girdle is elevated a little with the chiropractor's left arm, allowing more space between the clavicle and the first rib for a secure contact to be made.

Procedure
Whilst maintaining a firm contact with the right hand, the patient's right arm is lowered into extension and tractioned. This achieves joint pre-load tension and also lowers the scapula against the treatment table to stabilize the shoulder girdle. An impulse from superior to inferior is made with the right hand whilst stabilizing with the left hand.

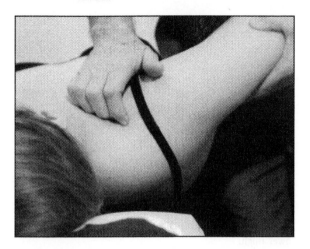

Fig. 8.2.7(a)

Stage I: The patient's arm and shoulder girdle are elevated (shown here without towel)

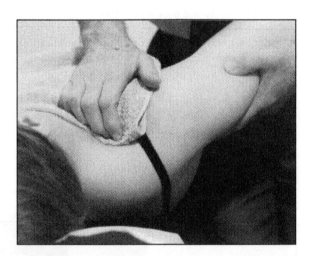

Fig. 8.2.7(b)

Stage II. The patient's arm is lowered and tractioned to stabilize the scapula and achieve joint pre-load tension

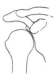

8.2.8 Supine acromio-clavicular joint superior to inferior pull technique

Application
Joint play glide loss from superior to inferior of the clavicle on the acromion process.

Patient's position
The patient is placed supine with the shoulder abducted to 60° or 70°.

Chiropractor's stance
The chiropractor stands on the affected side facing cephalad.

Contact
a) The left hand is placed around the lateral upper arm to grasp around the triceps and the patient's lower arm is held firmly between the chiropractor's ribs and elbow.
b) The right hand is placed over the distal clavicle, hooking all fingers over the superior aspect.

Procedure
Joint pre-load tension is achieved by drawing both contacts caudad. Without releasing the tension, a substantial impulse is made in a caudad direction, because the scapula is not well stabilized in this technique and the shoulder girdle absorbs a considerable amount of the thrust.

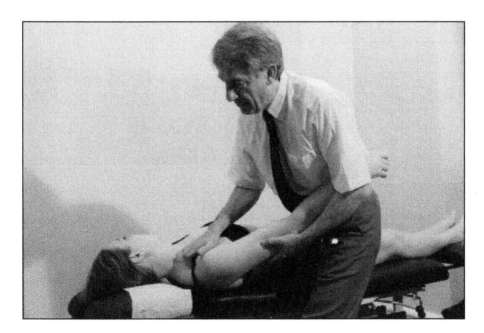

Fig. 8.2.8

The contact on the clavicle is made with all fingers hooked around the superior border

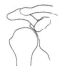

8.2.9 Prone acromio-clavicular joint superior to inferior and anterior to posterior pull technique

Application
Joint play glide loss from superior to inferior and anterior to posterior of the clavicle on the acromion process.

Patient's position
The patient is placed prone with the shoulder on the affected side abducted to approximately 45° and the elbow flexed to approximately 90°.

Chiropractor's stance
The chiropractor stands facing obliquely cephalad on the affected side holding the patient's elbow between the knees.

Contact
a) The right hand contacts the superior border of the clavicle just proximal to the joint, using the junction of the 2nd and 3rd phalanx of the right middle finger as the contact point. The remaining fingers close up to support the contact.
b) The left hand is wrapped over the top of the right hand as support. The left forearm is placed over the scapula to stabilize it.

Procedure
Holding the trunk flexed forwards to maintain pressure on the scapula, the chiropractor draws the patient's clavicle inferior to produce joint pre-load tension. Without slackening the tension, the impulse is made towards the chiropractor in an oblique superior to inferior direction.

REFERENCE

Gray, H. (1959) *Anatomy of the Human Body*. 27th centennial edn. Philadelphia, Lea and Febiger.

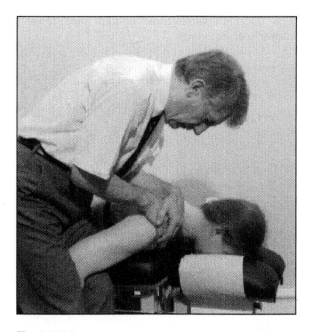

Fig. 8.2.9(a)

The patient's elbow is held between the chiropractor's knees

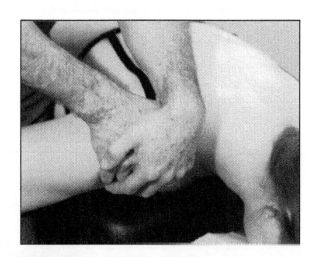

Fig. 8.2.9(b)

Detail showing contact. The left forearm is used to stabilize the patient's scapula

The glenohumeral joint

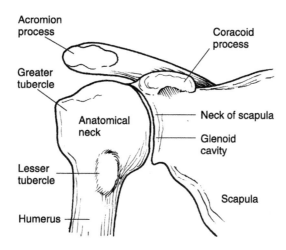

Acromion process

Coracoid process

Greater tubercle

Anatomical neck

Neck of scapula

Glenoid cavity

Lesser tubercle

Scapula

Humerus

Glenohumeral joint anterior to posterior techniques
8.3.A Joint play evaluation of the anterior to posterior glide of the humerus in the glenoid cavity
8.3.1 Sitting glenohumeral joint anterior to posterior flexion pull technique
8.3.2 Supine glenohumeral joint anterior to posterior flexion thrust technique
8.3.3 Prone glenohumeral joint anterior to posterior technique with abduction and external rotation
8.3.4 Supine glenohumeral joint anterior to posterior recoil technique with abduction and external or internal rotation
8.3.5 Supine glenohumeral joint anterior to posterior thrust technique with abduction and rotation

Glenohumeral joint superior to inferior techniques
8.3.B Joint play evaluation of the superior to inferior glide of the humerus in the glenoid cavity
8.3.6 Supine glenohumeral joint superior to inferior technique with abduction
8.3.7 Side reclining glenohumeral joint superior to inferior pull technique with abduction
8.3.8 Sitting glenohumeral joint superior to inferior mobilization technique with abduction
8.3.9 Prone glenohumeral joint superior to inferior pull technique with abduction
8.3.10 Prone glenohumeral joint superior to inferior mobilization technique with abduction

Glenohumeral joint inferior to superior techniques
8.3.C Joint play evaluation of the inferior to superior glide of the humerus in the glenoid cavity
8.3.11 Sitting glenohumeral joint inferior to superior pull technique
8.3.12 Sitting glenohumeral joint inferior to superior pull technique with flexion and internal rotation
8.3.13 Sitting glenohumeral joint inferior to superior pull technique with flexion and external rotation
8.3.14 Prone glenohumeral joint inferior to superior pull technique with abduction and external rotation

Glenohumeral joint medial to lateral techniques
8.3.D Joint play evaluation of the medial to lateral glide of the humerus in the glenoid cavity
8.3.15 Supine glenohumeral joint medial to lateral mobilization technique

Glenohumeral joint circumduction mobilization technique
8.3.16 Prone or supine glenohumeral joint circumduction mobilization technique with traction and abduction

Glenohumeral joint abduction mobilization technique
8.3.17 Supine glenohumeral joint abduction mobilization technique

Glenohumeral joint anterior to posterior techniques

8.3.A Joint play evaluation of the anterior to posterior glide of the humerus in the glenoid cavity

Procedure

Method I
The patient sits with the arm on the affected side relaxed and hanging down. The heel of the right hand contacts the anterior of the humeral head and presses firmly from anterior to posterior into joint play. The left hand stabilizes the scapula from the posterior.

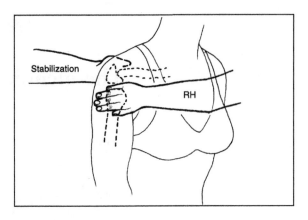

Fig. 8.3.AI

Anterior to posterior glide of the humerus in the glenoid cavity – Method I

Method II
The same test may be performed with the patient supine and the shoulder abducted on the affected side, the arm stabilized against the crest of the chiropractor's pelvis and held there with the elbow. The test should be performed as above, with either external or internal rotation added.

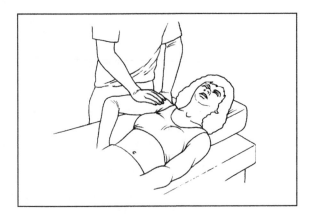

Fig. 8.3.AII

Anterior to posterior glide of the humerus in the glenoid cavity – Method II

Method III
A third alternative is to have the patient lying supine, stabilizing the scapula on the affected side from the posterior with the left hand and pressing anterior to posterior on the anterior of the humeral head with the right hand. External or internal rotation components may be added to the anterior to posterior test.

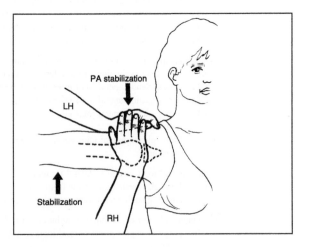

Fig. 8.3.AIII

Anterior to posterior glide of the humerus in the glenoid cavity – Method III

8.3.1 Sitting glenohumeral joint anterior to posterior flexion pull technique

Application
Joint play loss of anterior to posterior glide of humeral head in the glenoid fossa.

Patient's position
The patient sits with the affected arm flexed forwards to about 90°, the elbow flexed.

Chiropractor's stance
The chiropractor stands behind the patient, favouring the side of involvement, with the sternum held against the patient's scapula.

Contacts
a) The left hand is placed around the distal end of the elbow with the arm around the left side of the patient's neck.
b) The right hand reinforces the left by clasping it under the distal end of the olecranon process.

Procedure
Joint pre-load tension is achieved by pulling the elbow from anterior to posterior, stabilized by the chiropractor's sternum without releasing the tension. The impulse is delivered smartly from anterior to posterior. Only minimal depth of thrust is required.

Care must be taken not to pull the patient's hand into the face during this procedure.

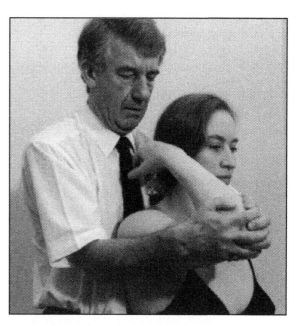

Fig. 8.3.1(a)

View 1: the chiropractor stabilizes the patient's scapula by pressing the sternum against it

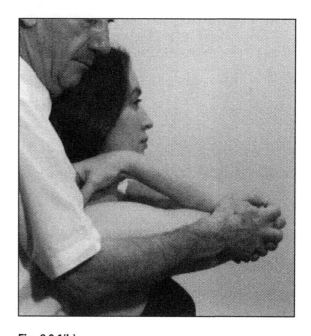

Fig. 8.3.1(b)

View 2: minimal depth of thrust is needed if correct joint pre-load tension is first achieved

8.3.2   Supine glenohumeral anterior to posterior flexion thrust technique

Application
Joint play glide loss of the humerus from anterior to posterior in the glenoid fossa when the joint is flexed.

Patient's position
The patient is placed supine with the elbow on the affected side fully flexed and the humerus elevated to a vertical position

Chiropractor's stance
The chiropractor stands on the affected side facing cephalad adjacent to the patient's shoulder. The trunk is flexed forwards over the contact and the right elbow is kept close to the side.

Contact
a)   The left hand stabilizes the patient's shoulder by holding around the anterior of the humeral head.
b)   The right hand is cupped over the patient's elbow, palm downwards, using the heel of the hand as the contact. The fingers point headwards.

Procedure
Joint pre-load tension is produced by the chiropractor stiffening the contact arm at the shoulder and elbow and leaning the trunk forwards against the contact. The impulse is made by using swift body drop (see Chapter 2) technique with minimal depth of thrust.

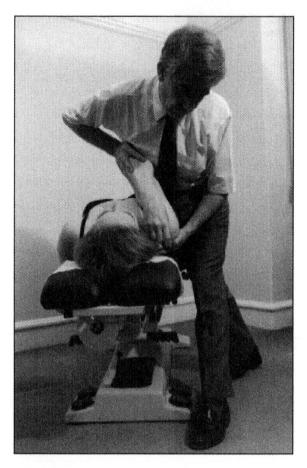

Fig. 8.3.2(a)

Joint pre-load tension is produced by flexing the trunk forwards and leaning gently into the contacts. Very little depth of thrust is required

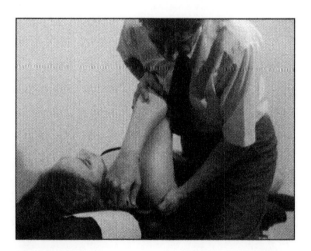

Fig. 8.3.2(b)

The left hand stabilizes the scapula

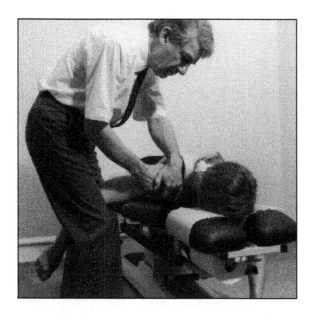

Fig. 8.3.3(a)

Initial position facing the patient, straddling the elbow with the knees

8.3.3 Prone glenohumeral joint anterior to posterior pull technique with abduction and upward rotation

Application
Joint play glide loss from anterior to posterior of the humerus in the glenoid fossa.

Patient's position
The patient is placed prone with the shoulder on the affected side abducted and the elbow flexed to about 90°. The patient's forearm hangs vertically down.

Chiropractor's stance
The chiropractor stands facing the patient opposite the affected shoulder and straddles the patient's elbow between the knees.

Contact
a) The right hand is placed over the proximal end of the humerus as close to the humeral head as possible, with the fingers cupped around the anterior.
b) The left hand is placed over the right hand.

Procedure
The chiropractor now turns cephalad. This places the patient's right forearm in contact with the posterior of the chiropractor's right lower leg and also abducts the patient's humerus a little. By lifting the right foot clear of the floor and flexing the knee, the patient's shoulder can be rotated internally and held downwards. The chiropractor's left forearm is now placed firmly over the patient's scapula to stabilize it. Joint pre-load tension is achieved by bringing the humeral head from superior to inferior and without releasing the tension, an impulse is made by pulling swiftly in the same direction.

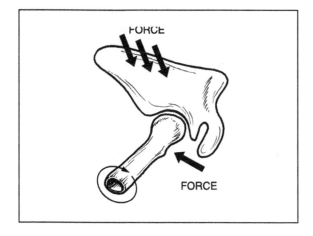

Fig. 8.3.3(b)

The adjustive forces exerted on the glenohumeral joint. By rotating the humerus with the leg, torsion is applied to the joint

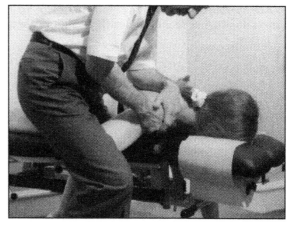

Fig. 8.3.3(c)

Final position. The chiropractor uses his lower leg to internally rotate the patient's arm. The patient's position and scapula are stabilized by forearm pressure

8.3.4 Supine glenohumeral joint anterior to posterior recoil technique

Application
Joint play glide loss of the humerus from anterior to posterior in the glenoid fossa.

Patient's position
The patient is placed supine with the affected shoulder abducted to approximately 45° with the elbow extended. The thoracic section on the treatment table is lightly set for the patient's weight, and cocked.

Chiropractor's stance
The chiropractor stands on the homolateral side facing cephalad, close up to the patient's axilla. The right hip is flexed and the anterior lower thigh just proximal to the knee is placed just under and against the lateral border of the scapula to stabilize it.

Contact
a) The left hand holds around the posterior of the patient's elbow, elevates and tractions it.
b) The right hand is placed over the anterior of the tibial head, using a heel of hand contact. The fingers are wrapped around the superior border of the tibial head.

Procedure
The left hand tractions the shoulder a little further, together with a light downward pressure on the humeral head to produce joint pre-load tension. The impulse is a light unilateral high velocity recoil type thrust (see Chapter 2) delivered with the right arm.

Note
An internal or external shoulder rotation component can be added, if required.

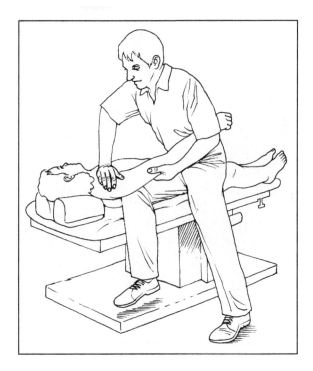

Fig. 8.3.4

The chiropractor's right hip is flexed and the right foot is lifted off the floor. The right anterior thigh stabilizes the lateral border of the scapula. Joint pre-load tension is produced by light anterior to posterior contact pressure on the humeral head with the right hand. The left contact elevates and tractions the arm

8.3.5 Supine glenohumeral joint anterior to posterior thrust technique with abduction and rotation

Application
Joint play glide loss of the humerus in the glenoid fossa from anterior to posterior with either an external or internal rotation component.

Patient's position
The patient is placed supine with the head well supported and the shoulder abducted approximately 45° and the elbow flexed to approximately 90°.

Chiropractor's stance
The chiropractor stands on the homolateral side facing cephalad, with the left leg ahead of the right, and the anterior of the thigh tight against the patient's axilla. The trunk is rotated to the left, away from the involved shoulder.

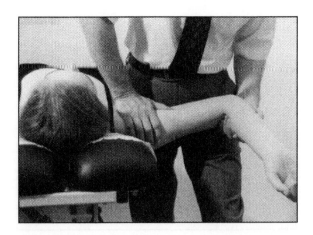

Fig. 8.3.5(a)

The chiropractor, using this stance may rotate the patient's shoulder externally as shown, or internally as required (see Fig. 8.3.5(b))

Contact

a) The left hand supports under the patient's elbow and rotates the shoulder externally or internally as required.

b) The right hand is placed over the anterior of the proximal humerus as close to the humeral head as possible, using the pisiform and 5th metacarpal as the contact.

Procedure

To achieve joint pre-load tension, the chiropractor rotates the trunk a few degrees further away from the involved shoulder whilst maintaining a firm contact. At the same time, the left hand elevates the elbow a little. The chiropractor may now either use a light body drop technique (see Chapter 2) or use a drop technique by cocking the thoracic section on the treatment table.

Glenohumeral joint superior to inferior techniques

8.3.B   Joint play evaluation of the superior to inferior glide of the humerus in the glenoid cavity

This assessment may be carried out with the patient sitting, standing, or lying supine.

Procedure

Method I

Both hands are laced together over the superior border of the humeral head, the patient's shoulder is abducted to 90° and the distal humerus is stabilized from the inferior with the chiropractor's shoulder. As the humeral head is depressed, the scapula will also move with it, therefore all slack must be taken up before joint play can be assessed.

Method II

Alternatively, the chiropractor stands behind the seated patient. The patient's shoulder is abducted to 90° and the distal humerus is stabilized from the inferior with the right hand. The lateral border of the left hand is placed over the proximal humerus as close to the humeral head as possible. The left hand exerts a pressure downwards into joint play after ensuring that all slack has been removed from the scapula. This manoeuvre should be repeated with external and internal rotation of the shoulder in turn.

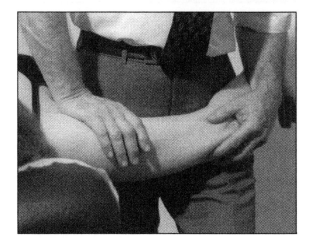

Fig. 8.3.5(b)

Using a similar stance to that seen in Fig. 8.3.5(a) the chiropractor rotates the patient's shoulder internally

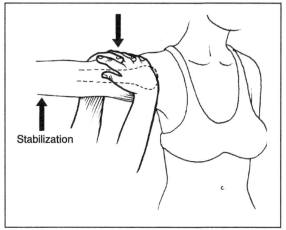

Fig. 8.3.B

Joint play evaluation of the superior to inferior glide

8.3.6 Supine glenohumeral joint superior to inferior techniques with abduction

Method I – Pull technique

Application
Joint play glide loss from anterior to posterior of the humeral head in the glenoid fossa.

Patient's position
The patient is placed supine with the shoulder abducted to about 90° or to tolerance.

Chiropractor's stance
The chiropractor stands on the homolateral side facing cephalad, adjacent to the patient's shoulder.

Contact
a) The left hand supports the patient's elbow and holds the patient's shoulder in abduction.
b) The right hand, palm upwards, contacts around under the proximal end of the humerus as close as possible to the humeral head from the posterior, with all fingers holding the superior aspect.

Procedure
As the left hand stabilizes the patient's arm, the right arm tensions the joint in a superior to inferior direction. Without slackening the tension, the impulse is delivered superior to inferior as a swift pull from superior to inferior. An external or internal shoulder rotation component can be added as required.

Method II – Thrust technique

Application
As for Method I.

Patient's position
As for Method I.

Chiropractor's stance
The chiropractor stands on the homolateral side facing caudad, standing level with the patient's head.

Contact
a) The left hand is placed over the proximal end of the humerus with all fingers wrapped around the anterior aspect.
b) The right hand supports the patient's elbow and maintains the arm at 90° abduction.

Procedure
Joint pre-load tension is achieved with the left hand pressing superior to inferior. Without slackening the tension, the impulse is delivered as a swift unilateral left arm thrust. An external or internal shoulder rotation component can be added as required.

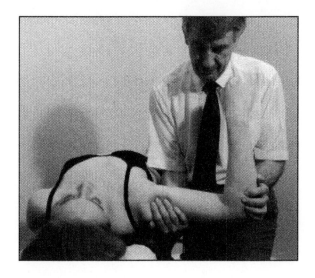

Fig. 8.3.6(a)

Method I – pull technique

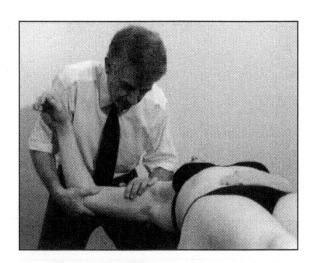

Fig. 8.3.6(b)

Method II – thrust technique

8.3.7 Side reclining glenohumeral joint superior to inferior pull technique with abduction

Application
Joint play glide loss from superior to inferior of the humerus in the glenoid fossa.

Patient's position
The patient is placed in the side reclining position with the affected side up and the shoulder abducted to about 45°.

Chiropractor's stance
The chiropractor stands behind the patient facing cephalad with the trunk inclined forwards.

Contact
The patient's right arm is held in abduction by passing the chiropractor's right arm beneath it, contacting elbow to elbow. Both hands are then laced together and the lateral border of the 5th metacarpal of either hand contacts the lateral superior border of the humerus as close to the humeral head as possible.

Procedure
Joint pre-load tension is obtained by gently pulling the humeral head from superior to inferior, abducting the arm at the same time. Without releasing the tension, a swift impulse is given in the same direction. Minimal depth of thrust is required.

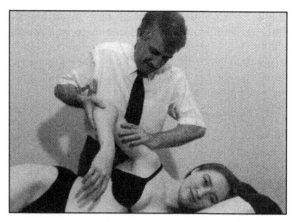

Fig. 8.3.7(a)

This technique may, by rotating the arm, be adapted for joint play loss of external or internal rotation

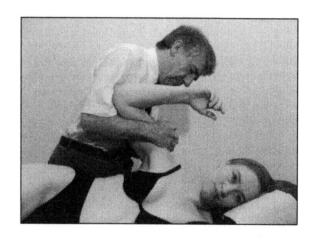

Fig. 8.3.7(b)

Superior to inferior, external rotation

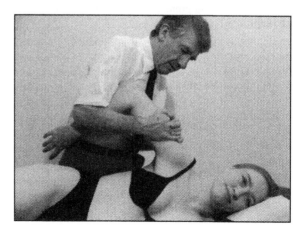

Fig. 8.3.7(c)

Superior to inferior, internal rotation

8.3.8 Sitting glenohumeral joint superior to inferior mobilization technique with abduction

Application
Joint play glide loss of the humeral head from superior to inferior in the glenoid fossa.

Patient's position
The patient sits with the affected arm abducted.

Chiropractor's stance
The chiropractor kneels adjacent to the patient's affected side facing towards the patient with the head placed behind the patient's shoulder. The patient's upper arm is placed over the chiropractor's right shoulder with the forearm pointing downwards as much as possible.

Contact
The chiropractor places **both hands** linked together over the proximal end of the humerus as close to the humeral head as possible.

Procedure
With the chiropractor's shoulder as a fulcrum on the humerus, the chiropractor pulls the hands gently but firmly downwards and then releases the pressure, repeating this action in a rhythmical fashion. The patient is instructed to steadily pull the scapula upwards, matching the pressure each time the humerus is pulled downwards by the chiropractor.

8.3.9 Prone glenohumeral joint superior to inferior pull technique with abduction

Application
Joint play glide loss from superior to inferior of the humeral head in the glenoid fossa.

Patient's position
The patient is placed prone with the affected shoulder abducted to 90° or to tolerance.

Chiropractor's stance
The chiropractor stands on the homolateral side facing the patient, adjacent to the affected shoulder. The trunk is flexed forwards.

Contact
a) The **left hand** holds and supports the patient's arm, holding under the distal end of the humerus and keeping it in abduction.
b) The **right hand** contacts the superior aspect of the proximal end of the humerus with all the fingers wrapped around it.

Procedure
The right hand presses superior to inferior until joint pre-load tension is felt. Without slackening the tension, the impulse is then delivered swiftly from superior to inferior.

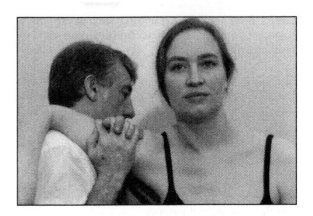

Fig. 8.3.8(a)

The chiropractor kneels very close to the patient. The forearm should point downwards vertically, if mobility will allow

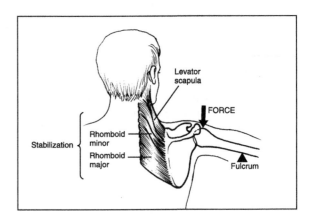

Fig. 8.3.8(b)

The scapula is stabilized by the levator scapula and rhomboid muscles

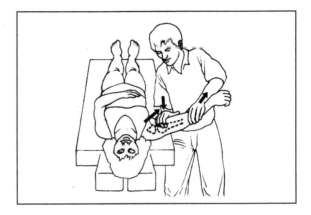

Fig. 8.3.9

The patient's shoulder is abducted with the right arm, held with the humerus horizontally and stabilized in that position. The left hand delivers the impulse

8.3.10 Prone glenohumeral joint superior to inferior mobilization technique with abduction

Application
Joint play glide loss of the humerus in the glenoid fossa from superior to inferior with abduction and joint rotation.

Patient's position
The patient is placed prone with the affected arm abducted to comfort and the forearm held as near vertically downwards as possible.

Chiropractor's stance
The chiropractor stands facing the patient with the lumbar spine semi-flexed over the patient and straddling the patient's elbow on the affected side with semi-flexed knees. It is important that the knees remain semi-flexed (see procedure below).

Contact
a) The left hand, palm downwards, contacts the lateral border of the scapula on the lower third of its length.
b) The right hand wraps around the superior border of the humerus as close to the humeral head as possible.

Procedure
In a smooth, co-ordinated, rhythmical motion, the procedure is as follows:

1 *The inferior tip of the scapula is moved medially with the left hand.*
2 *The humeral head is pressed towards the inferior with the right hand.*
3 *As the inferior angle of the scapula is moved medially, the shoulder is further abducted by using the semi-flexed knees in a caudad sideways swaying movement, with the trunk moving towards the patient's head.*

The procedure is repeated several times as required and always to the patient's tolerance.

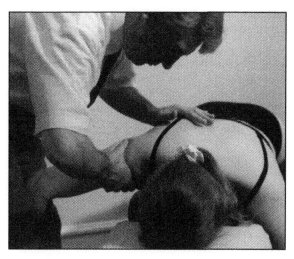

Fig. 8.3.10(a)
The chiropractor's knees should remain flexed throughout

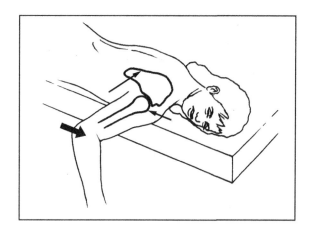

Fig. 8.3.10(b)

The directions of adjustive forces applied to the joint

Glenohumeral joint inferior to superior techniques

8.3.C   Joint play evaluation of the inferior to superior glide of the humerus in the glenoid cavity

Procedure

Method I

The patient is placed supine to help stabilize the scapula. The left hand holds the elbow around the superior border and the right hand contacts the inferior aspect of the upper humerus, close into the axilla. All joint slack must first be removed by pressing the right hand towards the head before joint play can be assessed. Pressure from inferior to superior is then applied firmly into joint play.

Method II

This manoeuvre can also be carried out with the patient in the sitting position. The chiropractor stands behind the patient. The left hand is placed over the superior border of the scapula and the clavicle to anchor them firmly. The right hand grasps under the proximal humerus as close to the humeral head as possible and pulls superiorly into joint play, ensuring that all shoulder girdle slack has first been removed.

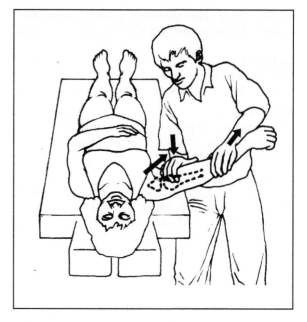

Fig. 8.3.C(a)

Joint play evaluation. Inferior to superior glide of the humerus in the glenoid cavity

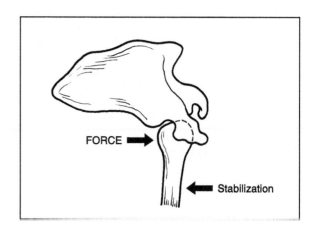

Fig. 8.3.C(b)

Inferior to superior glide of the humerus in the glenoid cavity. The direction of forces applied to elicit joint play

8.3.11 Sitting glenohumeral joint inferior to superior pull technique

Application
Joint play glide loss from inferior to superior of the humeral head in the glenoid fossa.

Patient's position
The patient sits on a stool with the elbow on the affected side flexed and the upper arm relaxed. Although the technique can be managed on a chair with a back rest, in the author's experience it is best done without one. The patient flexes the trunk slightly forwards.

Chiropractor's stance
The chiropractor stands facing the patient from behind, close up, favouring the side to be treated.

Contacts
a) The left hand reaches over past the left side of the patient's neck, around the front of the chest and grasps the underside of the elbow.
b) The right hand also grasps the underside of the elbow by reaching down the lateral side of the patient's upper arm.

Procedure
The chiropractor flexes the trunk forwards and presses the sternum against the upper aspect of the patient's right scapula and maintains this contact. The patient's elbow is elevated until joint pre-load tension is felt. Without releasing the tension, a swift upward impulse is then delivered with minimal depth of thrust, pulling from inferior to superior.

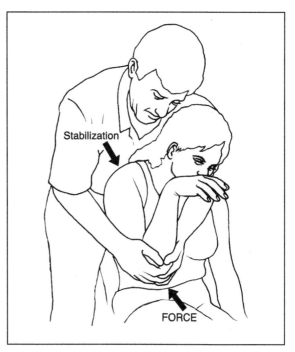

Fig. 8.3.11(a)

To brace the patient's shoulder, the chiropractor holds it against the sternum

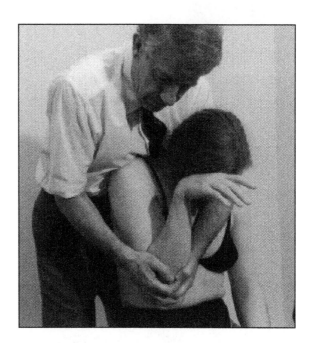

Fig. 8.3.11(b)

The patient is flexed slightly forward and the forearm is placed vertically

8.3.12 Sitting glenohumeral joint inferior to superior pull technique with flexion and internal rotation

Application
Joint play glide loss of the humerus in the glenoid fossa from inferior to superior with flexion and internal rotation.

Patient's position
This differs from technique 8.3.11 by rotating the shoulder internally so that the patient's forearm and hand are placed across the body.

Chiropractor's stance
As for technique 8.3.11.

Contact
As for technique 8.3.11.

Procedure
As for technique 8.3.11.

8.3.13 Sitting glenohumeral joint inferior to superior pull technique with flexion and external rotation

Application
Joint play glide loss of the humerus in the glenoid fossa from inferior to superior with external rotation.

Patient's position
This differs from technique 8.3.12 by rotating the patient's shoulder externally so that the patient's hand and forearm are pointing away from the body.

Chiropractor's stance
As for technique 8.3.11.

Contact
As for technique 8.3.11.

Procedure
As for technique 8.3.11.

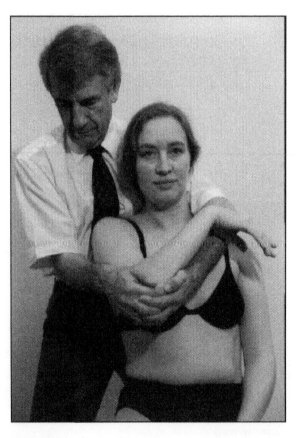

Fig. 8.3.12

The shoulder is rotated internally

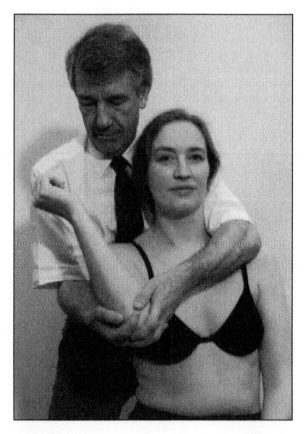

Fig. 8.3.13

The shoulder is rotated externally

8.3.14 Prone glenohumeral joint inferior to superior pull technique with abduction and rotation

Application
Joint play glide loss from inferior to superior of the humerus in the glenoid fossa in abduction and external rotation.

Patient's position
The patient is placed prone with the arm on the affected side abducted as close to 90° as possible. The forearm is allowed to hang downwards.

Chiropractor's stance
The chiropractor stands on the homolateral side superior to the patient's affected shoulder, facing caudad.

Contact
a) The left hand holds the patient's right elbow and stabilizes it.
b) The right hand is placed over the posterior of the upper arm, close to the humeral head, with all the fingers wrapped around the inferior of the humerus.

Procedure
The joint pre-load tension is produced by the left hand pushing towards the foot a little, matched by a pull towards the head with the right hand. Without slackening the tension, a swift headward pull is made with the right arm. Because the scapula is not stabilized in this position, extra depth of thrust may be required.

Glenohumeral joint medial to lateral techniques

8.3.D Joint play evaluation of the medial to lateral glide of the humerus in the glenoid cavity

Procedure
The patient either sits or reclines supine and the chiropractor faces the patient's affected side. The right hand contacts the medial proximal border of the humerus and pulls it laterally. The elbow is held to the patient's side with the chiropractor's trunk to stabilize it. The palm of the left hand is placed against the patient's rib cage high into the axilla with the fingers placed to stabilize the lateral border of the scapula. There is normally a wide excursion of the joint before joint play is reached.

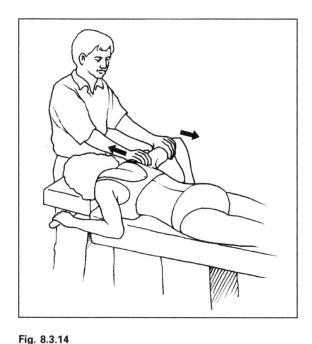

Fig. 8.3.14

The scapula is not stabilized in this position. This is overcome by increased depth of thrust and speed of delivery

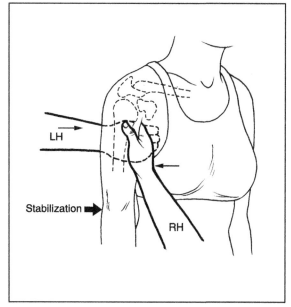

Fig. 8.3.D

Joint play evaluation of the medial to lateral glide of the humerus in the glenoid cavity

8.3.15 Supine glenohumeral joint medial to lateral mobilization technique

Application
Joint play glide loss from medial to lateral of the humerus in the glenoid fossa.

Patient's position
The patient is placed supine with the shoulder on the affected side abducted to approximately 40°.

Chiropractor's stance
The chiropractor stands on the homolateral side facing the patient, adjacent to the affected shoulder, with a hand towel wound around the left forearm to form a soft pad.

Contact
a) The left forearm is placed with the soft pad into the patient's axilla to act as a fulcrum against the upper medial humerus.
b) The right hand contacts the lateral border of the patient's elbow.

Procedure
The patient's right elbow is pressed towards the chest wall and then released. This movement is repeated several times in a rhythmical fashion and performed both requirement and to patient tolerance.

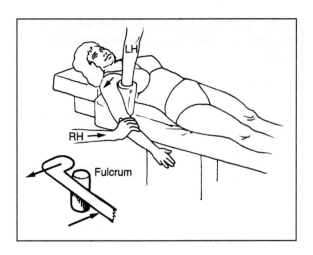

Fig. 8.3.15

A hand-towel is wrapped around the chiropractor's left forearm which acts as a padded fulcrum. The right arm presses the patient's elbow medially and rhythmically and repetitively, in a pressure–release–pressure sequence

Glenohumeral joint circumduction mobilization technique

8.3.16 Prone or supine circumduction mobilization technique with traction and abduction

Application
Loss of multidirectional joint play glide and intercapsular adhesions between the humerus and the glenoid fossa.

Patient's position
The patient is placed prone or supine with the affected shoulder abducted to 90° or to the patient's tolerance and the forearm pointing downwards.

Chiropractor's stance
The chiropractor stands on the homolateral side facing the patient, flexing the trunk forwards and supporting the patient's elbow between the knees.

Contact
Both hands grasp around the proximal end of the humerus as close to the humeral head as possible, with the fingers laced together at the anterior, affording a firm hold on the humerus.

Procedure
The chiropractor leans the weight backwards, to traction the patient's shoulder into long axis extension. Whilst maintaining the traction, the humeral head is moved in circumduction several times to the patient's tolerance.

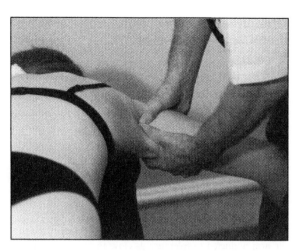

Fig. 8.3.16(a)

The patient is placed prone. The chiropractor's hands clasp around the upper humerus with the fingers laced together

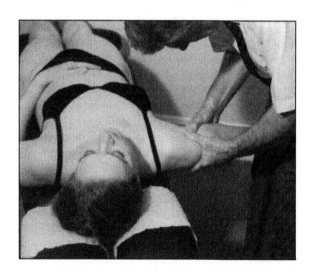

Fig. 8.3.16(b)

The same traction mobilization technique may also be used with the patient lying supine

Glenohumeral joint abduction mobilization technique

8.3.17 Supine glenohumeral joint abduction mobilization technique with external or internal rotation

Application
Joint play glide loss of abduction of the humerus in the glenoid fossa with an external and/or internal component. This condition is frequently encountered in patients with chronic adhesive capsulitis.

Patient's position
The patient is placed supine, with the head supported and the arm abducted to tolerance as close to 90° as possible.

Chiropractor's stance
The chiropractor either sits or stands facing the patient, adjacent to the affected shoulder. If the chiropractor is sitting the patient's elbow is rested on the knees.

For external rotation:

Contact
a)   The right hand is placed palm upwards under the patient's elbow.
b)   The left hand is placed over the volar surface of the patient's wrist.

Procedure
The patient's shoulder is rotated gently upwards to its limit and held for a few seconds, stretched a little and released. This is repeated gently several times.

For internal rotation:

Contact
The hands are reversed.
a)   The right hand is placed over the dorsum of the patient's wrist.
b)   The left hand is placed under the patient's elbow.

Procedure
The patient's shoulder is rotated gently downwards to the point of joint resistance and even more gently stretched in the same direction, held for a few seconds and then released. This procedure may be repeated several times.

Caution
Careful attention must be paid to the patient's tolerance when using this technique.

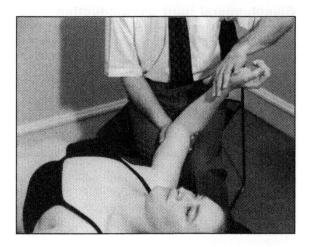

Fig. 8.3.17(a)

Upward rotation. The patient's relaxed elbow is placed on the chiropractor's knees

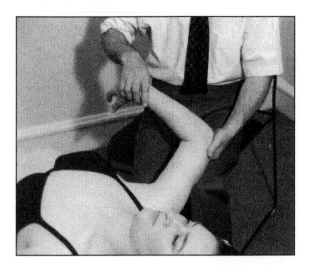

Fig. 8.3.17(b)

Downward rotation

The scapulo-thoracic articulation

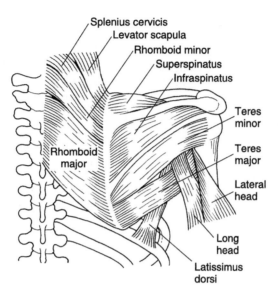

Splenius cervicis
Levator scapula
Rhomboid minor
Superspinatus
Infraspinatus
Teres minor
Teres major
Lateral head
Rhomboid major
Long head
Latissimus dorsi

8.4.1 Prone scapulo-thoracic inferior to superior mobilization technique

Application
Stiffness and tightness of the scapula on the rib cage.

Patient's position
The patient is placed prone with the shoulder on the affected side abducted to approximately 45°, with the forearm hanging downwards and the elbow flexed to approximately 90°.

Chiropractor's stance
The chiropractor stands on the homolateral side facing the treatment table straddling the patient's right elbow with the knees.

Contact
a) The left hand is placed over the mid-scapula region with a flat hand contact. The heel of the hand is over the medial part of the scapular spine.
b) The right hand is cupped around the superior borders of the acromion and coracoid processes.

Procedure
With an oscillating rhythmical motion, the scapula is moved superiorly and laterally with the left hand then checked and brought inferiorly again with the right hand by elevating the right shoulder girdle and pulling it inferiorly. This movement is repeated as often as necessary and performed to patient tolerance.

8.4.2 Prone scapulo-thoracic lateral to medial mobilization technique

Utilizing the same contacts as described above, the scapula can also be mobilized from lateral to medial and vice versa.

Application
Stiffness and tightness of the scapula on the rib cage from medial to lateral.

Patient's position
The patient is placed prone or sitting, with the hand on the affected side placed behind the back.

Chiropractor's stance
The chiropractor stands on the affected side.

Contact
a) The left hand grasps the medial border of the scapula.
b) The right hand holds the anterior of the glenohumeral joint.

Procedure
The right hand lifts the shoulder girdle from anterior to posterior enabling the left fingers to slide under the medial border of the scapula. The left hand alternately moves the scapula laterally and then, as it returns medially, the fingers are pressed under it again to stretch the tissues. The movement is repeated as often as necessary and performed to patient tolerance.

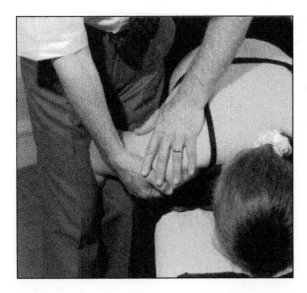

Fig. 8.4.1

The articulation is mobilized by the oscillating movements of the scapula on the rib cage

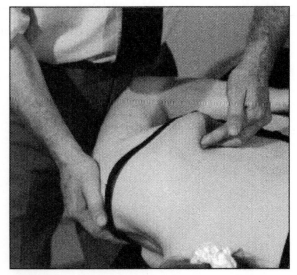

Fig. 8.4.2

The patient is placed prone and the shoulder is elevated from anterior to posterior, enabling the fingers to press under the scapula and stretch it laterally

8.4.3   Prone scapulo-thoracic rotation mobilization technique

Application
Stiffness and tightness of rotation of the scapula on the rib cage.

Patient's position
The patient is placed prone.

Chiropractor's stance
The chiropractor stands facing cephalad on the homolateral side.

Contact
a)   The left hand is placed over the medial angle of the scapula with the heel of the hand pressed firmly against it.
b)   The right hand is placed over the lateral aspect of the inferior angle using a heel of hand contact.

Procedure
The left hand stabilizes the scapula by pressing the medial angle laterally. The right hand moves the inferior angle medially and superiorly in an oscillating manner. The manoeuvre may need to be repeated a number of times to stretch the muscles, and must be performed carefully to patient tolerance.

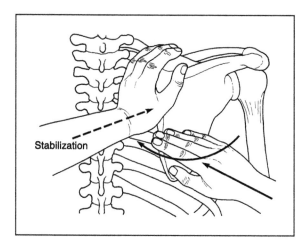

Fig. 8.4.3

The inferior angle is pressed medially and superiorly and stabilized on the medial angle

The elbow

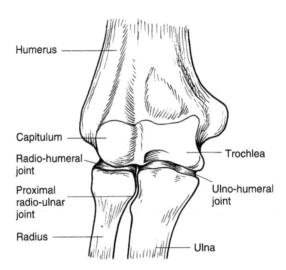

Humerus

Capitulum

Radio-humeral joint

Proximal radio-ulnar joint

Radius

Trochlea

Ulno-humeral joint

Ulna

Ulno-humeral joint techniques

8.5.A Joint play evaluation of the ulno-humeral joint

Procedure

The patient reclines, stands or sits with the shoulder on the affected side flexed and abducted a little and the elbow also slightly flexed, with the palm facing upwards.

a)   Lateral to medial glide

The index finger of the left hand is flexed and the lateral distal end of the first phalanx is placed against the lateral border of the olecranon process and presses the elbow medially into valgus stress. The right hand holds the distal end of the radius and ulna over the volar aspect with the fingers around the ulna and simultaneously pulls the forearm laterally. Joint play should be felt as an elasticity at the end of the range of joint motion.

b)   Medial to lateral glide

The patient's wrist is supinated and the chiropractor's hands are reversed. The left hand holds the forearm in varus stress and the first phalanx of the right hand presses laterally on the medial border of the olecranon process into joint play.

8.5.B Joint play evaluation of the ulno-humeral joint: long axis distraction

Procedure

The patient's elbow is flexed to approximately a right-angle with the palm facing upwards. The web of the left hand is placed against the proximal tip of the olecranon process of the ulna. The web of the right hand is placed over the anterior of the upper arm just distal to the elbow joint, avoiding the bulk of the biceps muscle. Both hands press firmly in opposing directions until all tissue slack is removed. Without releasing the tension, further opposing pressure is exerted to elicit joint play.

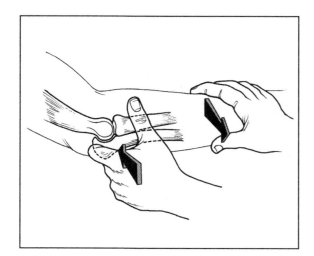

Fig. 8.5.A

Lateral to medial and medial to lateral glide of the ulno-humeral joint. The patient's palm faces upwards

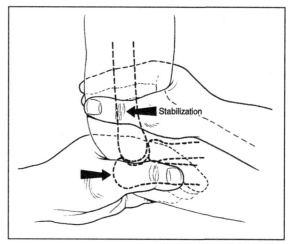

Fig. 8.5.B

The patient's elbow is flexed to a right angle with the palm facing upwards

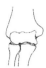

8.5.1 Supine, sitting or standing ulno-humeral medial to lateral short lever thrust technique – Method I

Application
Joint play glide loss from medial to lateral of the ulna on the humerus.

Patient's position
The patient stands, sits or reclines supine with the shoulder on the affected side a little flexed and slightly rotated externally. The palm of the hand faces upwards and the elbow is kept slightly flexed.

Chiropractor's stance
The chiropractor stands on the lateral side of the patient's affected arm adjacent to the elbow, turning with the back towards the patient.

Contact
a) The left hand is placed along the medial aspect of the ulna close to the elbow joint using a heel of hand (see Glossary of Terms, p. 285) contact.
b) The right hand is placed along the lateral side of the distal end of the forearm just proximal to the wrist and grasps the radius and ulna from the posterior.

Procedure
The lateral border of the distal humerus is placed against the left side of the chiropractor's trunk to stabilize the elbow. The patient's forearm is held slightly flexed, gently tractioned in long axis with the chiropractor's right arm, and the distal end of it is pressed minimally towards the patient to achieve joint pre-load tension. Without slackening the tension, the left hand makes a light, swift impulse from medial to lateral using only minimal depth of thrust.

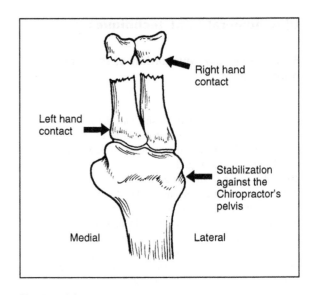

Fig. 8.5.1(a)

Anterior view of the elbow showing the contacts and point of humeral stabilization

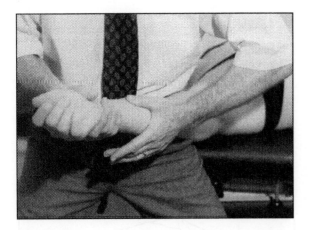

Fig. 8.5.1(b)

Joint tension is achieved by tractioning the patient's forearm. The patient is lying supine

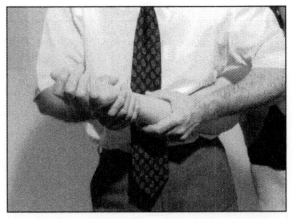

Fig. 8.5.1(c)

Ulnohumeral technique medial to lateral. The alternative patient position – Method I

8.5.2 Supine, sitting or standing ulno-humeral medial to lateral short lever thrust technique – Method II

Application
Joint play glide loss from medial to lateral of the ulna on the humerus.

Patient's position
The patient sits, stands or reclines supine with the shoulder on the affected side slightly abducted and externally rotated and the forearm supinated. The elbow is held slightly flexed.

Chiropractor's stance
The chiropractor stands facing the patient, favouring the side of the involvement.

Contact
a) The left hand grasps around the posterior of the forearm just proximal to the wrist ensuring that the patient's hand remains facing palm upwards.
b) The right hand with the thumb facing upwards, is placed along the proximal end of the medial aspect of the ulna. The anterior of the first phalanx of the first finger contacts along the medial edge of the olecranon process.

Procedure
The patient's elbow is kept slightly flexed throughout the procedure. To achieve joint pre-load tension, the left arm distracts and medially flexes the elbow. The impulse is delivered with the right hand from medial to lateral swiftly with minimal depth, still ensuring that the elbow remains flexed.

8.5.3 Supine, sitting or standing ulno-humeral lateral to medial short lever thrust technique – Method I

Application
Joint play glide loss from lateral to medial of the ulnar on the humerus.

Patient's position
The patient sits, stands or reclines supine with the shoulder on the affected side flexed, abducted and slightly rotated externally. The palm of the hand faces upwards and the elbow is also kept slightly flexed.

Chiropractor's stance
The chiropractor stands on the medial side of the patient's affected arm and adjacent to the elbow, turning the back towards the patient.

Contact
a) The left hand is placed along the distal end of the forearm just proximal to the wrist and grasps the radius and ulna from the posterior, ensuring that the patient's hand remains supinated.
b) The right hand is placed along the lateral aspect of the ulnar close to the elbow using a heel of hand (see Glossary of Terms, p. 285) contact.

Procedure
The medial border of the distal humerus is placed against the right side of the chiropractor's trunk to stabilize the humerus. The patient's forearm is held slightly flexed, gently tractioned in long axis with the chiropractor's left hand and the distal end of it is pressed minimally away from the patient to achieve joint pre-load tension. Without slackening the tension, the right hand makes a light, swift impulse from lateral to medial using minimal depth of thrust.

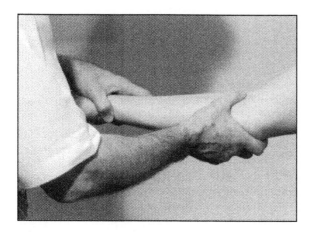

Fig. 8.5.2

Method II: as the impulse is delivered by the right arm, the left arm maintains the tension by slightly distracting and flexing the elbow medially

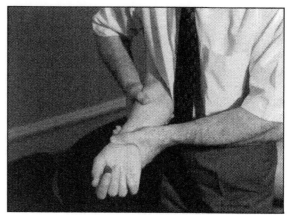

Fig. 8.5.3

Method I: for this technique, the patient may stand, sit or recline supine. The contact on the lateral side of the olecranon and the medial pressure exerted serves to stabilize the humerus against the right side of the chiropractor's pelvis

8.5.4 Supine, sitting or standing ulno-humeral lateral to medial short lever thrust technique – Method II

Application
Joint play glide loss from lateral to medial of the ulna on the humerus.

Patient's position
The patient stands, sits or reclines supine with the shoulder on the affected side abducted, slightly flexed and externally rotated. The palm of the hand is placed facing upwards.

Chiropractor's stance
The chiropractor stands on the affected side adjacent to the elbow on the lateral side of the arm facing the patient.

Contact
a) With the thumb facing upwards, the left hand is placed along the lateral proximal aspect of the ulna. The anterior of the first phalanx of the first finger contacts the lateral edge of the olecranon process.
b) The right hand grasps around the posterior of the forearm just proximal to the wrist, ensuring that the patient's hand remains supinated.

Procedure
Joint pre-load tension is achieved by using the right hand to press the patient's forearm laterally and then maintains the tension throughout the procedure. The impulse is made from lateral to medial solely with the left arm, utilizing minimal depth of thrust.

8.5.5 Sitting or standing ulno-humeral long axis distraction technique

Application
Joint play glide loss of the ulna with the humerus from proximal to distal.

Patient's position
The patient stands or sits with the affected elbow flexed to approximately 90°.

Chiropractor's stance
The chiropractor stands or sits at the side of the patient adjacent to the affected elbow.

Contact
a) The left hand is wrapped around the medial aspect of the distal humerus using an anterior middle phalanx middle finger contact on the anterior of the distal humerus, as close to the joint as possible. The remaining fingers support it closely.
b) The right hand is wrapped around the medial aspect of the proximal ulna. A middle digit middle finger contact is used on the proximal tip of the olecranon process, with the remaining fingers supporting it closely.

Procedure
The patient's shoulder is slightly abducted and extended to achieve a firmer contact on the olecranon process. The lateral border of the patient's humerus is held firmly against the chiropractor's chest. Joint pre-load tension is produced by drawing the elbows to the sides. The impulse is made by swiftly pulling both hands in equal and opposite directions, away from each other.

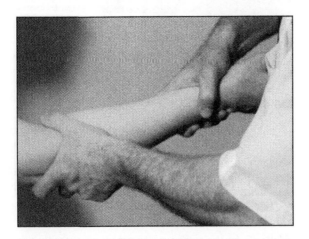

Fig. 8.5.4

The arm holding the patient's wrist is used as a stabilizer. The thrust is made solely with the contact on the proximal ulna

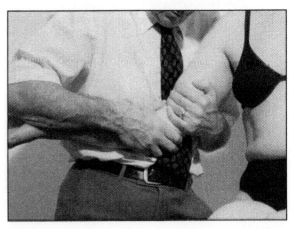

Fig. 8.5.5

The patient's elbow is extended slightly to increase the firmness of the contact on the olecranon

8.5.6 Sitting, standing or supine ulno-humeral circumduction mobilization technique

Procedure

The patient is seated, standing or placed supine and is instructed to keep the affected arm in a relaxed state throughout the duration of the manoeuvre. The arm is not quite fully extended, with the palm facing and held upwards.

The chiropractor's left hand grasps under the patient's elbow with the thumb on the lateral border of the olecranon process and the lateral aspect of the first finger contacts the medial border of the olecranon to stabilize it. The chiropractor's right hand holds the anterior of the patient's wrist and maintains the patient's forearm in supination. By using both hands, the patient's elbow is then flexed a little and the wrist is gently made to describe a circle, to patient tolerance, in a clockwise direction. For counter-clockwise mobilization, the chiropractor's hands are best reversed.

8.5.7 Sitting or supine ulno-humeral anterior to posterior stretch mobilization technique

Procedure

With the patient seated or lying supine, the chiropractor places the ulnar side of the right forearm obliquely over the antecubital fossa, favouring the medial side of the patient's elbow, producing a soft contact. The chiropractor's **left hand** grasps the patient's right wrist and gently flexes the patient's elbow until tension is felt. The patient's elbow is then gently and rhythmically flexed to tolerance, then released. The action is repeated several times as necessary.

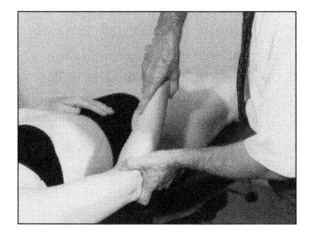

Fig. 8.5.6

The elbow is gently mobilized in a clockwise direction until the motion limitation is felt or patient tolerance is reached. For counter-clockwise movement, the hands are reversed

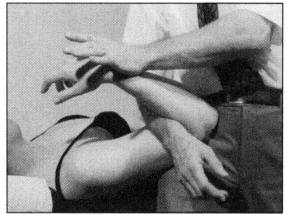

Fig. 8.5.7

The chiropractor's right forearm is placed obliquely over the patient's elbow, favouring the medial side, to contact the ulna

8.5.8 Standing, sitting or prone ulno-humeral extension mobilization stretch technique

Procedure

This technique is also known as the Mills manoeuvre. The patient may stand, sit or lie prone. The chiropractor medially rotates the patient's shoulder, pronates the patient's right forearm and flexes the wrist, holding it in this position with the right hand against the back of the patient's hand. The finger and thumb of the left hand are placed on either side of the proximal ulna close to the olecranon.

The patient's elbow is gently extended to tolerance, releasing the tension and repeating the procedure several times. The patient frequently feels very apprehensive in this position and much care must be taken not to overstress the joint.

Proximal radio-ulnar joint techniques

8.5.C Joint play evaluation of the radio-ulnar joint

Procedure

a) External to internal rotation

The patient sits or reclines supine and the elbow is flexed to 90°, with the wrist also flexed. The thumb of the left hand is placed against the lateral border of the radial head. The right hand holds the wrist, maintaining it in flexion and then pronates the forearm by rotating the wrist. The left thumb simultaneously rotates the radio-ulnar joint internally and at the end of the travel, presses it further into joint play.

b) Internal to external rotation

The patient sits or reclines supine as above. The elbow and wrist remain flexed and the forearm is rotated externally. The contacts are reversed. The thumb of the right hand contacts the radial head and at the end of the travel, presses it externally into joint play as the left hand simultaneously rotates the forearm still further.

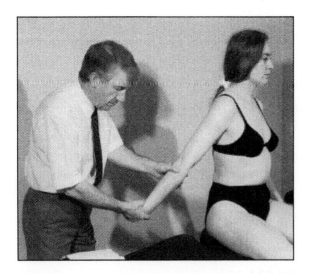

Fig. 8.5.8

The patient's elbow is gently stretched as the thrust is applied

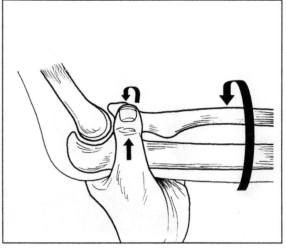

Fig. 8.5.C

External to internal rotation of the radio-ulnar joint

8.5.D Joint play evaluation of the radio-ulnar joint posterior to anterior glide

Procedure
The patient sits, stands or reclines prone with the shoulder on the affected side slightly abducted, extended and with the elbow flexed to a right angle. The patient's shoulder and elbow must remain relaxed. The thumb of the left hand contacts the posterior of the radial head and the thumb of the right hand contacts the anterior proximal end of the ulna. By applying firm thumb pressure in equal and opposite directions, joint play can be detected as a feeling of elasticity in the joint. Joint play glide loss is detected by a hard end feel to pressure.

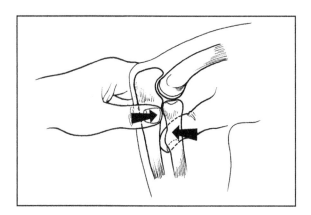

Fig. 8.5.D

Radio-ulnar joint posterior to anterior glide

8.5.9 Sitting, standing or supine radio-ulnar joint external to internal rotation pull technique

Application
Joint play glide loss of rotation of the radius from external to internal on the ulna.

Patient's position
The patient sits, stands, or reclines supine with the elbow and the wrist on the affected side flexed to about 90°. The wrist is then fully rotated in pronation.

Chiropractor's stance
The chiropractor stands on the side of involvement, facing the patient medial to the patient's arm.

Contact
a) The left hand holds the patient's hand and wrist, rotating the forearm externally until tension is felt at the patient's elbow.

b) The right hand slides over the anterior of the patient's elbow from the medial side. The middle phalanx of the middle finger contacts the lateral border of the radius supported closely by the other fingers.

Procedure
Joint pre-load tension is further achieved using both hands to further rotate the patient's forearm. Without releasing the tension a rapid impulse is made with the right hand pulling the radial head internally, using minimal depth of thrust.

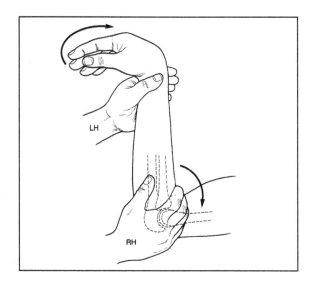

Fig. 8.5.9(a)

The left hand externally rotates the patient's wrist and forearm until tension is felt at the elbow

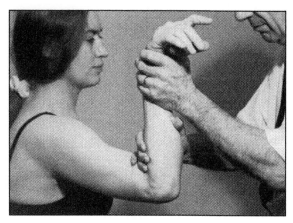

Fig. 8.5.9(b)

With a middle finger contact on the radius, the rotational thrust is made with minimal depth

8.5.10 Supine or sitting radio-ulnar joint internal to external rotation thrust technique

Application
Joint play glide loss of internal to external rotation of the radius on the ulna.

Patient's position
The patient is either seated or reclining supine. The elbow and wrist on the affected side are flexed to a right-angle.

Chiropractor's stance
The chiropractor stands medial to the patient's forearm.

Contact
a)   The left hand holds the patient's wrist and hand over the dorsum and maintains and stabilizes the wrist and elbow in flexion.
b)   The anterior aspect of the distal phalanx of the thumb on the right hand contacts the medial aspect of the radial head and all the fingers are wrapped under the posterior of the proximal end of the ulna.

Procedure
The left hand rotates the wrist and forearm externally into supination until joint pre-load tension is reached. At the moment full tension is reached, the right thumb exerts a rapid shallow-depth impulse from medial to lateral.

Alternative method
The hands may be reversed. The middle phalanx of the middle finger of the left hand is placed against the medial border of the radial head supported by the remaining fingers. The right hand holds the patient's wrist and hand in flexion and rotates the forearm externally into supination. The left contact exerts an external rotation pull impulse just as the right hand reaches the point of tension as it externally rotates the forearm.

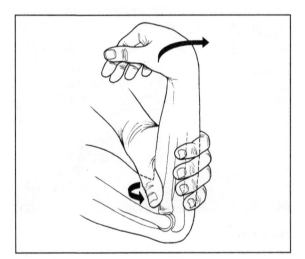

Fig. 8.5.10

The wrist is held in flexion with the left hand. A rapid shallow impulse is delivered by the right thumb from internal to external

8.5.11 Prone radio-ulnar joint posterior to anterior recoil technique

Application
Joint play glide loss from posterior to anterior of the radius on the ulna.

Patient's position
The patient is placed prone. The shoulder on the affected side is rotated externally and the elbow is semi-flexed. The distal end of the humerus is supported by a high-density padded wedge-block placed with the apex facing cephalad.

Chiropractor's stance
The chiropractor stands alongside the affected elbow, facing cephalad.

Contact
a)   The left hand is placed against the inferior margin of the radial head with a pisiform contact. Using a low arch (see Glossary of Terms, p. 285), the fingers wrap loosely around the lateral border of the elbow.
b)   The right hand is placed over the dorsum of the left distal carpals and proximal metacarpals. The fingers wrap around the medial side of the elbow to help stabilize the narrow available contact.

Procedure
The thoracic section of the treatment table is set for the patient's weight and cocked. The impulse is a light high velocity shallow recoil thrust (see p. 8) of minimal depth.

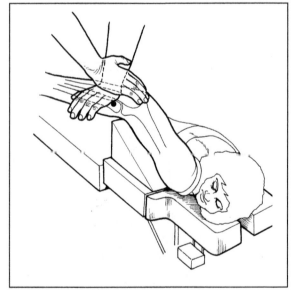

Fig. 8.5.11

The wide end of the wedge block is placed at the distal end of the anterior humerus to maintain the elbow in flexion. The dorsum of the hand rests on the treatment table. A light rapid shallow-depth recoil thrust is used in conjunction with the treatment table thoracic drop section

8.5.12 Sitting, standing or supine radio-ulnar joint long axis thrust technique

Application
Joint play glide loss of the radius on the ulna from distal to proximal.

Patient's position
The patient sits, stands or is placed supine with the shoulder and elbow on the affected side flexed and the wrist rotated, with the thumb facing upwards.

Chiropractor's stance
The chiropractor stands on the side of involvement, facing the patient and lateral to the patient's arm.

Contact
a) The left hand is placed against the lateral side of the patient's proximal radial shaft. The left thumb takes the tissue slack proximally and is pressed firmly against the neck of the radius, just distal to the head. The thumb is held stiffly and flattened against the shaft.
b) The right hand grasps the patient's distal ulna from the anterior with the fingers holding under the lateral side of the ulna.

Procedure
The adjustment is made with a swift proximal impulse with the stiff left thumb. At the same time, to achieve joint pre-load tension, the right hand tractions the ulna swiftly distally. These combined movements have the effect of slightly extending the elbow joint. The thrust must be completed before the patient's elbow reaches full extension.

Radio-humeral joint techniques

8.5.E Joint play evaluation of the radio-humeral joint: Anterior to posterior glide

Procedure
The patient is placed supine with the elbow flexed to a right-angle with the upper arm resting on the treatment table to stabilize the humerus. The thumb of the left hand contacts the anterior border of the radial head and presses from anterior to posterior into joint play until ligamentous resistance is felt. Further pressure is then exerted. The right hand stabilizes the forearm by holding it firmly to prevent ulno-humeral movement.

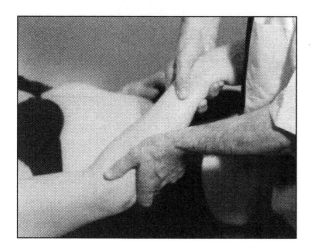

Fig. 8.5.12

When the thrust is made, the patient's elbow must not reach full extension

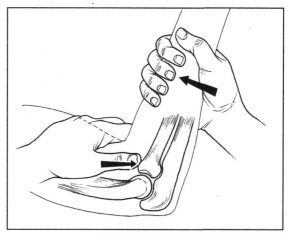

Fig. 8.5.E

Anterior to posterior glide of the radio-humeral joint

8.5.13 Prone radio-humeral anterior to posterior distraction technique

Application
Joint play glide loss of the radius from anterior to posterior on the humerus.

Patient's position
The patient is placed prone with the shoulder abducted, the affected arm extended and the elbow flexed to about 90°.

Chiropractor's stance
The chiropractor stands adjacent to the patient's affected side facing cephalad. If variable height equipment is used, it is raised until the chiropractor's elbows are approximately at right-angles when the contacts are made. The left foot is placed ahead of the right one, so that the thigh is close to the patient's axilla.

Contact
a) The right hand is placed around the lateral side of the upper arm to contact the anterior aspect of the distal humerus with the first finger as close to the joint as possible, with the remaining fingers supporting it.
b) The left hand is placed around the forearm to contact the anterior aspect of the proximal radius with the first finger over the head of the radius and the remaining fingers supporting it.

Procedure
Joint pre-load tension is achieved by the chiropractor bringing the elbows to the sides. The medial side of the patient's elbow is held firmly against the chiropractor's lower sternum. The impulse is made with a rapid 'scissor-type' movement, both arms simultaneously distracting the joint in equal and opposite directions. Only minimum depth of thrust is required.

8.5.14 Sitting or prone radio-humeral anterior to posterior mobilization stretch technique

Procedure
With the patient seated or lying supine, the chiropractor places the left forearm against the proximal radius, as close to the joint as possible. The patient's forearm is pronated until the thumb faces upwards. The chiropractor's right hand grasps the patient's right wrist and flexes the forearm until joint pre-load tension is felt. The patient's elbow is then gently and rhythmically flexed to the patient's tolerance, then released. This is repeated several times as necessary.

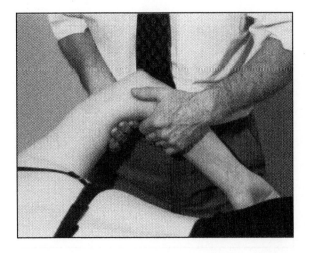

Fig. 8.5.13

The thrust is made with both arms in equal and opposite directions

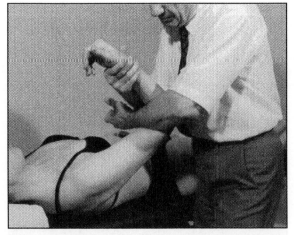

Fig. 8.5.14

The chiropractor's left forearm is placed over the patient's right proximal radius and the elbow is gently flexed to tolerance, released and flexed again

The wrist and hand

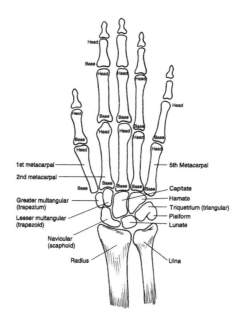

Interphalangeal techniques
8.6.A   Joint play evaluation of the interphalangeal joints
8.6.1   Interphalangeal joint posterior to anterior and anterior to posterior short lever pull techniques
8.6.2   Interphalangeal joint lateral to medial and/or medial to lateral short lever traction techniques

Metacarpo-phalangeal techniques
8.6.B   Joint play evaluation of the metacarpo-phalangeal joints
8.6.3   1st to 3rd metacarpo-phalangeal posterior to anterior extension/distraction technique
8.6.4   4th and 5th metacarpo-phalangeal posterior to anterior extension/distraction technique
8.6.5   Metacarpo-phalangeal anterior to posterior flexion/distraction technique

Intermetacarpal techniques
8.6.C   Joint play evaluation of the intermetacarpal joints
8.6.6   Intermetacarpal mobilization clasp technique

Metacarpo-carpal techniques
8.6.D   Joint play evaluation of the metacarpo-carpal joints
8.6.7   1st metacarpo-carpal lateral to medial with long axis distraction
8.6.8   1st metacarpo-carpal posterior to anterior short lever pull technique
8.6.9   1st metacarpo-carpal anterior to posterior technique
8.6.10   2nd or 3rd metacarpo-carpal posterior to anterior technique – Method I
8.6.11   2nd or 3rd metacarpo-carpal posterior to anterior technique – Method II
8.6.12   2nd or 3rd metacarpo-carpal anterior to posterior technique
8.6.13   4th or 5th metacarpo-carpal posterior to anterior technique
8.6.14   4th or 5th metacarpo-carpal anterior to posterior technique

Intercarpal techniques
8.6.E   Joint play evaluation of the intercarpal joints
8.6.15   Greater multangular (trapezium) on the navicular (scaphoid) anterior to posterior short lever pull technique.
8.6.16   Greater multangular (trapezium) on the navicular (scaphoid) posterior to anterior short lever pull technique.
8.6.17   Capitate on the navicular (scaphoid) posterior to anterior short lever pull technique
8.6.18   Capitate on the navicular (scaphoid) anterior to posterior short lever pull technique
8.6.F   Joint play evaluation of adjacent intercarpal joints
8.6.19   Pisiform on the triangular (triquetrum) lateral to medial short lever pull technique
8.6.20   Pisiform on the triangular (triquetrum) medial to lateral short lever pull technique
8.6.21   Triangular (triquetrum) on the hamate posterior to anterior recoil technique

Radio-carpal techniques
8.6.G   Joint play evaluation of the radio-navicular (scaphoid) and radio-lunate joints
8.6.22   Radio-navicular (scaphoid) posterior to anterior technique
8.6.23   Radio-navicular (scaphoid) anterior to posterior technique
8.6.24   Radio-navicular (scaphoid) posterior to anterior wrist extension technique
8.6.H   Joint play evaluation of the navicular (scaphoid) on the radius
8.6.25   Radio-navicular (scaphoid) lateral to medial technique
8.6.J   Joint play evaluation of the radio-carpal joint in long axis extension
8.6.26   Radio-lunate posterior to anterior technique
8.6.27   Radio-lunate anterior to posterior technique

Distal radio-ulnar techniques
8.6.K   Joint play evaluation of the distal radio-ulnar joint
8.6.28   Distal radio-ulnar posterior to anterior technique
8.6.29   Distal radio-ulnar anterior to posterior technique

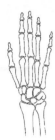

Interphalangeal techniques

8.6.A   Joint play evaluation of the interphalangeal joints

Procedure
Each of the phalanges is held in turn between the fingers and thumbs. The joints are pressed firmly into flexion, extension, rotation, distraction and lateral flexion, ensuring that full travel of the joint is first reached before further pressure is exerted to detect the joint play in each of the directions of normal joint movement. Joint play is felt as a perception of elasticity at the end of joint travel.

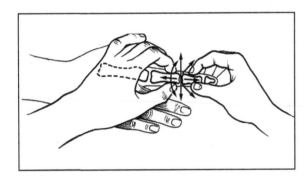

Fig. 8.6.A

Posterior view of the right hand

8.6.1   Interphalangeal posterior to anterior and anterior to posterior short lever pull technique

Application
Joint play glide loss of the interphalangeal joints from anterior to posterior or posterior to anterior.

Patient's position
The patient sits, stands or reclines supine. The shoulder on the affected side is abducted and slightly flexed, with the wrist supinated and the palm of the hand facing upwards. The fingers are semi-flexed.

Chiropractor's stance
The chiropractor stands or sits beside the patient on the affected side, lateral to the patient's arm and with the patient's hand adjacent to the chiropractor's body mid-line.

Contact
For **posterior to anterior** short lever pull technique:
a)   The left hand is placed over the patient's palm and the first finger curls around the posterior of the phalanx distal to, and close up to, the joint to be adjusted. The thumb supports it by contacting the anterior distal end of the same phalanx.
b)   The right hand is placed so that the first finger (and also the second finger if there is room) is curled around the anterior of the joint to be adjusted, with the contact as close to the joint as possible.

For **anterior to posterior** short lever pull technique the hands are reversed:
a)   The left first finger curls around the posterior phalanx proximal to the joint to be adjusted.
b)   The right first finger curls around the anterior of the phalanx distal to the joint to be adjusted.

Procedure
Standard short lever pull technique (see Chapter 2) is used. Joint pre-load tension is achieved by lowering the elbows to the sides and slightly backwards. The impulse is given in equal and opposite directions. Only minimal depth of thrust is required. See Figs 8.6.1(a,b,c,d).

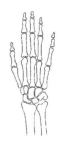

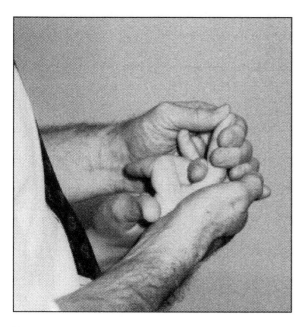

Fig. 8.6.1(a)

Interphalangeal joint posterior to anterior, between the first and second row on the middle finger. The technique is similar on all the interphalangeal articulations

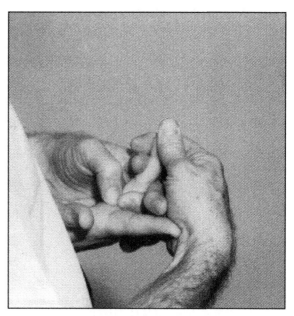

Fig. 8.6.1(c)

Interphalangeal joint anterior to posterior technique showing the reversal of the hand positions

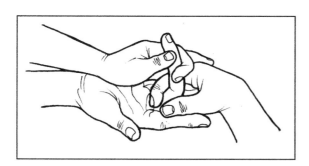

Fig. 8.6.1(b)

This technique is similar for all the interphalangeal articulations. Shown here are the hand positions used between the proximal and middle phalanges of the middle finger

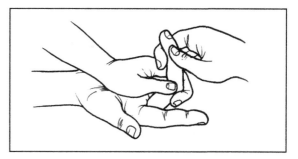

Fig. 8.6.1(d)

Close-up showing hand positions for interphalangeal joint anterior to posterior

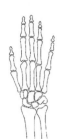

8.6.2 Interphalangeal lateral to medial and/or medial to lateral short lever traction techniques

Application
Joint play glide loss of the interphalangeal joints from lateral to medial and/or medial to lateral.

Patient's position
The patient sits, stands or reclines, with the affected arm relaxed, the elbow slightly flexed and the palm facing down with the fingers extended.

Chiropractor's stance
The chiropractor stands beside and facing towards the patient's forearm on the affected side.

Contact
a) The left hand reaches over the dorsum of the patient's hand and holds, between the thumb and first finger, the digit proximal to the joint being treated.
b) The right hand reaches over the posterior of the patient's finger tips and holds, with the thumb and first finger, the digit distal to the joint being treated.

Procedure
The left hand acts as a stabilizer while the right hand tractions the joint a little, then rapidly moves the digit distal to the articulation with a combination of lateral flexion and lateral translation across the joint and then immediately, equally rapidly, reverses the movement to medial flexion and medial translation the opposite way across the joint.

Metacarpo-phalangeal techniques

8.6.B Joint play evaluation of the metacarpo-phalangeal joints

Procedure
The distal metacarpals are stabilized between the chiropractor's finger and thumb. The proximal phalanges are contacted at the bases with the fingers and on the bodies by the thumb. Pressure is exerted in flexion, extension, rotation, distraction and lateral flexion, fully through the available free movement and then into joint play, when further firm pressure is applied to reach the end play.

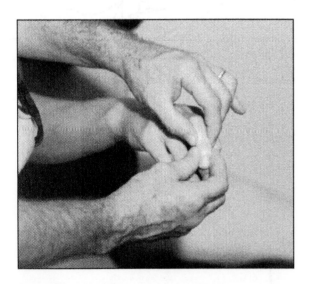

Fig. 8.6.2

The digit distal to the joint is first tractioned then moved rapidly into lateral, then medial flexion, each with a component of translation in opposite directions across the joint. This adjustment can be applied to all of the interphalangeal joints

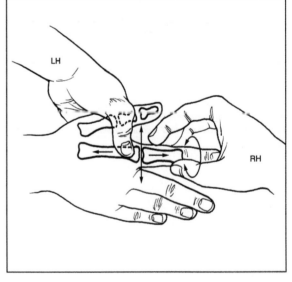

Fig. 8.6.B

Left hand, posterior view showing the directions in which the articulations of the metacarpo-phalangeal joints are moved

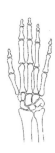

8.6.3 1st to 3rd metacarpo-phalangeal posterior to anterior short lever extension/distraction technique

Application
Joint play glide loss from posterior to anterior of the proximal row of phalanges on the metacarpals.

Patient's position
The patient sits, stands or reclines supine. The shoulder on the affected side is flexed, the elbow held extended with the hand held palm downwards and the fingers extended.

Chiropractor's stance
The chiropractor stands on the affected side, sideways on to the patient lateral to the patient's arm, holding the patient's hand across the body at about mid-sternal height.

Contact
a) The left hand stabilizes the metacarpals by holding the dorsal surface, wrapping the fingers from the lateral to the medial side right around to the anterior reaching as far around as the first three metacarpals if possible.

b) The right hand is passed under the patient's hand from the lateral side to reach around to the medial side, enabling the first and middle fingers to contact the posterior of the base of the appropriate phalanx, as close to the joint as possible. The thumb contacts and presses against the anterior distal end of the same phalanx.

Procedure
The phalanx is extended backwards with the right thumb. Joint pre-load tension is achieved by this extension and by distracting the joint in long axis extension with the right hand. This is frequently all that is necessary to achieve cavitation. If not, then a light, swift impulse of minimal depth using standard short lever pull technique (see Chapter 2) is applied. The right hand distracts and takes the joint slightly further into extension and the left hand stabilizes the metacarpals.

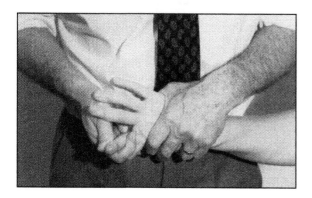

Fig. 8.6.3

The technique shown is being applied to the second metacarpo-phalangeal articulation

8.6.4 4th and 5th metacarpo-phalangeal posterior to anterior short lever extension/distraction technique

Application
Joint play glide loss from posterior to anterior of the 4th or 5th proximal phalanges on the metacarpals.

Patient's position
The patient stands, sits or reclines supine with the shoulder on the affected side flexed and slightly abducted. The elbow is extended and the palm faces downwards.

Chiropractor's stance
The chiropractor stands sideways on to the patient, facing laterally. The medial side of the affected forearm is placed across the chiropractor's chest. The medial border of the patient's hand is pressed against the mid-sternum and the chiropractor's elbows are held approximately at right-angles.

Contact
a) The left hand passes under the patient's hand from the medial side and the middle and 4th fingers reach around to contact either the 3rd or 4th posterior proximal phalanx whichever is appropriate. On the anterior aspect, the thenar eminence contacts the distal end of the same phalanx.

b) The right hand wraps over the dorsum of the wrist and metacarpals from the medial side. All fingers are curled around the lateral border to the palmar surface of the hand, as close to the metacarpo-carpal joint as possible.

Procedure
Standard short lever pull technique (see Chapter 2) is applied taking the phalanx into extension and long axis distraction.

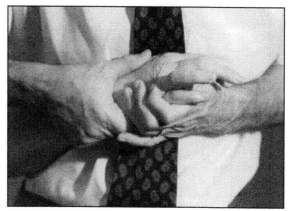

Fig. 8.6.4

Manipulations of the 1st proximal phalanx and the 5th metacarpal from posterior to anterior. The 5th proximal phalanx is extended and distracted with the chiropractor's index finger

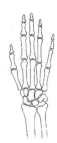

8.6.5   2nd to 5th metacarpo-phalangeal anterior to posterior (A–P) and posterior to anterior (P–A) flexion/distraction technique

Application
Joint play loss from anterior to posterior of the proximal phalanges on the metacarpals.

Patient's position
The patient sits, stands or reclines supine, the shoulder on the affected arm is flexed and the elbow is also held flexed. The palm of the hand is held downwards and the forearm is held horizontally.

Chiropractor's stance
The chiropractor stands facing the patient with the patient's forearm placed across the mid-sternal region. The chiropractor's elbows are held approximately at right-angles.

Contact
a)   The right hand is placed palm down over the dorsum of the patient's hand. All the fingers are wrapped around to permit contact on the distal end of the 1st or 2nd metacarpal on the posterior. The thumb is placed around the anterior distal metacarpals.

b)   The thumb on the left hand is placed over the posterior of the base of the patient's 2nd to 5th proximal phalanx. All the fingers contact the anterior of the same phalanx.

Procedure for A–P technique
Joint pre-load tension is attained by first flexing the joint and simultaneously distracting it. When the joint slack is removed, a rapid, light impulse is made in the same direction.

Procedure for P–A technique
The joint pre-load tension is achieved by moving the phalanx into full extension and, without slackening the tension, a swift impulse, distracting the joint in long axis extension, is applied with minimum depth.

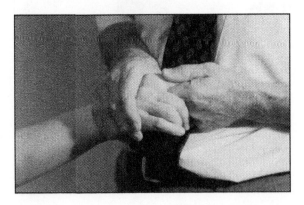

Fig. 8.6.5

The patient's finger is swiftly distracted in long axis extension and at the same time, fully flexed. This technique can be applied to all the metacarpo-phalangeal joints

Intermetacarpal techniques

8.6.C   Joint play evaluation of the intermetacarpal joints

The 2nd, 3rd, 4th and 5th metacarpals articulate with each other at their bases. They are also connected by the volar ligaments, the dorsal ligaments and the interosseous ligaments. The joint evaluation of the intermetacarpals therefore has two objectives: first the evaluation of the joint play between the articulations at the bases and secondly the assessment of the intermetacarpal ligaments for laxity or shortening.

Procedure
The patient's hand is placed palm downwards. The adjacent metacarpal bases are held between the fingers and thumbs of both hands. As one metacarpal base is pressed firmly from posterior to anterior with the finger and thumb of one hand, the pressure is opposed by the finger and thumb of the other hand.

Next, the adjacent metacarpals are held between the fingers and thumbs of both hands, mid-way along the shafts of the metacarpals, and by using see-saw movements with each hand in opposing directions, the motion can be assessed for ligamentous shortening or laxity.

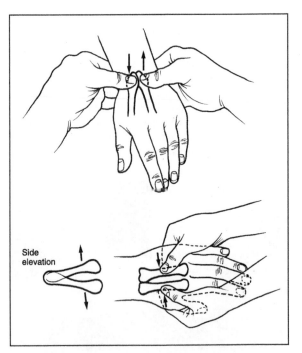

Side
elevation

Fig. 8.6.C

Adjacent metacarpals are held between the fingers and thumbs and pressed from posterior to anterior and from anterior to posterior

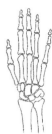

8.6.6 Intermetacarpal clasp mobilization technique

Application
Stiffness and restriction of motion between adjacent metacarpals.

Patient's position
The patient may sit, stand or recline supine. The shoulder and the elbow on the affected side are extended and the palm faces downwards.

Chiropractor's stance
The chiropractor sits or stands on the homolateral side, adjacent to the patient's affected hand.

Contact
The fingers of both hands are interlaced.
a) The left hand is placed over the dorsal surface of the metacarpals so that the heel of the hand is placed against the lateral one of the two adjacent affected metacarpals.
b) The right hand is placed around the anterior of the metacarpals so that the heel of the hand contacts the medial of the two adjacent affected metacarpals.

Procedure
The heels of the hands are first separated and then brought very rapidly together again with the heel of the right hand striking the palm of the left hand. This has a shearing and stretching effect between the adjacent metacarpals. The procedure may be repeated several times as necessary. The strike bias can also be reversed on clinical demand.

Note
This method may also be utilized in similar fashion as intermetatarsal mobilization techniques (8.10.8 and 8.10.9). For the description of this technique see Chapter 2.

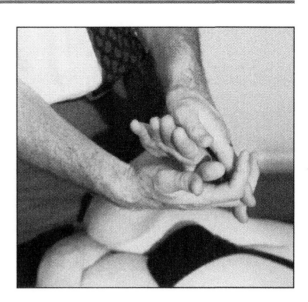

Fig. 8.6.6(a)

The fingers are laced together and the heels of the hands are separated

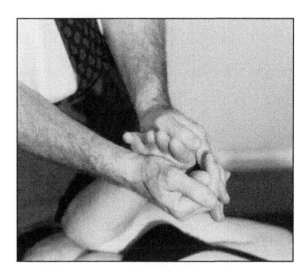

Fig. 8.6.6(b)

The fingers remain interlaced and the heels of the hands are brought rapidly together. The heel of the right hand strikes the palm of the left producing a shearing of the two adjacent metacarpals placed between them

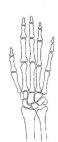

Metacarpo-carpal techniques

8.6.D   Joint play evaluation of the metacarpo-carpal joints

Procedure

a)   With one hand, the distal carpal is held on the anterior and posterior between the finger and thumb and prevented from moving. With the other hand, the proximal phalanx is contacted on the anterior and posterior of the base and pressed firmly into joint play in anterior to posterior glide, then flexion, extension, rotation, distraction and lateral flexion. There is usually very little rotation of the 2nd and 3rd metacarpo-carpal joints.

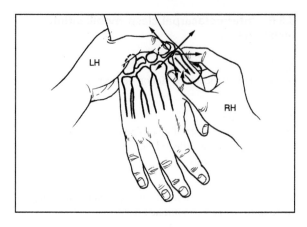

Fig. 8.6.D(a)

Right hand, posterior view showing the directions into which the chiropractor's thumb and index finger move the patient's 1st metacarpal

b)   The carpals are stabilized from the posterior with the laced fingers. A double thumb contact is used on the anterior base of the metacarpal and presses each one in turn into full extension then the movement is continued into joint play.

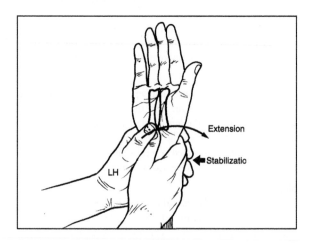

Fig. 8.6.D(b)

Extension of the metacarpo-carpal joints

c)   The carpals are each in turn stabilized from the anterior with a thumb contact. The other thumb contacts the posterior of the metacarpal base and presses the metacarpal into full flexion. Extra pressure is then firmly applied to test for joint play in each joint.

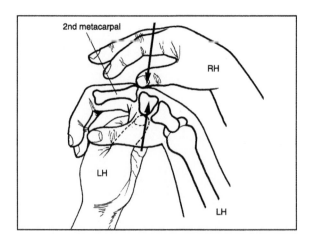

Fig. 8.6.D(c)

Flexion of the metacarpo-carpal joints

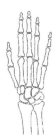

8.6.7 1st metacarpo-carpal lateral to medial short lever pull technique with long axis distraction

Application
Joint play glide loss from lateral to medial of the 1st metacarpal on the greater multangular (trapezium).

Patient's position
The patient sits, stands or reclines supine, with the affected hand held with the thumb upwards.

Chiropractor's stance
The chiropractor stands facing the patient favouring the affected side.

Contact
a)   The left hand is placed over the dorsum of the wrist with the index finger over the greater multangular (trapezium), close up against the base of the thumb. All the remaining fingers are wrapped around to the palmar side of the patient's hand to support the contact.

b)   The fourth finger of the right hand is placed from the palmar side around the lateral border of the base of the 1st metacarpal; the other fingers support closely by also firmly contacting around the body of the 1st metacarpal. The right thumb is placed against the anterior aspect of the distal end of the patient's metacarpal and abducts it.

Procedure
Tension is achieved by tractioning the patient's thumb into long axis extension with the right hand whilst abducting it with the chiropractor's right thumb. The left hand acts as a stabilizer. Standard short lever pull technique (see Chapter 2) is applied with minimal depth of thrust. The impulse is made in equal and opposite directions.

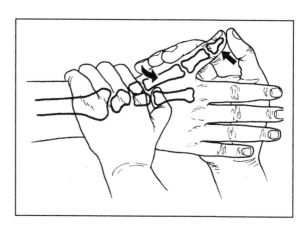

Fig. 8.6.7(a)

The left hand stabilizes the greater multangular. The fourth finger of the right hand contacts the lateral base of the 1st metacarpal

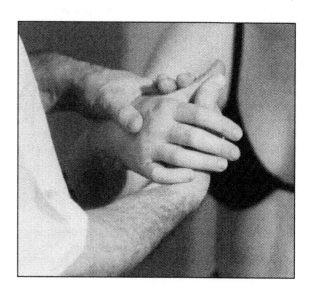

Fig. 8.6.7(b)

Before the impulse is made, the chiropractor's elbows are relaxed and held to the sides of the body

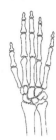

8.6.8   1st metacarpo-carpal posterior to anterior short lever pull technique

This is a variant of technique 8.6.7 and the hand positions are identical. The difference is that the line of thrust is made from posterior to anterior.

8.6.9   1st metacarpo-carpal anterior to posterior short lever pull technique

Application
Joint play glide loss from anterior to posterior loss of the first metacarpal on the greater multangular (trapezium).

Patient's position
The patient sits, stands or reclines supine, with the forearm on the affected side pointing obliquely upwards and the thumb extended.

Chiropractor's stance
The chiropractor stands facing the patient on the affected side with the right shoulder adjacent to the patient's sternum.

Contact
a)   The left hand: the fourth finger wraps around the base of the 1st metacarpal from the lateral side and is supported by the other fingers. The left thumb contacts the anterior of the body of the patient's first phalanx and holds it in extension.
b)   The right hand: the first finger contacts the dorsal surface of the greater multangular (trapezium) and is supported by the other fingers.

Procedure
Joint pre-load tension is achieved by further extending the patient's 1st metacarpal, bringing the elbows to the sides, thus tractioning the joint, and then applying standard short lever pull technique (see Chapter 2). The impulse is of minimal depth and made in equal and opposite directions.

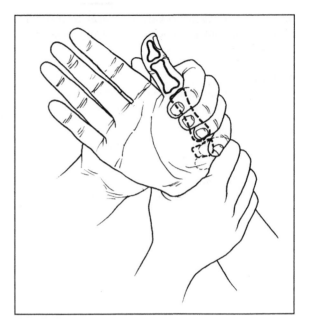

Fig. 8.6.9(a)

To attain joint pre-load tension, the chiropractor's thumb holds the patient's thumb in extension

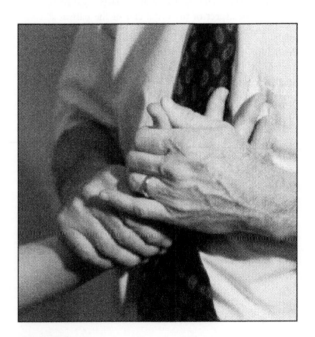

Fig. 8.6.9(b)

The chiropractor faces the patient, who may be sitting, standing or reclining supine. Note that the chiropractor's left thumb is pressed against the distal end of the patient's thumb

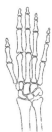

8.6.10 2nd or 3rd metacarpo-carpal posterior to anterior short level pull technique – Method I

Application
This technique may be selected for the following two fixations:

1) *Joint play glide loss from posterior to anterior of the second metacarpal on the greater and lesser multangulars (trapezium and trapezoid).*

2) *Joint play glide loss from posterior to anterior of the third metacarpal on the capitate.*

Patient's position
The patient sits, stands or reclines supine with the forearm on the affected side held vertically.

Chiropractor's stance
The chiropractor stands facing the patient, with the ulnar side of the patient's affected forearm held against the sternum.

Contact
a) The left hand is placed around the anterior of the patient's wrist from the radial side with a middle finger contact along the anterior distal row of carpals. The remaining fingers support it by closing up around the wrist. The thumb is placed around the posterior of the wrist.

b) The right hand, with an anterior middle phalangeal middle finger contact, is placed around the posterior of the proximal end of the 2nd or 3rd metacarpal (whichever is applicable) from the thumb side, as close to the joint as possible. The remaining fingers close up around the contact for support. The thumb is placed against the anterior distal end of the relevant metacarpal and holds it in extension.

Procedure
Joint pre-load tension is achieved by dorsiflexing the wrist and hand. The adjustment is delivered by applying standard short lever pull technique (see Chapter 2), using minimal depth of thrust. The impulse is made in equal and opposite directions along the arms, respecting the plane line of the joints.

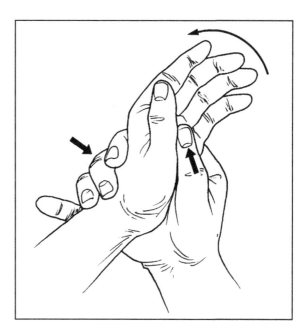

Fig. 8.6.10(a)

Joint pre-load tension is achieved by extending the wrist with the right thumb contact against the anterior distal metacarpal

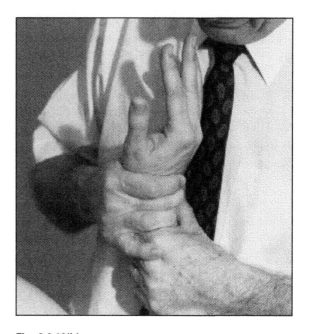

Fig. 8.6.10(b)

The patient's forearm is placed vertically along the chiropractor's sternum

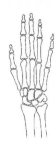

8.6.11 2nd or 3rd metacarpo-carpal posterior to anterior short lever pull technique – Method II

Application
Joint play glide loss of the 2nd metacarpal from posterior to anterior on the greater and lesser multangulars (trapezium and trapezoid) or the 3rd metacarpal from posterior to anterior on the capitate.

Patient's position
The patient sits, stands or reclines supine with the shoulder and elbow on the affected side semi-flexed and the hand held palm downwards.

Chiropractor's stance
The chiropractor sits or stands facing the patient on the affected side with the 5th metacarpal of the patient's hand held along the mid-line, against the sternum at a position which allows the elbows to remain at approximately 90°.

Contact
a) The left hand is placed over the dorsum of the wrist with the 1st phalanx of the first finger over the posterior of the greater multangular (trapezium), lesser multangular (trapezoid) and the capitate. The distal phalanx is pressed against the ventral surface of the greater and lesser multangulars, blocking all movement of these carpals. The remaining fingers support the contact and stabilize the wrist, radius and ulna.

b) The right hand is placed against the palmar surface of the patient's hand. The middle phalanx of the middle finger is placed over the posterior of the distal end of the 2nd or 3rd metacarpal (whichever is fixated) as close to the joint as possible. The remaining fingers support the contact. The thumb is placed against the anterior surface of the distal end of the affected 2nd or 3rd metacarpal.

Procedure
Joint pre-load tension is achieved by flexing the wrist backwards with the right hand and flexing the 2nd or 3rd metacarpal, as appropriate, backwards with the right thumb. Whilst maintaining the tension, standard short lever pull technique (see Chapter 2) is applied from posterior to anterior with the right hand and with equal pressure exerted in the opposite direction with the left hand.

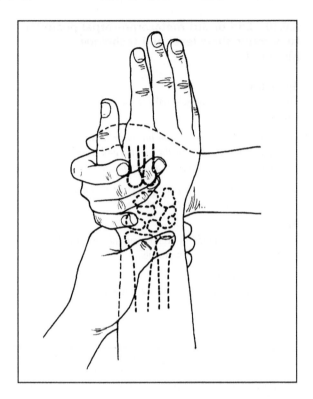

Fig. 8.6.11

The chiropractor's elbows are flexed to approximately 90°. The patient's wrist is flexed back and held by thumb pressure on the anterior of the appropriate metacarpal. The left hand stabilizes the carpals

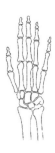

8.6.12 2nd or 3rd metacarpo-carpal anterior to posterior short lever pull technique

Application
Joint play glide loss of the 2nd or 3rd metacarpal joints from anterior to posterior on the carpals.

Patient's position
The patient sits, stands or reclines supine with the shoulder flexed and the forearm on the affected side held vertically and supinated. The fingers are flexed.

Chiropractor's stance
The chiropractor stands sideways on to the patient, facing the medial side of the patient's extended arm with the right shoulder adjacent to the patient's sternum. The patient's hand is held against the chiropractor's lower sternum.

Contact
a) The left hand is placed over the posterior surface of the metacarpals to hold them in flexion. The second and third row of the third and fourth phalanges are held stiffly in extension. Using the finger tips as contacts, they are placed over the anterior base of the appropriate (2nd or 3rd) metacarpal. The remaining fingers close up together to support the contact.
b) The right hand is placed over the ventral surface of the wrist with the fingers wrapped over the medial border to reach around to the posterior surfaces of the greater multangular, lesser multangular (trapezium and trapezoid) and capitate, stabilizing the distal row of carpals.

Procedure
Joint pre-load tension is achieved by further flexing the metacarpal to be adjusted. Standard short lever pull technique (see Chapter 2) is applied with equal pressure from the left and right arms. Little depth of thrust is required.

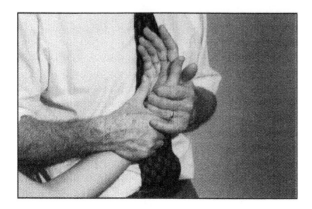

Fig. 8.6.12

The chiropractor stands alongside the patient, facing the medial side of the patient's forearm. The third and fourth contact fingers of the left hand are held stiff and straight between the 2nd/3rd phalangeal rows and pressed firmly against the anterior base of the 2nd or 3rd metacarpals. The right hand stabilizes the distal row of carpals

8.6.13 4th or 5th metacarpo-carpal posterior to anterior short lever pull technique

Application
This technique may be selected for the following two fixations:
a) Joint play glide loss from posterior to anterior of the fourth metacarpal on the hamate.
b) Joint play glide loss from posterior to anterior of the fifth metacarpal on the hamate.

Patient's position
The patient sits, stands or reclines supine. The arm is held out with the elbow semi-flexed and the palm of the hand facing downwards.

Chiropractor's stance
The chiropractor stands sideways on to the patient, facing the medial border of the forearm and hand with the right shoulder adjacent to the patient's sternum. The thumb side of the patient's hand is held against the lower sternum.

Contact
a) The left hand is placed around the back of the patient's hand with the second, third and fourth fingers curling around the 5th metacarpal to reach the posterior of the 4th or 5th metacarpal base as appropriate. These fingers are held close together and the second and third row of phalanges are held stiff and straight. The left thumb is placed on the anterior distal end of the appropriate metacarpal.
b) The right hand is used to stabilize the distal row of carpals by placing it over the dorsum of the wrist. The first finger extends around the ulnar side of the wrist to contact the hamulus of the hamate on the volar surface.

Procedure
Joint pre-load tension is achieved by extending the metacarpal being treated backwards with the left thumb. Whilst maintaining the pre-load tension, standard short lever pull technique (see Chapter 2) is applied from posterior to anterior with the left hand and equal pressure exerted in the opposite direction with the right, while respecting the plane lines of the joints.

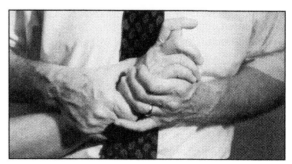

Fig. 8.6.13

The third and fourth fingers of the left hand contact the posterior base of the 4th or 5th metacarpal as appropriate and the right hand stabilizes the distal row of carpals. The index finger of the left hand contacts the hamulus on the volar surface of the hamate

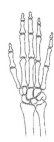
8.6.14 4th or 5th metacarpo-carpal anterior to posterior short lever pull technique

The technique is performed in the same manner as the preceding manoeuvre except that the chiropractor's hands are reversed. The left middle finger contacts the relevant anterior proximal metacarpal and the right anterior middle finger contacts the posterior distal row.

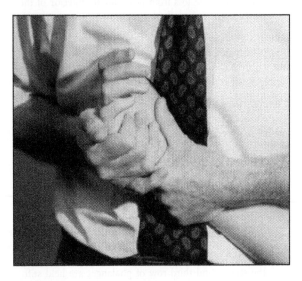

Fig. 8.6.14

The chiropractor stands sideways on to the patient on the lateral side of the affected arm. The patient turns the palm upwards and flexes the wrist. The left hand is placed under the dorsal surface of the distal carpal row to stabilize it. The third and fourth fingers of the right hand reach under and around the lateral side of the hand to contact the 4th or 5th metacarpal

Intercarpal techniques

8.6.E Joint play evaluation of the intercarpal joints

Procedure 1

Evaluation of anterior to posterior glide of the distal row of carpals on the proximal row:
The patient's forearm is held vertically and pronated so that the palm faces the chiropractor. The chiropractor's right index finger contacts horizontally across the posterior of the proximal row to prevent movement. A double thumb contact is placed on the anterior of each of the distal carpals in turn and pressure into wrist extension is exerted. After full free movement is reached, further pressure is then exerted into joint play.

Procedure 2

Evaluation of posterior to anterior glide of the distal row of carpals on the proximal row:
The hands are reversed from the positions described above. The double thumb contact is placed over the posterior of each of the distal carpals in turn and the wrist taken into flexion. The proximal row is stabilized with the right first finger placed horizontally across the anterior of the proximal row. After full free movement is reached, further pressure is then exerted into joint play, which is perceived as an elastic end-feel.

Procedure 3

Anterior to posterior and posterior to anterior joint play evaluation:
Integrity of the distal carpals on the proximal row as a group (the mid-carpal joint) may be tested by holding the proximal row with one hand and pressing firmly to the anterior, whilst the other hand, holding the distal row firmly, opposes the motion and vice versa.

Procedure 4

Posterior to anterior and anterior to posterior intercarpal joint play evaluation:
Further intercarpal joint play assessment can be made by placing the patient's hand, palm downwards or upwards, and by using the lateral border of the head of the chiropractor's 1st phalanx of the flexed index finger against the volar surface of one carpal, and a double thumb contact on the dorsal surface of an adjacent articulating carpal. A squeezing pressure with the double thumb contact is exerted.

An example of this is to place the patient's hand palm downwards. The chiropractor's left index finger is flexed and the lateral border is placed under the volar surface of the navicular (scaphoid) to prevent any movement of that carpal. A double thumb contact is then placed over the posterior surface of the capitate and firm pressure from posterior to anterior is exerted to elicit joint play between the two. This method can be employed with careful placement of the contacts across the carpals from posterior to anterior and vice versa.

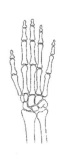

An alternative method to detect and isolate which intercarpal joints show loss of anterior to posterior joint play glide, uses opposing thumb pressures in a similar manner to the examination of the tarsal complex of joints. For example, the tip of one thumb is placed on the posterior of the navicular (scaphoid) and held firmly against it. The other thumb is placed in turn on the anterior of each of the carpals which articulate with it (lunate, capitate, greater multangular and lesser multangular).

With consideration for the plane lines of the joints, firm squeezing pressures are exerted on each joint in turn by the thumbs in opposing directions to elicit joint play. The thumbs are then reversed with one thumb tip pressed and held firmly against the anterior of the navicular while the other thumb is placed in turn on the posterior of each of the carpals which articulate with it, pressing firmly in opposing directions to elicit joint play. As well as for evaluating all of the intercarpal joints, this method can be adapted for examining the metacarpo-carpals and radio-carpal joints.

8.6.15　Greater multangular (trapezium) on the navicular (scaphoid) anterior to posterior short lever pull technique

Application
Joint play glide loss from anterior to posterior of the greater multangular (trapezium) on the navicular (scaphoid).

Patient's position
The patient sits, stands or reclines supine with the affected wrist and hand held vertically.

Chiropractor's stance
The chiropractor either sits or stands facing the patient with the ulnar side of the patient's affected wrist and hand resting firmly against the sternum. The elbows are held at approximately 90°.

Contact
a)　The left hand closes around the dorsum of the wrist on the radial side so that the 2nd phalanx of the middle finger contacts the anterior of the greater multangular (trapezium), with the remaining fingers closed against it for support, also anchoring the distal end of the radius.

b)　The right hand closes around the radial side of the wrist so that the first finger contacts the posterior of the navicular (scaphoid). The remaining fingers support the contact.

Procedure
Typical short lever pull technique (see Chapter 2) is applied using minimal depth of thrust. The chiropractor's elbows remain relaxed at the sides. Joint pre-load tension is achieved by keeping the wrists rigid and drawing the elbows back a little.

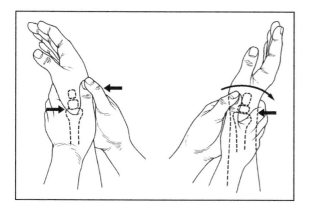

Fig. 8.6.E

Anterior to posterior glide of the intercarpal joints. To test posterior to anterior glide, the hands are reversed and the thumbs press from the posterior

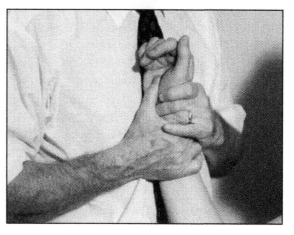

Fig. 8.6.15

The patient's hand and wrist are held with the ulnar side vertically against the chiropractor's sternum

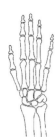

8.6.16 Greater multangular (trapezium) on the navicular (scaphoid) posterior to anterior short lever pull technique

Application
Joint play glide loss from posterior to anterior of the greater multangular (trapezium) on the navicular (scaphoid).

Patient's position
The patient sits, stands or reclines supine with the affected wrist and hand held vertically.

Chiropractor's stance
The chiropractor either sits or stands facing the patient with the ulnar side of the patient's affected wrist and hand resting against the mid-sternum.

Contact
a) The left hand is placed around the radial side of the wrist from the anterior. The middle finger contacts the posterior of the greater multangular (trapezium) supported by the other fingers.
b) The right hand is placed around the radial side of the wrist from the posterior. The second digit of the first finger contacts the anterior of the navicular (scaphoid) supported by the other fingers.

Procedure
Typical short lever pull technique is applied using minimal depth of thrust. The elbows are relaxed at the sides and joint pre-load tension is achieved by holding the wrists and hands rigid while drawing the elbows backwards a little.

8.6.17 Capitate on the navicular (scaphoid) posterior to anterior extension short lever pull technique

Application
Joint play glide loss from posterior to anterior of the capitate on the navicular (scaphoid).

Patient's position
The patient sits, stands or reclines supine with the arm, elbow and hand on the affected side extended and the palm is placed facing downwards.

Chiropractor's stance
The chiropractor faces the patient and is close enough to ensure that both elbows are semi-flexed.

Contact
The fingers of both hands are laced together and flexed. The first finger of the right hand is on top. This is placed on the anterior surface of the navicular (scaphoid) to prevent any movement. A double thumb contact is made on the posterior of the capitate.

Procedure
The patient's wrist is gently extended until joint pre-load tension is felt. Without releasing the tension, a gentle quick impulse, with minimal depth of thrust, is made on the capitate taking the wrist into further extension. Very little force is required.

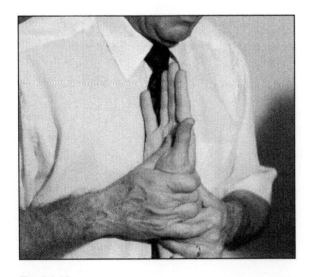

Fig. 8.6.16

The hands are reversed compared with the anterior to posterior technique shown in Fig. 8.6.15

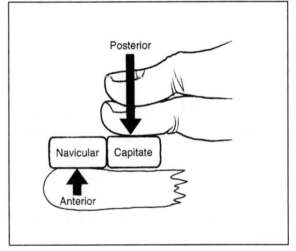

Fig. 8.6.17(a)

A double thumb contact is used on the posterior of the capitate

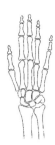

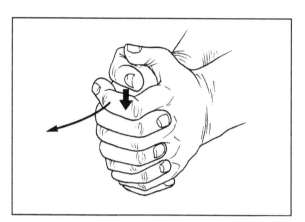

Fig. 8.6.17(b)

The lateral border of the index finger of the right hand, supported by the remaining fingers, contacts the anterior aspect of the navicular

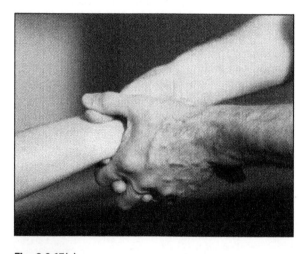

Fig. 8.6.17(c)

The chiropractor flexes the elbows. The patient extends the arm and wrist

8.6.18 Capitate on the navicular (scaphoid) anterior to posterior flexion short lever pull technique

Application
Joint play glide loss from anterior to posterior of the capitate on the navicular (scaphoid).

Patient's position
The patient stands, sits or is placed supine with the affected arm and wrist extended and the palm held facing upwards.

Chiropractor's stance
The chiropractor faces the patient with both elbows flexed.

Contact
All fingers on both hands are flexed and laced together, the left first finger on top. This is placed under the posterior surface of the navicular (scaphoid). A double thumb contact is made on the anterior of the capitate.

Procedure
The patient's wrist is flexed and, at the same time, gently laterally flexed to the ulnar side to achieve joint pre-load tension. Without releasing the tension, a quick anterior to posterior impulse, with minimal depth, is made into further wrist flexion.

Note
The previous two techniques may be applied to joint play glide loss of the other intercarpal articulations from posterior to anterior and anterior to posterior, as listed below, by altering the contacts as appropriate:
- *Greater multangular (trapezium) – lesser multangular (trapezoid)*
- *Capitate – hamate*
- *Hamate – triangular (triquetrum)*
- *Triangular (triquetrum) – lunate*
- *Lunate – navicular (scaphoid)*

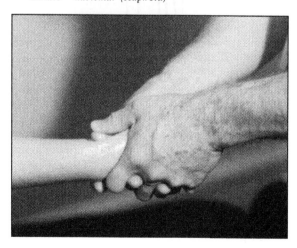

Fig. 8.6.18

The patient's forearm is supinated, the palm upwards and the wrist is flexed and laterally flexed to the ulnar side

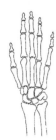

8.6.F Joint play evaluation of adjacent intercarpal joints

Procedure 1
Evaluation of anterior to posterior glide of the proximal row of carpals:
By contacting adjacent carpals between fingers and thumbs, pressure is exerted in opposite directions. Care must be taken to exert sufficient pressure at the end of the joint travel to elicit joint play. This is perceived as an elastic end-feel as the joint reaches its normal limit of motion.

Procedure 2
Evaluation of lateral to medial glide of the pisiform on the triangular (triquetrum):
Using a double thumb contact on the lateral border of the pisiform a lateral to medial pressure is exerted. The triangular (triquetrum) is stabilized by the fingers laced around the other carpals. Considerable motion of the joint is normally elicited before joint play can be assessed.

Procedure 3
Evaluation of medial to lateral glide of the pisiform on the triangular (triquetrum):
A double thumb contact is placed on the medial border of the pisiform which is pressed firmly laterally. The triangular (triquetrum) is stabilized with the right first finger. All of the remaining fingers of the right hand close up to support this contact. As with the lateral to medial motion described above, considerable passive movement is elicited before the elasticity of joint play can be assessed on this articulation.

8.6.19 Pisiform on the triangular (triquetrum) lateral to medial short lever pull technique

Application
Joint play glide loss of the pisiform on the triangular (triquetrum) from lateral to medial.

Patient's position
The patient sits, stands or reclines. The forearm on the affected side is held vertically, with the lateral border of the hand held towards the chiropractor.

Chiropractor's stance
The chiropractor stands facing the patient's mid-line with the elbows flexed to approximately 90°.

Contact
a) The left hand is placed around the dorsum of the wrist from the lateral side and the fingers contact around the wrist to hold it securely. The anterior of the distal digit of the left thumb contacts the lateral border of the pisiform.
b) The right hand is placed around the ventral side of the wrist, around the fingers of the left hand. The right thumb is placed over the left thumb.

Procedure
First the joint pre-load is achieved by pressing the thumbs towards the mid-line of the patient's wrist until joint pre-load tension is felt. Without releasing the tension, a rapid shallow thrust with the thumbs is employed in an oblique direction from lateral to medial and posterior to anterior.
Note: This thrust direction on the pisiform is necessary because of the oval-shaped articular facet with the triangular (triquetrum) bone.

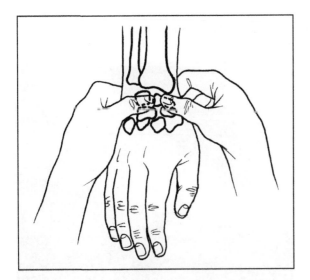

Fig. 8.6.F

Evaluation of anterior to posterior glide of the proximal row of carpals, excepting the pisiform on the triquetrum

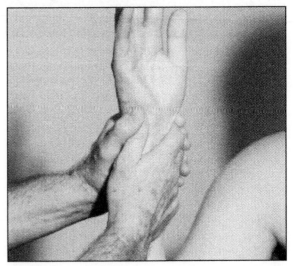

Fig. 8.6.19

The direction of the thrust is obliquely from lateral to medial and posterior to anterior

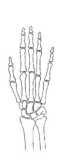

8.6.20 Pisiform on the triangular (triquetrum) medial to lateral short lever pull technique

This technique utilizes a similar method of delivery to the pisiform technique described above except that the patient's wrist is rotated so that the palm faces the chiropractor. A double-thumb contact is made on the medial aspect of the pisiform and the thrust is medial to lateral and obliquely from anterior to posterior.

8.6.21 Triangular (triquetrum) on the hamate posterior to anterior recoil technique

Application
Joint play glide loss from posterior to anterior of the triangular (triquetrum) on the hamate.

Patient's position
The patient sits or stands and places the affected hand upon a convenient treatment table drop-piece (see Glossary of Terms, p. 285), palm downwards with the wrist in a neutral position.

Chiropractor's stance
The chiropractor stands beside the patient shoulder to shoulder, facing in the same direction as the patient.

Contact
a) The left hand is placed over the posterior surface of the triangular (triquetrum) using a pisiform low arch contact (see Glossary of Terms, p. 285).
b) The right hand is placed over the left wrist with the fingers clasping over the dorsum to the lateral side.

Procedure
With the drop-piece cocked, a recoil adjustment (see Chapter 2) is delivered using a high velocity pectoralis triceps anconius thrust with very low amplitude.

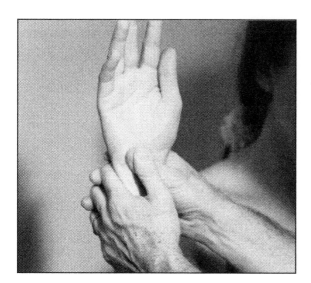

Fig. 8.6.20

The patient's palm is turned towards the chiropractor and a double thumb contact is used on the medial aspect of the pisiform

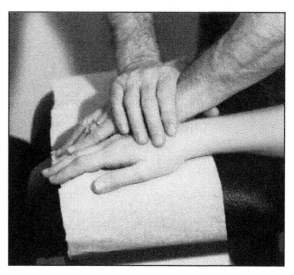

Fig. 8.6.21

The patient's hand is placed palm down on the treatment table drop-piece and the wrist is kept in a neutral position. The drop-piece is cocked, set for tension and a recoil adjustment is used with high velocity and very low amplitude

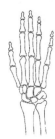

Radio-carpal techniques

8.6.G   Joint play evaluation of the radio-navicular and radio-lunate joints

Procedure 1
Evaluation of posterior to anterior glide of the radio-navicular (scaphoid) and radio-lunate articulations:
The index finger of the right hand is placed across the anterior of the head of the ulna and the distal extremity of the radius to immobilize them. A double thumb contact is placed on the posterior of the navicular (scaphoid).

Pressure is applied, taking the wrist into flexion and then further pressure is exerted to elicit joint play. Careful assessment is necessary because of the normal considerable free motion of this joint. By maintaining the contact on the radius and ulna with the right hand and by sliding the double thumb contact medially on to the lunate, joint play can be similarly assessed on the lunate radial articulation.

Procedure 2
Evaluation of anterior to posterior glide of the radio-navicular (scaphoid) and radio-lunate articulations:
The hands are reversed, with a double thumb contact on the anterior of the navicular (scaphoid) or lunate and the first finger on the posterior of the distal radius and ulnar. The wrist is taken into extension.

Procedure 3
Evaluation of the radio-carpals in long axis distraction:
The patient sits or stands, with the affected arm extended and the hand held palm downwards. The left hand is placed around the dorsum of the wrist, ensuring that the first finger and thumb contact the proximal carpal row. The remaining fingers close up around the contact to support it. The right hand is also placed around the dorsum of the wrist ensuring that the first finger and thumb contact the styloid process of the radius and ulna. It has been clinically observed that frequently if long axis distraction fixation is present in conjunction with an anterior to posterior or posterior to anterior fixation of either the navicular (scaphoid) or lunate, it has been observed that correcting the latter will usually correct the former as well. Careful re-evaluation of joint function is necessary to assess the effects of each manipulation.

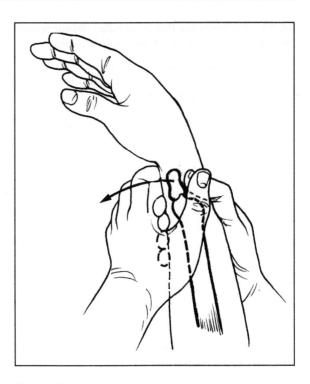

Fig. 8.6.G

Medial view of the right hand, showing posterior to anterior glide of the navicular (scaphoid) on the radius

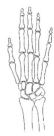

8.6.22 Radio-navicular (scaphoid) posterior to anterior short lever pull technique

Application
Joint play glide loss from posterior to anterior of the navicular on the radius.

Patient's position
The patient sits, stands or reclines supine. The forearm on the affected side is held vertically.

Chiropractor's stance
The chiropractor stands or sits, facing the patient with the ulnar side of the patient's wrist and hand on the affected limb placed against the sternum.

Contact
a)   The left hand wraps right around the distal radius from the posterior with the first finger contacting firmly against the anterior of the radius and the remaining fingers closed up beside it for support. The web of the left thumb contacts the posterior of the distal ulna and the thumb wraps around it to grasp the anterior.

b)   The right hand approaches from the anterior and the middle finger wraps around the wrist to contact the posterior aspect of the navicular; the remaining fingers close up to support it.

Procedure
To enhance the joint pre-load tension, the patient's wrist is slightly extended and then distracted in long axis with the chiropractor's right hand. Standard short lever pull technique (see Chapter 2) is employed with the elbows drawn to the sides and the thrust given in equal and opposite directions across the joint. The right hand thrusts posterior to anterior on the navicular and the left hand stabilizes the radius.

Note
Clinically, it has been observed that this fixation is very frequently encountered in cases of wrist pain of mechanical origin.

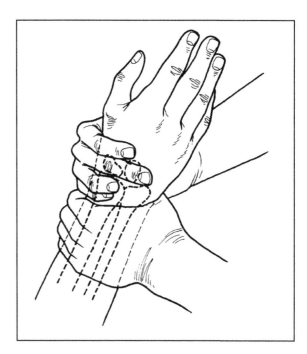

Fig. 8.6.22(a)

Radio-navicular (scaphoid) posterior to anterior short lever technique

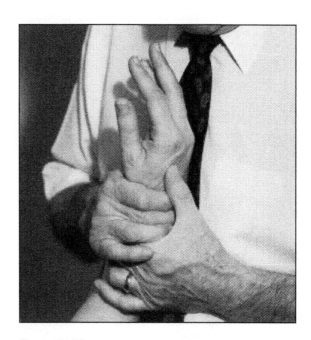

Fig. 8.6.22(b)

To enhance the joint pre-load tension, the patient's wrist is slightly extended and then distracted in long axis with the right hand

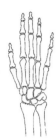

8.6.23 Radio-navicular (scaphoid) anterior to posterior short lever pull technique

Application
Joint play glide loss from anterior to posterior of the navicular (scaphoid) on the radius.

Patient's position
The patient sits, stands or reclines supine, with the forearm on the affected side held vertically and the wrist rotated so that the ulnar side of the wrist is directed away from the body.

Chiropractor's stance
The chiropractor either sits or stands facing the patient with the ulnar side of the patient's wrist and hand on the affected side placed against the mid-sternal area.

Contact
a)   The middle finger of the left hand contacts the anterior of the navicular (scaphoid) and is supported by the remaining fingers.
b)   The first finger of the right hand contacts around the posterior of the distal end of the radius as close to the joint as possible, supported closely by the remaining fingers.

Procedure
To achieve joint pre-load tension, the wrist is flexed a little forwards and distracted in long axis. Standard short lever pull technique (see Chapter 2) is then employed, impulsing in equal and opposite directions, the right hand stabilizing the radius and ulna and the left thrusting with minimal depth from anterior to posterior.

8.6.24 Radio-navicular (scaphoid) posterior to anterior wrist extension technique

Application
Joint play glide loss from posterior to anterior of the navicular (scaphoid) on the radius.

Patient's position
The patient sits with the arm on the affected side slightly abducted and the palm of the hand resting flat on the treatment table.

Chiropractor's stance
The chiropractor stands behind the patient with the mid-line of the body directly above the contact.

Contact
a)   The left hand – a pisiform contact is used with the wrist held in extension.
b)   The right hand grasps the left wrist as close as possible to the distal ends of the radius and ulna, with the fingers wrapped around the ulna.

Procedure
Either a light body drop technique (see Chapter 2) using minimal depth of thrust or recoil technique (see Chapter 2) with or without a drop mechanism (see Glossary of Terms, p. 285) may be used. The patient's wrist is placed in extension and the direction of thrust is at approximately 90° to the radius.

Note
The radio-lunate joint may also be adjusted using this procedure – see technique 8.6.26.

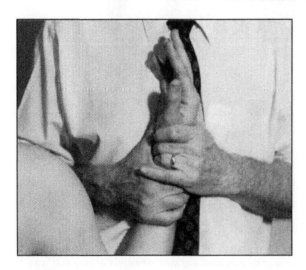

Fig. 8.6.23

To assist in achieving joint pre-load tension, the patient's wrist is slightly flexed and then distracted in long axis

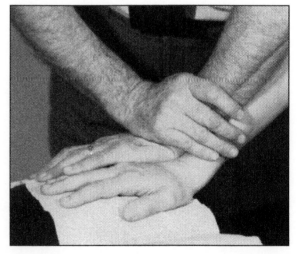

Fig. 8.6.24

The thrust line is oblique to comply with the plane line of the joint. This procedure may also be used to adjust the radio-lunate joint

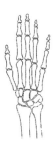

8.6.H   Joint play evaluation of the navicular (scaphoid) on the radius

Procedure 1
Evaluation of the lateral to medial glide of the navicular (scaphoid) on the radius:
The patient's wrist is first deviated to the ulnar side. The tip of the chiropractor's index finger of the right hand is then placed over the 'anatomical snuff box' to contact the navicular (scaphoid). The wrist is then radially deviated with the chiropractor's left hand, and the navicular (scaphoid) is pressed medially. Contact with the navicular (scaphoid) must be maintained and, with normal motion, it will be felt to slide away medially from the index finger. At the end of the travel, firm but gentle pressure is used to assess joint play.

Procedure 2
Evaluation of joint play of the medial to lateral and lateral to medial glide of the navicular (scaphoid) and the lunate on the radius is tested together as a group:
Evaluation of the medial to lateral and lateral to medial joint play of the radio-carpals as a group may be carried out by holding the distal radius and ulna with one hand, and holding around the proximal row with the other. Lateral to medial motion is made with one hand whilst being firmly opposed by the other. Joint play can be assessed at the end of the joint travel by applying further firm pressure in the same direction. Joint play is felt as an elastic end-feel.

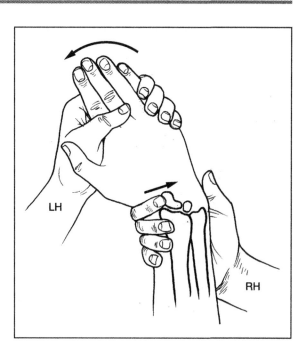

Fig. 8.6.H

Lateral to medial glide of the navicular (scaphoid) on the radius

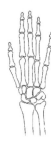

8.6.25 Radio-navicular (scaphoid) lateral to medial short lever pull technique

Application
Joint play glide loss of lateral to medial of the navicular (scaphoid) on the radius.

Patient's position
The patient sits, stands or reclines supine, with the affected hand held vertically, the palmar side facing towards the patient and with slight lateral flexion of the wrist to the radial side.

Chiropractor's stance
The chiropractor stands facing the patient.

Contact
a) The left hand wraps around the volar aspect of the wrist from the radial side and all the fingers grasp the posterior of the distal end of the ulna. The thumb is placed over the dorsum of the wrist.

b) The middle finger of the right hand contacts the lateral aspect of the navicular from the volar side, and the index and fourth fingers support it closely. The thumb is placed around the back of the hand.

Procedure
i) The patient's hand is flexed medially towards the thumb to achieve joint pre-load tension.

ii) The elbows are held relaxed down to the sides.

iii) Short lever pull technique (see Chapter 2) is then applied with the impulse of minimal depth generated by swiftly contracting the rhomboid muscles. The thrust is a scissor-type action with equal and opposite pressure applied to the contacts.

Note
Very little depth of thrust is needed to produce cavitation of the joint.

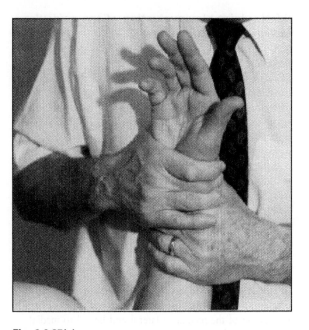

Fig. 8.6.25(a)

The elbows are flexed to approximately 90°. The back of the patient's hand is held firmly against the sternum

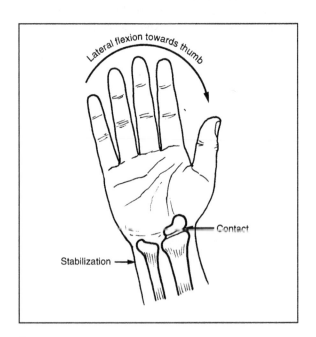

Fig. 8.6.25(b)

The anterior of the middle phalanx of the right middle finger contacts the lateral surface of the navicular (scaphoid)

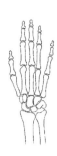

8.6.J   Joint play evaluation of the radio-carpal joint in long axis extension

Procedure

The patient sits, stands or reclines supine with the elbow on the affected side flexed to approximately 90° and the palm facing downwards. The chiropractor faces the patient and the left hand is placed around the dorsum of the patient's wrist, carefully placing the index finger and thumb to contact the proximal carpal row. The right hand is also placed around the dorsum of the wrist ensuring that the index finger and thumb contact the styloid process of the radius and ulna. Whilst holding the contacts firmly, the chiropractor pulls the hands apart to distract the joint. When the slack has been taken up, further shallow but firm pressure is applied to assess the integrity of the joint play. Normal joint play is felt as a perception of elasticity at the end of the joint travel.

It is worthy of note that it has been clinically observed that if long axis distraction fixation is present in conjunction with an anterior to posterior or posterior to anterior fixation of either the navicular (scaphoid) or lunate, correcting these latter fixations will frequently also correct the former.

8.6.26   Radio-lunate posterior to anterior short lever pull technique

Application

Joint play glide loss from posterior to anterior of the lunate on the radius.

Patient's position

The patient sits, stands or reclines supine with the forearm on the affected side held vertically and the elbow flexed. The hand and wrist are rotated so that the ulnar side faces away from the patient.

Chiropractor's stance

The chiropractor stands facing the patient with the ulnar side of the patient's forearm and wrist placed against the lower sternum.

Contact

a)   The left hand wraps around the distal radius from the posterior, with the anterior of the first finger pressed tightly against the anterior of the radius. The remaining fingers close up against it for support.

b)   The right hand approaches from the anterior of the patient's wrist. The anterior of the distal phalanx of the middle finger reaches right around the medial side of the wrist to contact the posterior aspect of the hamate and is held stiffly against it. The remaining fingers support it by closing up on either side of it.

Procedure

Joint pre-load tension is enhanced by using the web of the right hand to first extend the wrist backwards several degrees and then by distracting the joint. Standard short lever pull technique (see Chapter 2) is then employed. The impulse is applied in equal and opposite directions. The role of the left hand is to stabilize the wrist, blocking any movement proximal to the contact, and the direction of the right hand thrusts is from posterior to anterior utilizing minimal depth of thrust.

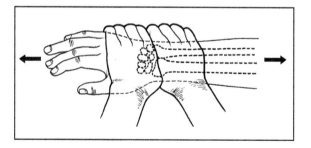

Fig. 8.6.J

Posterior to anterior view of the right hand

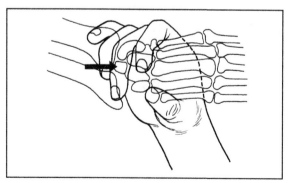

Fig. 8.6.26

The middle phalanx of the middle finger of the right hand presses against the lunate and keeps the distal phalanx extended with a firm contact. The wrist is then extended several degrees backwards. A measure of long axis distraction is employed to achieve joint pre-load tension

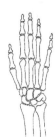

8.6.27 Radio-lunate anterior to posterior short lever pull technique

Application
Joint play glide loss from anterior to posterior of the lunate on the radius.

Patient's position
The patient sits, stands or reclines supine. The forearm on the affected side is held vertically, the elbow flexed. The ulna is turned to face away from the patient.

Chiropractor's stance
The chiropractor stands facing the patient, favouring the affected side. The patient's forearm and wrist are placed against the chiropractor's lower sternum.

Contact
a) The anterior surface of the distal digit of the middle finger of the left hand contacts the anterior of the lunate.
b) The anterior surface of the first finger of the right hand contacts around the posterior of the distal radius as close to the joint as possible, supported by the remaining fingers.

Procedure
Joint pre-load tension is achieved by flexing the patient's wrist forwards and by drawing the elbows gently to the sides. Short lever pull technique is then applied utilizing minimal depth of thrust. The thrust direction is in equal and opposite directions across the joint, respecting the plane line of the joint.

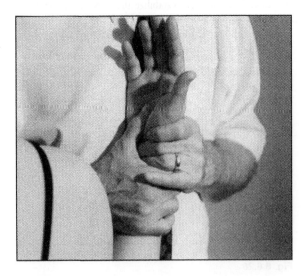

Fig. 8.6.27

The ulnar side of the patient's wrist and hand are held vertically and firmly against the sternum. The wrist is then slightly flexed and distracted to achieve joint pre-load tension prior to the delivery of the thrust

Distal radio-ulnar techniques

8.6.K Joint play evaluation of the distal radio-ulnar joint

Procedure 1
Evaluation of posterior to anterior glide of the radius on the ulna:
The patient sits, stands or reclines supine. The elbow on the affected side is extended and the palm faces downwards. A double thumb contact is placed over the posterior of the distal radius and the lateral side of the left first phalanx is placed under the anterior of the ulna to stabilize it and prevent any motion. A downward pressure exerted by the thumbs on the radius first removes the slack in the joint, then further firm pressure is applied to assess the joint play.

Procedure 2
Evaluation of anterior to posterior glide of the radius on the ulna:
The patient sits, stands or reclines supine. The elbow on the affected side is extended and the palm faces downwards. A double thumb contact is placed over the posterior of the distal ulna and the lateral side of the right first phalanx is placed under the anterior of the radius to stabilize it and prevent any motion. A downward pressure is then exerted by the thumbs on the ulna to remove all slack in the joint before further pressure is applied to assess joint play.

Procedure 3
Evaluation of outward and inward rotation of the radius and the ulna:
The patient is placed sitting, standing or reclining supine with the elbow on the affected side extended and the hand held palm downwards. A first finger and thumb contact is made on the anterior and posterior of the radius with the left hand and a first finger and thumb contact on the anterior and posterior of the ulna is made with the right hand. Outward and inward rotational pressure is exerted until all slack is removed from the joint. Further firm pressure is then applied to assess the joint play. Normal joint play is perceived as an elasticity at the end range of motion.

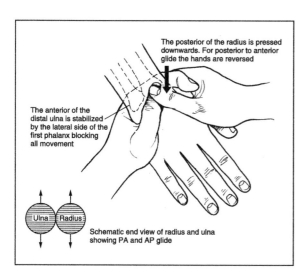

Fig. 8.6.K(a)

Right hand, posterior to anterior view. Distal radio-ulnar joint play evaluation posterior to anterior and anterior to posterior glide of the radius on the ulna

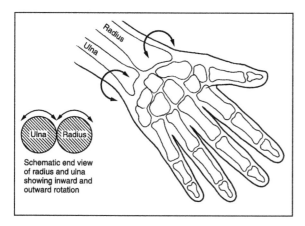

Fig. 8.6.K(b)

Distal radio-ulnar outward and inward joint play evaluation. Held between fingers and thumbs, the distal radius are rotated externally and internally.

8.6.28 Distal radio-ulnar posterior to anterior short lever pull technique

Application
Joint play glide loss from posterior to anterior of the distal radius on the ulna.

Patient's position
The patient sits, stands or reclines supine with the forearm on the affected limb held vertically. The patient rotates the wrist so that the ulnar side of the forearm is placed against the chiropractor's sternum.

Chiropractor's stance
The chiropractor stands or sits facing the patient favouring the side of the affected limb.

Contact
a) The left hand wraps around the radius from the posterior to allow all four finger tips, which are held stiffly and close up together, to press in a line along the anterior of the distal ulna, fingers close up together.

b) The right hand wraps around the radial side of the wrist to make a middle finger contact using the middle and distal phalanx against the posterior of the distal radial head. The remaining fingers close right up against it for support.

Procedure
The chiropractor's hands and wrists are held stiffly. Joint pre-load tension is achieved by drawing the elbows to the sides. Short lever pull technique is then applied in equal and opposite directions across the joint, utilizing minimum depth of thrust.

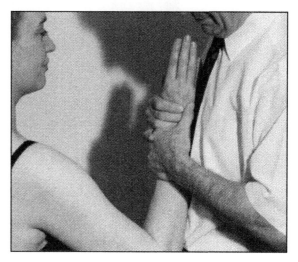

Fig. 8.6.28

The ulnar side of the wrist and hand is held firmly against the chiropractor's sternum

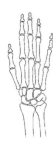

8.6.29   Distal radio-ulnar anterior to posterior short lever pull technique

Application
Joint play glide loss from anterior to posterior of the distal radius on the ulna.

Patient's position
The patient sits, stands or reclines supine with the forearm on the affected side held vertically. The wrist is rotated to allow the ulna to be placed against the chiropractor's sternum.

Chiropractor's stance
The chiropractor stands or sits facing the patient, favouring the side of involvement.

Contact
a)   The left hand wraps around the radial side of the wrist from the posterior to allow a middle finger contact on the anterior distal radius. The remaining fingers close up against it for support.
b)   The right hand also wraps around the distal end of the radius, proximally to the left hand, to allow all four finger tips to press in a line along the posterior of the distal end of the ulna.

Procedure
The chiropractor's fingers, hands and wrists are held stiffly. Joint pre-load tension is achieved by drawing the elbows to the sides. Short lever pull technique is then applied in equal and opposite directions across the joint. Only minimal depth of thrust is required.

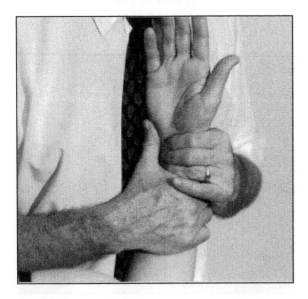

Fig. 8.6.29

This technique is similar to 8.6.28 except that the hand positions are reversed and the force vector is from anterior to posterior. All four fingers of the chiropractor's right hand are pressed in a line along the posterior of the distal end of the ulna

Section

2

The Lower Extremity

The hip joint

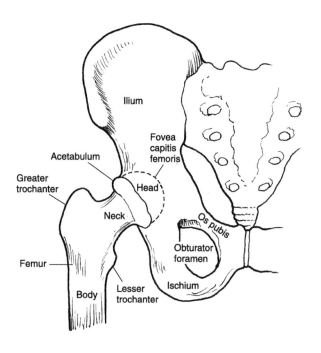

Ilium

Fovea
capitis
femoris

Acetabulum

Greater
trochanter

Head

Neck

Os pubis

Obturator
foramen

Femur

Ischium

Body

Lesser
trochanter

Joint play evaluation of the hip

8.7.A   Long axis extension
8.7.B   Superior to inferior glide with hip joint flexion
8.7.C   Superior to inferior glide with flexion and internal rotation
8.7.D   Superior to inferior glide with flexion and external rotation
8.7.E   Posterior to anterior glide with extension rotation
8.7.F   Anterior to posterior glide with flexion
8.7.G   Internal to external glide
8.7.H   Long axis extension with abduction
8.7.I   Adduction

Iliofemoral techniques

8.7.1   Supine iliofemoral flexion abduction/adduction mobilization technique
8.7.2   Supine iliofemoral superior to inferior mobilization technique
8.7.3   Supine iliofemoral flexion/abduction/rotation mobilization technique
8.7.4   Supine iliofemoral anterior to posterior springing mobilization technique

8.7.5   Prone iliofemoral posterior to anterior springing technique
8.7.6   Side reclining iliofemoral abduction mobilization technique
8.7.7   Side reclining iliofemoral circumduction mobilization technique
8.7.8   Prone iliofemoral abduction/internal rotation mobilization technique
8.7.9   Supine iliofemoral internal to external mobilization technique
8.7.10   Supine iliofemoral anterior to posterior flexion mobilization technique
8.7.11   Supine iliofemoral external to internal rotation mobilization technique
8.7.12   Supine iliofemoral internal to external rotation mobilization technique
8.7.13   Supine iliofemoral abduction mobilization technique
8.7.14   Supine iliofemoral adduction mobilization technique
8.7.15   Supine iliofemoral flexion/abduction/external rotation mobilization technique
8.7.16   Supine iliofemoral long axis extension mobilization technique
8.7.17   Prone iliofemoral long axis extension mobilization technique

Joint play evaluation of the hip

8.7.A Long axis extension

Procedure
The patient is placed supine with the hip extended and knee on the affected side flexed, with the lower leg placed to about 90° over the side of the treatment table. The chiropractor's right arm, hooked under the patient's knee, pulls the right femur firmly caudad to its full extent and into joint play and the left hand palpates the hip joint for the movement.

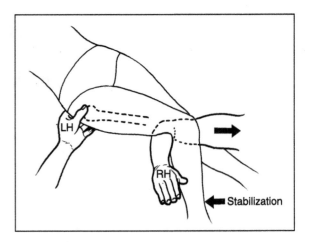

Fig. 8.7.A

Long axis extension

8.7.B Superior to inferior glide with hip joint flexion

Procedure
The patient is placed supine with the leg on the affected side flexed at the knee and the hip. The foot can be placed over and supported on the chiropractor's shoulder. Both hands are laced together around the anterior of the proximal thigh, as close to the joint as possible. Pressure in an inferior direction is exerted first to remove all tissue slack and then with further pressure, to pull the hip into joint play, which is perceived as an elastic end-feel at the end of the travel.

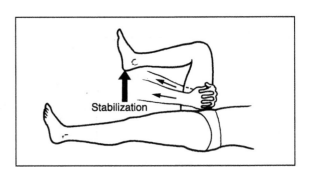

Fig. 8.7.B

Superior to inferior glide with flexion

8.7.C Superior to inferior glide with flexion and internal rotation

Procedure
The patient is placed supine with the leg on the affected side flexed at the knee and hip. The left elbow is placed under the patient's lower leg with the left hand reaching around under the knee, past the lateral lower thigh, to the anterior of the thigh. The chiropractor's trunk is rotated caudad to internally rotate the hip joints. Both hands are laced together at the anterior of the proximal thigh. The tissue slack is removed by pulling inferiorly with both hands. Without slackening the tension, and while maintaining the internal rotation, further pressure is exerted in an inferior direction into joint play, which is perceived as an elastic sensation at the fullest extent of the joint travel.

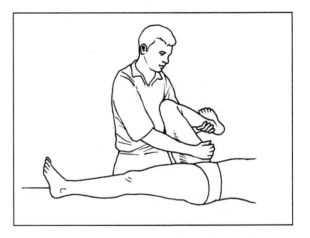

Fig. 8.7.C

Superior to inferior glide with flexion and internal rotation

8.7.D   Superior to inferior glide with flexion and external rotation

Procedure

The patient is placed supine with the affected leg flexed at the knee and hip. The chiropractor stands on the homolateral side facing the patient's mid-line. The hip is rotated externally by placing the right elbow under the patient's lower leg. The hand is then passed under the patient's knee and the distal medial thigh to reach the other hand at the anterior aspect of the distal thigh. Both hands are laced together at the anterior of the proximal thigh and the trunk is rotated cephalad. The tissue slack is removed by pulling inferiorly. Without slackening the tension, further pressure is exerted in an inferior direction into joint play.

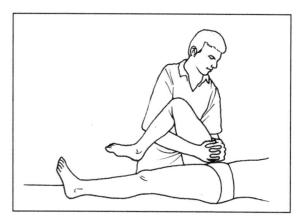

Fig. 8.7.D

Superior to inferior glide with flexion and external rotation

8.7.E   Posterior to anterior glide with extension

The patient is placed prone and the chiropractor stands on either side, according to preference, facing the affected hip. As one hand at the knee lifts the leg into extension, the other presses the hip joint anteriorly to the full extent of joint travel and then into joint play.

8.7.F   Anterior to posterior glide with flexion

The patient is placed supine. With one hand the chiropractor lifts the affected hip a few degrees into flexion and with the other, contacting the anterior of the greater trochanter, the hip is pressed downwards posteriorly into joint play.

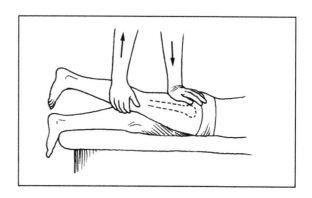

Fig. 8.7.E

Posterior to anterior glide with extension

8.7.G   Internal to external glide

The patient is placed supine with the hip flexed to 90° and the practitioner stands on the contralateral side. As the left hand stabilizes the patient's femur at the distal end, a heel of right hand contact presses the proximal end of the femur from the medial side firmly in a lateral direction into joint play.

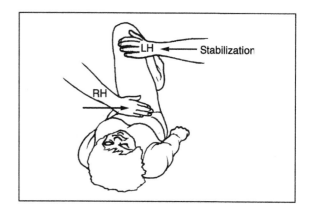

Fig. 8.7.G

Internal to external glide

8.7.H Long axis extension with abduction

Procedure

The patient is placed in a side reclining position on the non-affected side. With the practitioner standing behind the patient, the right hand abducts the hip and the left hand pushes the greater trochanter inferiorly. A firm pressure is used to take the joint through the full extent of its travel. A perception of elasticity should be present at the end of the joint movement, if joint play is normal.

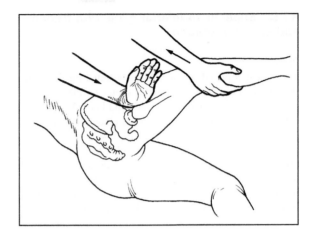

Fig. 8.7.H

Long axis extension with abduction

8.7.I Adduction

Procedure

The patient is placed supine with the hip on the affected side slightly flexed. The chiropractor stands on the affected side. The right hand contacts the distal end of the femur and pushes the hip joint past the patient's mid-line firmly into full adduction. Extra pressure is then exerted into joint play. The left hand palpates for movement of the joint, which is perceived as an elasticity when the joint has reached the full extent of its motion.

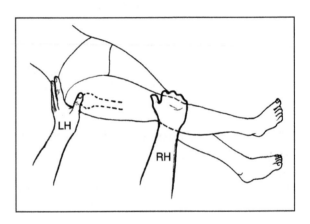

Fig. 8.7.I

Adduction

Iliofemoral techniques

8.7.1 Supine iliofemoral flexion abduction/adduction mobilization technique

Application
Hip flexion joint play glide loss and gross movement restriction with or without an abduction or an adduction component.

Patient's position
The patient is placed supine in a comfortable position, with the hip flexed to tolerance on the affected side and the knee fully flexed.

Chiropractor's stance
The chiropractor stands facing cephalad on the homolateral side, legs apart with the left leg ahead of the right. The right leg is placed approximately level with the patient's right knee.

Contact
a) The left hand is placed over the anterior aspect of the proximal tibia, close to the knee joint.
b) The right hand grasps the anterior aspect of the tibia just proximal to the ankle.

Procedure 1
The patient's knee is held flexed. The hip joint is flexed until the ligamentous barrier is felt. From this position, the hip is gently further flexed to the patient's tolerance, held for a few seconds and released. The procedure is repeated several times, as necessary.

Procedure 2
If joint play is also restricted in adduction, the same procedure as above is repeated with the patient's knee taken towards the contralateral shoulder.

Procedure 3
If joint play is also restricted in abduction, the same procedure as above is repeated with the patient's knee taken towards the homolateral shoulder.

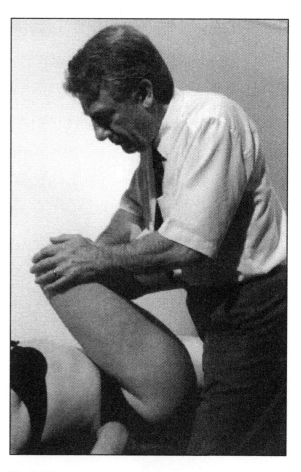

Fig. 8.7.1

With the patient supine and relaxed, the affected hip is passively flexed

8.7.2 Supine iliofemoral superior to inferior joint mobilization technique

Application
Joint play glide loss of the hip from superior to inferior.

Patient's position
The patient is placed supine with the hip and knee on the affected side each flexed to about 40°. The knee is placed over the chiropractor's shoulder.

Chiropractor's stance
The chiropractor faces cephalad and kneels. The right buttock rests back on the right heel. The left foot is placed forwards flat on the floor approximately level with the patient's hip joint. The left knee is semi-flexed.

Contact
The fingers of both hands are laced together and a middle finger contact from either hand grasps the anterior proximal aspect of the femur as close to the hip joint as possible.

Procedure
The patient's hip is tractioned by the chiropractor firmly pulling the trunk up in a cephalad direction with the contact until the left lower leg is approximately vertical and the patient's hip and knee are flexed to about 90°. Without releasing the tension, an impulse is then applied in a caudad direction.

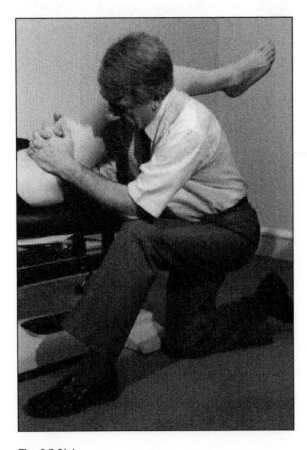

Fig. 8.7.2(a)

Starting position – hip semi-flexed

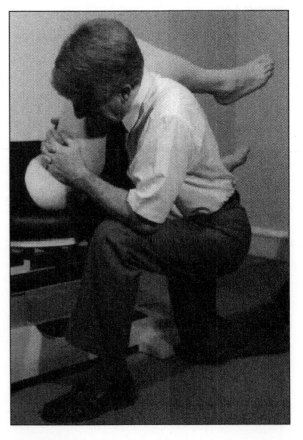

Fig. 8.7.2(b)

Final position

8.7.3   Supine iliofemoral flexion/abduction/rotation technique

Application
Joint play glide loss of the hip on flexion, abduction and external rotation.

Patient's position
The patient is placed supine with the hip and knee on the affected side flexed with the foot placed flat on the treatment table.

Chiropractor's stance
The chiropractor stands on the affected side facing the patient's midline approximately opposite the patient's hip.

Contact
a)   The left hand grasps the medial side of the patient's right knee.
b)   The right hand reaches over the patient and contacts the left anterior superior spine (ASIS) to stabilize the pelvis.

Procedure
The patient's hip is held in flexion with the chiropractor's right hand then pushed laterally into external rotation until ligamentous tension is felt. The hip is then gently pushed further into external rotation and held to the patient's tolerance, for several seconds. After releasing the pressure, the procedure is repeated several times. The patient's foot remains on the surface of the treatment table.

8.7.4   Supine iliofemoral anterior to posterior springing mobilization technique

Application
Joint play glide loss from anterior to posterior of the femur head in the acetabulum.

Patient's position
The patient is placed supine with the knee and hip flexed on the affected side. The other leg remains fully extended.

Chiropractor's stance
The chiropractor stands on the contralateral side, facing the patient and adjacent to the hip joints.

Contact
a)   The left hand is placed around the lateral part of the patient's right knee holding with all fingers around the posterior aspect of the knee.
b)   The heel of the right hand is placed on the right femur as close to the hip joint as possible, with the pisiform towards the greater trochanter.

Procedure
The left hand supports the leg and flexes the hip joint. At the same time as the hip flexes, the right hand exerts pressure on the hip joint in an anterior to posterior direction. This is performed several times in a rocking motion, to patient tolerance. The joint is then reassessed and the procedure is repeated as necessary.

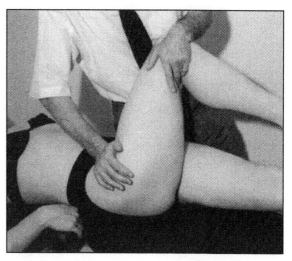

Fig. 8.7.4

A slow, stretching, rhythmical pressure is exerted on the hip joint

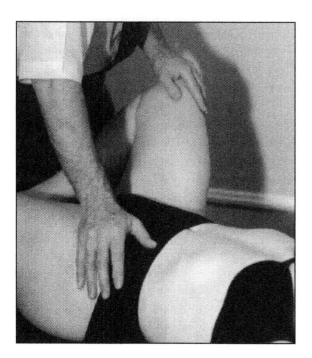

Fig. 8.7.3

The right hand reaches across to the patient's contralateral side and stabilizes the pelvis by contacting the anterior superior iliac spine

8.7.5 Prone iliofemoral posterior to anterior springing mobilization technique

Application
Joint play glide loss from posterior to anterior of the femoral head in the acetabulum.

Patient's position
The patient is placed prone with the knee on the affected side fully flexed.

Chiropractor's stance
The chiropractor stands on the homolateral side facing the mid-line of the patient.

Contact
a) From the medial side, the left hand is placed under the anterior of the distal end of the femur close to the knee joint. All fingers are used to make a firm contact.
b) The heel of the right hand is placed over the posterior of the patient's greater trochanter as close to the ilium as possible.

Procedure
The chiropractor turns the trunk slightly caudad, pressing rhythmically downwards on the hip joint with the right hand. The pressure exerted is slow and stretching with medium depth. As the right hand presses downwards, the left hand conversely elevates the patient's thigh in equal rhythmical pressures to maximize the posterior to anterior glide of the hip joint and utilizing an element of hip extension. The manoeuvre is performed to patient tolerance and repeated as necessary.

8.7.6 Side-reclining iliofemoral abduction mobilization technique

Application
Hip joint play glide loss of abduction and distraction.

Patient's position
The patient is placed in a side-reclining position with the hip on the affected side upwards and abducted. The knee on the affected side may be kept extended or flexed depending on the size of the patient and the chiropractor.

Chiropractor's stance
The chiropractor faces the patient from behind, standing just distal to the patient's greater trochanter.

Contact
a) The heel of the left hand is placed over the superior aspect of the patient's greater trochanter with the fingers over the lateral aspect of the femur.
b) The right hand – the right forearm is placed under the medial aspect of the patient's knee, cradling and supporting it in the abducted position. All the fingers of the right hand are placed around to the anterior of the lower thigh.

Procedure
Using the right arm, the patient's hip is abducted to the patient's tolerance in a firm but gentle motion, initiating the movement just before ligamentous tightness is felt. This action is synchronized with pressure from the left hand which exerts a caudad distraction pressure on the greater trochanter. The maximum pressure is exerted just as the patient's hip reaches maximum abduction. This manoeuvre is performed to patient tolerance and repeated several times, using a rocking motion.

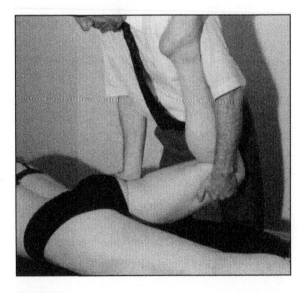

Fig. 8.7.5

The chiropractor turns the trunk caudad to effect the thrust

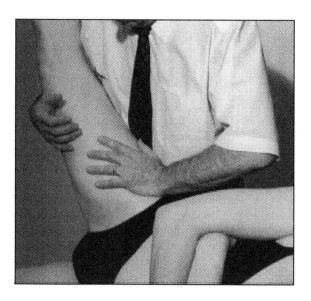

Fig. 8.7.6(a)

By leaning the trunk slightly cephalad, a greater pressure can be exerted on the greater trochanter

8.7.7 Side-reclining iliofemoral circumduction mobilization technique

Application
Joint play glide loss in hip flexion, abduction, extension and adduction.

Patient's position
The patient is placed in a side-reclining position with the affected hip upwards and the knee fully flexed.

Chiropractor's stance
The chiropractor stands behind the patient, just distal to the hip joint, with the upper thigh contacting the patient's buttock to stabilize the trunk.

Contact
a) The left heel of hand is placed over the superior aspect of the patient's greater trochanter with the fingers pointing along the femur.
b) The right forearm cradles the patient's knee from under the medial side and the right hand grasps the anterior of the patient's lower thigh on the medial side.

Procedure
Whilst stabilizing the patient's pelvis and hip with the left hand, the chiropractor moves the patient's hip into circumduction with the right arm starting towards the patient's midline then into adduction followed by flexion and finally into abduction and extension. Ligamentous tension is maintained throughout the manoeuvre. The procedure is repeated several times as necessary, and performed to patient tolerance.

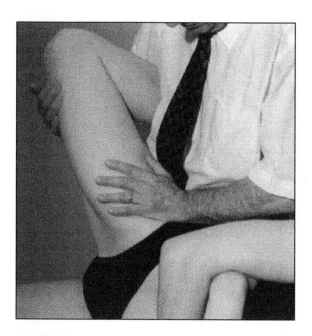

Fig. 8.7.6(b)

The alternative patient leg position with knee flexed. This effectively shortens the lever arm

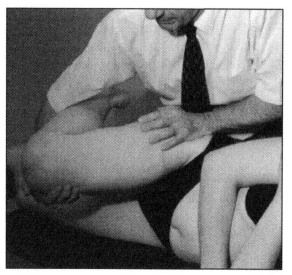

Fig. 8.7.7

The chiropractor's right forearm cradles the patient's knee

8.7.8 Prone iliofemoral abduction/internal rotation mobilization technique

Application
Internal rotation restriction of the hip with an abduction component.

Patient's position
The patient is placed prone with the leg on the affected side abducted to 20–25° and the knee flexed to about 120°.

Chiropractor's stance
The chiropractor stands on the homlateral side facing the midline of the patient and slightly caudad.

Contact
a) The left hand grasps around the medial side of the patient's right ankle with all four fingers wrapped around to the anterior aspect.
b) The right hand is placed palm downwards with the heel of the hand across to the left sacroiliac joint, with all four fingers wrapped around the mid-buttock region.

Procedure
The left hand brings the patient's hip into internal rotation by taking the foot away from the mid-line of the body and the iliofemoral ligament is gently stretched to tolerance. The pressure is then released and gently repeated several times. The right hand stabilizes the opposite side of the pelvis and prevents it from rising as internal rotation of the affected hip is applied.

8.7.9 Supine iliofemoral internal to external mobilization technique

Application
Joint play restriction of the hip joint in rotation from internal to external.

Patient's position
The patient is placed supine with the affected hip flexed as close to 90° from the horizontal as possible, or to patient tolerance. The knee on the affected side is also flexed.

Chiropractor's stance
The chiropractor stands between the patient's legs and facing cephalad. Alternatively, the chiropractor may sit between the patient's legs, turning the trunk cephalad.

Contact
a) The left lower arm is tucked under the patient's calf from the lateral side to support the leg and the leg pressed securely against left side of the chiropractor's trunk to stabilize it. The left hand is placed under the patient's proximal tibia, close to the knee joint on the medial side.
b) With the palm of the right hand against the medial side of the patient's upper thigh, the fifth metacarpal is placed against the proximal femur as close to the neck of the femur as possible. The fingers are pointed upwards over the anterior of the upper thigh.

Procedure
Rhythmical pressures are exerted to patient tolerance with the right hand, from internal to external against the joint resistance of the hip. The procedure is repeated as necessary.

Note
Because of the possibly compromising position of the chiropractor's right hand on the medial aspect of the patient's upper thigh, it would be wise to explain the procedure and seek express permission from the patient beforehand, and also to consider having a chaperone present during the manoeuvre.

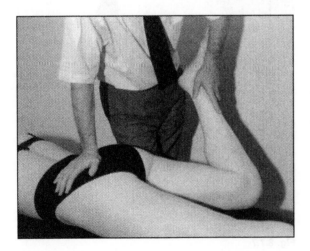

Fig. 8.7.8

The hip is abducted on the affected side and the chiropractor turns slightly caudad

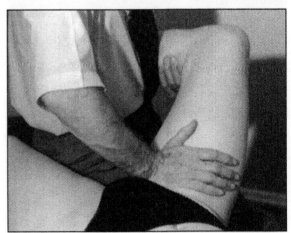

Fig. 8.7.9

Because of the possibly compromising position of the chiropractor's right hand on the medial aspect of the patient's upper thigh, express permission should be sought from the patient beforehand

8.7.10 Supine iliofemoral anterior to posterior flexion mobilization technique

Application
Hip joint play glide loss from anterior to posterior with a flexion component.

Patient's position
The patient is placed supine with the knee and hip flexed on the affected side.

Chiropractor's stance
The chiropractor stands on the homolateral side facing cephalad, level with the patient's hip, with the chest placed against the patient's lower leg.

Contact
With the elbows held low, both hands are laced together over the superior border of the patient's flexed knee.

Procedure
A downward compression is applied at various degrees of flexion until joint play loss is detected. At the degree of hip flexion where the anterior to posterior joint play restriction is felt, a swift, shallow downward impulse is given. The procedure may be repeated as a series of thrusts, until joint play is restored. The technique is performed to patient tolerance.

8.7.11 Supine iliofemoral external to internal rotation technique

Application
Joint play glide loss of internal rotation of the femoral head in the acetabulum.

Patient's position
The patient is placed supine with both the knee and the hip on the affected side flexed to 90°.

Chiropractor's stance
The chiropractor stands facing cephalad between the patient's legs.

Contact
Both hands are laced together and placed over the anterior of the patient's knee. The patient's lower leg from the ankle to the mid-calf is cradled over the chiropractor's left forearm.

Procedure
Joint pre-load tension is achieved by the chiropractor leaning forwards and rotating the trunk to the right. A series of gentle rotational thrusts from external to internal are then made, to the patient's tolerance. The manoeuvre is repeated as necessary.

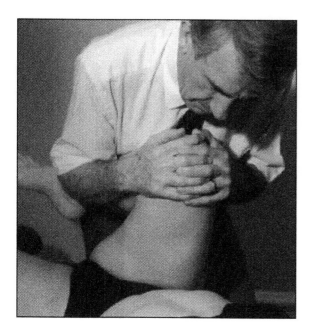

Fig. 8.7.10

The patient's lower leg is placed against the chiropractor's chest as an additional leverage against the hip joint

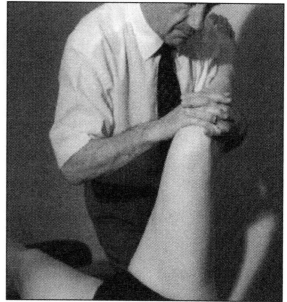

Fig. 8.7.11

To achieve joint pre-load tension, the chiropractor leans forwards and rotates the trunk to the left

8.7.12 Supine iliofemoral internal to external rotation mobilization technique

Application
Joint play glide loss of external rotation of the femoral head in the acetabulum.

Patient's position
The patient is placed supine with the knee and hip on the affected side flexed to 90°.

Chiropractor's stance
The chiropractor stands on the homolateral side facing cephalad adjacent to the hip joint.

Contact
The lower leg from the ankle to the mid-calf is cradled over the chiropractor's right forearm. Both hands are laced together over the anterior of the patient's leg just proximal to the knee. The left hand approaches from the lateral side and the right hand from the medial side.

Procedure
The chiropractor leans forwards a little, rotating the trunk to the left. Joint pre-load tension is achieved by further flexing the patient's hip. A series of gentle rotational thrusts from internal to external are then made, performed with the patient's tolerance.

8.7.13 Supine abduction mobilization technique

Application
Joint play glide loss of the femoral head in the acetabulum on abduction.

Patient's position
The patient is placed supine with the legs fully extended.

Chiropractor's stance
The chiropractor stands at the foot end of the table, facing cephalad.

Contact
The chiropractor stabilizes the unaffected leg with one hand and holds the lower tibia with the other hand, just proximal to the ankle on the affected side and abducts the patient's leg until ligamentous tension is felt.

Procedure
The hip joint is gently stretched into further abduction to the patient's tolerance. The knee on the affected side is kept fully extended. The technique is repeated as necessary.

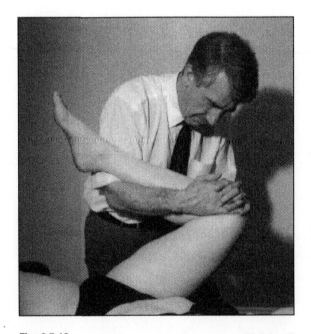

Fig. 8.7.12

The chiropractor's hands are laced together around the knee joint and the patient's lower leg is stabilized on the chiropractor's forearm

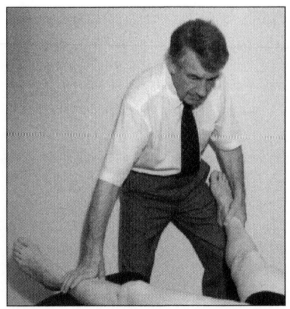

Fig. 8.7.13

The hip joint is gently stretched into further abduction

8.7.14 Supine iliofemoral adduction mobilization technique

Application
Joint play glide loss of the femur head in the acetabulum on adduction.

Patient's position
The patient is placed supine with both legs fully extended.

Chiropractor's stance
The chiropractor stands at the foot end of the table facing cephalad.

Contact
With one hand, the chiropractor holds the lower tibia on the affected side. The other hand stabilizes the unaffected side. The patient's affected hip is flexed approximately 15–20° with the knee still fully extended.

Procedure
The chiropractor adducts the affected hip and to patient tolerance, gently stretches the hip joint into further adduction. The technique is repeated as necessary.

8.7.15 Supine iliofemoral flexion/abduction/external rotation mobilization technique

Application
Joint play glide loss of the femur head in the acetabulum in combined flexion/abduction/external flexion.

Patient's position
The patient is placed supine with both legs flexed at the hips and knees, the feet placed flat on the treatment table. The knees are held apart.

Chiropractor's stance
The chiropractor stands facing cephalad on the homolateral side.

Contact
The chiropractor holds the patient's knees and pushes them further apart until ligamentous tension is felt.

Procedure
Further gentle outward pressure is then exerted with emphasis on the affected side. Pressure may be exerted bilaterally if the patient has evidence of this restriction in both hips. The technique is performed to patient tolerance and repeated as necessary.

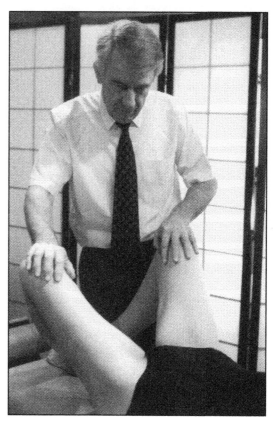

Fig. 8.7.15

Both legs are flexed at the hips and knees

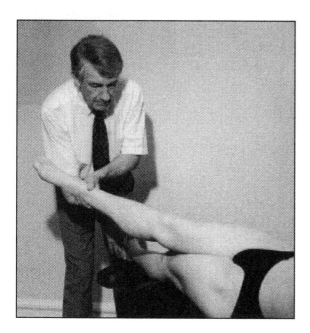

Fig. 8.7.14

The chiropractor gently stretches the hip joint into further adduction

8.7.16 Supine iliofemoral long axis extension mobilization technique

Application
Joint play glide loss of the femur head in the acetabulum in long axis extension.

Patient's position
The patient is placed supine with the leg on the affected side fully extended. The opposite leg may be flexed so that the patient can brace the foot against the table footplate or foot rest for support, if available. The patient is also advised to hold firmly on to the sides of the treatment table to prevent slipping footwards when pressure is applied.

Chiropractor's stance
The chiropractor stands on the homolateral side facing cephalad.

Contact
Both hands grasp around the patient's lower tibia.

Procedure
The chiropractor gently and firmly pulls caudad until ligamentous tension is felt. The traction is held for several seconds, relaxed then repeated. No sudden impulse is made. Several authors advocate the use of a towel, wrapped around the patient's ankle. Traction is then exerted on the towel ends, producing a more comfortable contact on the patient's lower leg.

Note
This is a long lever technique and caution must be exercised due to the stresses exerted up the entire limb extending to the low back and beyond.

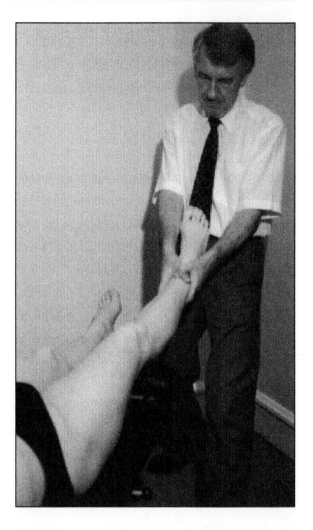

Fig. 8.7.16

The patient holds firmly onto the sides of the treatment table

8.7.17 Prone iliofemoral long axis extension mobilization technique

Application
Joint play glide loss of the femoral head in the acetabulum in extension.

Patient's position
The patient is placed prone with the leg on the affected side fully extended.

Chiropractor's stance
The chiropractor stands on the homolateral side.

Contact
Both hands grasp the patient's lower leg just proximal to the ankle joint.

Procedure
Traction is applied until ligamentous tension is felt then slightly increased to the patient's tolerance. The traction is maintained for several seconds, released and repeated as necessary. As described in the previous technique, a towel may be used around the patient's ankle to make the contact more comfortable.

Note
Caution must be exercised as this is a long lever technique, with stresses applied through the joints of the whole limb and throughout the kinematic chain.

Variation
A variation of this technique is for the chiropractor to face cephalad and straddle the patient's knee on the affected side with the lower thighs, the knees held semi-flexed. By leaning forwards at the waist, the chiropractor contacts the patient's pelvis on the posterior superior iliac spine. By bracing the patient's body with the hands, the chiropractor can now apply traction in long axis by gradually extending the previously semi-flexed knees.

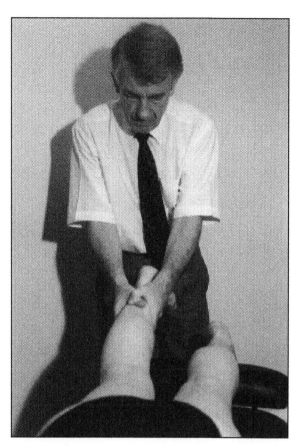

Fig. 8.7.17(a)

The chiropractor stands on the homolateral side

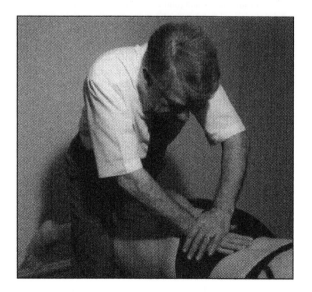

Fig. 8.7.17(b)

Alternatively, the chiropractor may straddle the patient's knee

The knee

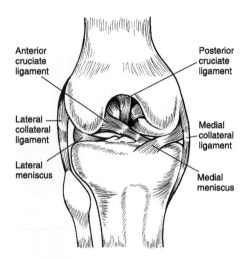

Anterior cruciate ligament

Posterior cruciate ligament

Lateral collateral ligament

Medial collateral ligament

Lateral meniscus

Medial meniscus

Tibio-femoral joint rotation techniques

8.8.A Joint play evaluation of the tibio-femoral joint in internal to external and external to internal rotation

Being an incongruent hinge joint, flexion of the knee allows the tibia to rotate (Segal, 1987). As the knee flexes, the intercondylar tubercles of the tibia move clear of the intercondylar notch of the femur (Kapandji, 1983).

Procedure
Internal and external rotation of the tibia on the femur – Method I:

The patient may be placed either supine or sitting, with the knee flexed to approximately 90° as in Fig. 8.8.A. The left hand holds around the lower leg and ankle and the knee joint is first rotated internally and then externally into joint play. The right hand is placed over the anterior of the patient's knee with the tips of the thumb and index finger straddling the lateral and medial aspects of the tibial and femoral condyles. As the tibia is rotated, the thumb and index finger palpate for joint play loss.

Procedure
Internal and external rotation of the tibia on the femur – Method II:

The patient is placed supine with the knee flexed to 30–40°. The chiropractor straddles the patient's lower leg and holds it just above the knee to stabilize it. The hands hold on the lateral and medial condyles of the tibia with the thenar eminences curling the fingers around to the posterior. Whilst maintaining the flexion, the knee is rotated internally or externally and then pressing firmly into joint play.

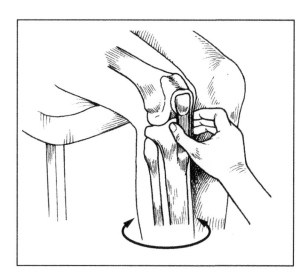

Fig. 8.8.A

Methods I and II. Internal and external rotation of the tibia on the femur

8.8.1 Supine tibio-femoral joint external to internal or internal to external rebound rotation technique

Application
Joint play glide loss of the tibia on the femur in external to internal rotation.

Patient's position
The patient is placed supine with the affected knee fully extended and the hip on the ipsilateral side abducted to about 20°.

Chiropractor's stance
The chiropractor stands on the affected side facing cephalad just distal to the patient's knee, legs astride with the left leg placed ahead of the right.

Contact
a) The right hand holds around the antero/medial border of the tibial condyle with all fingers around to the posterior.
b) The left hand is cupped around the lateral border of the tibia just distal to the knee joint with all fingers towards the posterior and with the thumb kept against the antero/lateral aspect.

Procedure
The adjustment is carried out in three fast, continuous, smooth, synchronous stages, beginning and finishing with the knee flexed to about 40° from the fully extended position. The patient's heel remains in contact with the treatment table throughout the manoeuvre and for an effective outcome it is essential that the entire leg remains relaxed at all times.

Stage I: Using both hands together, the patient's knee is drawn firmly up to approximately 40° of flexion. Internal rotation of the tibia is applied and maintained.

Stage II: Whilst still maintaining the internal rotation of the tibia, the patient's knee is very swiftly and deftly thrust downwards into full extension. At the moment of full extension, the left (lateral) hand releases its contact on the tibia.

Stage III: The knee rebounds back into flexion again assisted by the right hand which still also maintains the internal rotation.

The chiropractor's left hand now also rebounds upwards and strikes the posterior lateral aspect of the patient's tibia, bringing it into sudden further internal rotation and introducing an element of distraction.

Note
This technique may also be applied if the joint play glide loss of the tibia on the femur is in internal to external rotation. The patient's position, chiropractor's stance and the contacts are all similar to those described. The procedure differs only in that the adjustive thrust is made in the direction of external rotation with the chiropractor's right hand striking the posterior medial aspect of the patient's tibia.

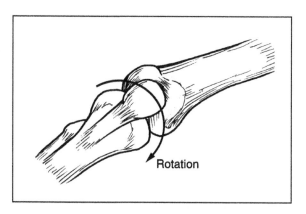

Fig. 8.8.1(a)

The arrows show the forces applied to the joint. The affected knee is drawn up into 40° of flexion and the hip is abducted 20–30°

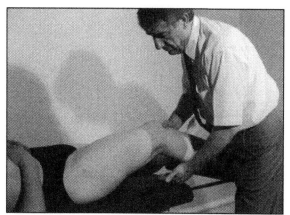

Fig. 8.8.1(b)

The starting position. The patient's knee is semi-flexed with both of the chiropractor's hands on the contact. The knee is rotated medially

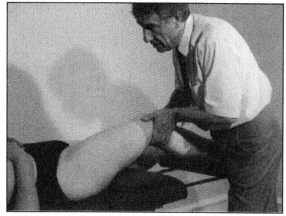

Fig. 8.8.1(d)

The knee joint rebounds into semi-flexion. The chiropractor's hand remains close to the cushion

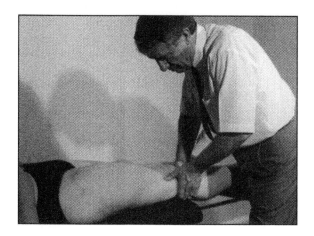

Fig. 8.8.1(c)

The knee joint is rapidly pressed into full extension maintaining medial rotation

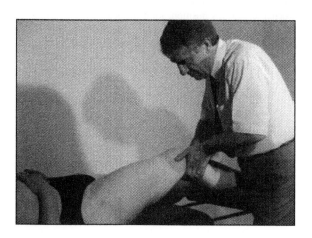

Fig. 8.8.1(e)

The final position. The chiropractor's left hand strikes the posterior of the tibia into further medial rotation

8.8.2 Supine tibio-femoral joint external to internal or internal to external flexion/rotation technique – Method I

Application
Rotational joint play glide loss from external to internal of the tibia on the femur.

Patient's position
The patient is placed supine with the affected knee flexed and the hip on the affected side flexed to approximately 90°.

Chiropractor's stance
Standing facing cephalad on the homolateral side, with the left leg placed forward of the right, about level with the patient's greater trochanter.

Contact
a) The left hand is mainly a support and is placed over the anterior of the knee with the first and middle fingers placed over the medial tibio-femoral joint line. It also further flexes the hip to about 100° and abducts it approximately 30°.

b) The right hand contacts the lateral border of the patient's hind foot, the fingers under the plantar surface and the thumb wrapped around the lateral border of the talus.

Procedure
The chiropractor flexes the patient's knee fully, rotates the patient's foot and ankle medially and maintains this rotation and flexion throughout the adjustment. The patient's heel is then made to describe a small circular motion beginning in the direction of the opposite greater trochanter. In this position, joint pre-load tension will be felt. At this point of tissue tension, the knee is gently hyperflexed and the circular motion is continued now towards the chiropractor as a moderately rapid impulse, whilst still maintaining the tissue tension. The fingers of the left hand will feel the release.

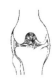

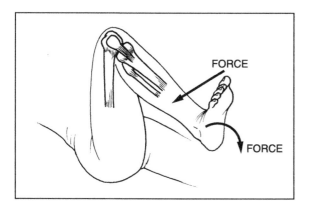

Fig. 8.8.2(a)

The directions of the adjustive forces applied to the tibio-femoral joint

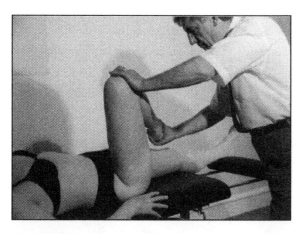

Fig. 8.8.2(b)

Starting position – external to internal flexion/rotation technique. The chiropractor stands on the ipsilateral side

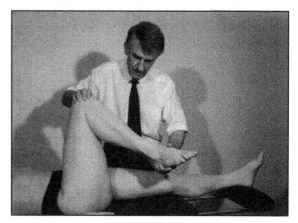

Fig. 8.8.2(d)

Starting position – internal to external flexion/rotation technique. The chiropractor stands on the contra-lateral side and rotates the patient's foot and ankle externally

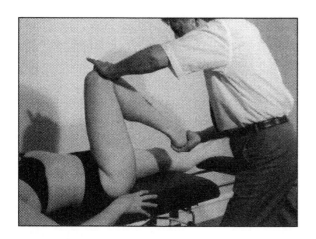

Fig. 8.8.2(c)

Final position – external to internal flexion/rotation technique. The foot and ankle are held in internal rotation and the knee is hyperflexed throughout the procedure

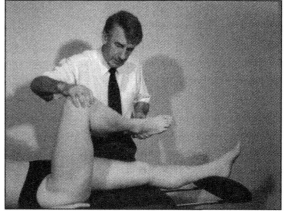

Fig. 8.8.2(e)

Final position – internal to external flexion/rotation technique. The knee and hip remain flexed and externally rotated. On joint pre-load tension a rapid shallow impulse into further rotation is made with the left hand, with due care

8.8.3 Supine tibio-femoral joint internal to external or external to internal flexion/rotation technique – Method II

Application
Rotational joint play glide loss of the tibia on the femur from lateral to medial or from medial to lateral.

Patient's position
The patient is placed supine with the leg on the affected side flexed to 90° at the hip and the knee. The patient then clasps around the posterior of the lower femur just proximal to the knee joint and laces the fingers together.

Chiropractor's stance
The chiropractor stands on the affected side facing cephalad adjacent to the patient's knee and semi-flexes the trunk forwards. The right foot is placed on the treatment table close up to the patient's right buttock. The knee, now at right angles, is placed against the patient's clasped hands just proximal to the knee joint. To cushion the contact a pad or folded towel is placed between them.

Contact
a) The right elbow is hooked around the patient's medial lower leg, ensuring that the contact is well away from the ankle (another pad and towel may be used here to cushion the contact). The right forearm is placed under the calf and the right hand reaches over to hold the left biceps.
b) The left arm reaches over the anterior of the patient's shin, contacting it firmly and the left hand holds on to the right biceps.

Procedure
By slowly leaning back and extending the lumbar spine, joint pre-load tension is felt on the knee. At the same time, the patient is asked to match this pressure by pulling the knee towards the chest. This distracts the knee joint. Without releasing the tension, the impulse is made with a swift backward impulse into lumbar extension, further distracting the joint. The chiropractor's trunk is simultaneously flexed laterally to the right to rotate the joint internally or flexed medially to the left to rotate the joint externally. **It is essential that the patient's knee remains relaxed throughout the procedure.**

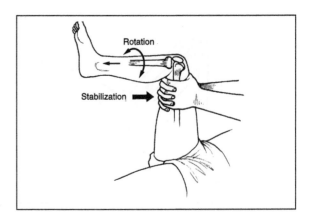

Fig. 8.8.3(a)

The adjustive forces applied to the tibio-femoral joint

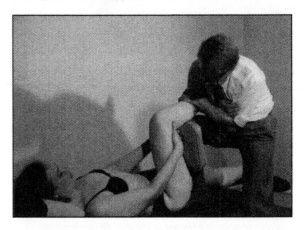

Fig. 8.8.3(b)

Initial patient/practitioner positions. The knee and hip are flexed to 90°, held by the patient with fingers laced together, just proximal to the knee joint. A pad is placed to cushion the contact against the knee

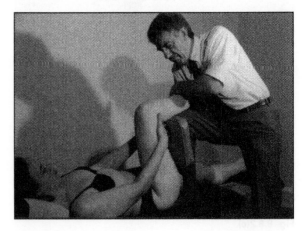

Fig. 8.8.3(c)

Viewed from the side, showing the practitioner laterally flexing the trunk to the right to achieve the rotational thrust from lateral to medial

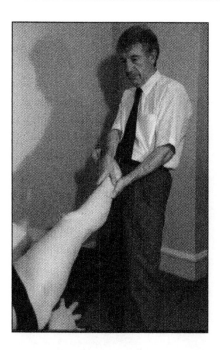

Fig. 8.8.4(a)

The final position before the adjustive thrust is applied. The practitioner maintains a straight back and leans backwards, distracting the knee. The left leading leg presses into the floor to stabilize the practitioner's position

8.8.4 Supine tibio-femoral joint external to internal rotation traction/leverage technique – Method III

Application
Rotational joint play glide loss of the tibia on the femur from external to internal.

Patient's position
The patient is placed supine and requested to stabilize the trunk by holding on to the sides of the treatment table. The affected leg is fully extended and relaxed.

Chiropractor's stance
Standing at the foot end of the table facing cephalad, with the left foot placed forward of the right foot.

Contact
a) The right hand is placed around the lower leg from the anterior, rotating it medially. The right forearm is placed against the lateral border of the patient's mid-foot, which also assists in rotating it internally.

b) The left hand clasps the right hand from the posterior of the patient's lower leg and the fingers of both hands are laced together.

Procedure
With the chiropractor holding the spine straight and leaning back, braced by the legs, internal rotation is maintained and traction applied. Without slackening the traction, a quick impulse is made towards the practitioner, distracting and medially rotating the joint.

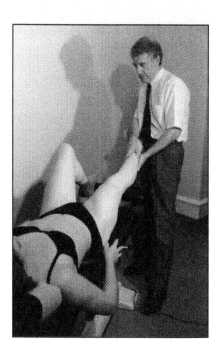

Fig. 8.8.4(b)

With long lever techniques, there is greater patient safety if high velocity with minimum depth of thrust is used. The patient may place the foot on the unaffected side against the footrest, for stability

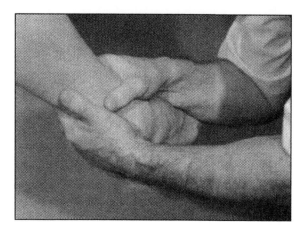

Fig. 8.8.4(c)

The right forearm presses against the lateral border of the patient's foot, gently rotating it internally

8.8.5 Supine tibio-femoral joint internal to external traction leverage rotation technique

Application
Rotational joint play glide loss from internal to external of the tibia on the femur.

Patient's position
The patient is placed supine with the affected leg fully extended and abducted about 20° and the feet well over the end of the treatment table. The patient is instructed to hold firmly on to the sides of the treatment table to prevent sliding, and to relax the affected leg.

Chiropractor's stance
The chiropractor stands at the foot end of the table facing cephalad and holds the patient's right leg at about waist height, with the left foot placed well ahead of the right.

Contact
a) The left hand grasps the medial side of the patient's right lower leg, proximal to the ankle, fingers wrapping around the lateral aspect of the distal tibia. The left lateral forearm is placed against the medial border of the patient's foot, rotating the foot externally until tissue tension is felt.
b) The right hand is placed around the posterior aspect of the lower leg from the medial side, fingers wrapped around to the lateral side, interlacing with the fingers of the left hand.

Procedure
The patient's leg is further rotated externally and tractioned by the chiropractor bracing and pushing backwards with the leading leg. At all times, a straight back is maintained. Without slackening the traction, a fast controlled-depth impulse is made straight backwards in long axis.

Note
Great caution must be exercised with long lever techniques because the force is exerted over several joints and it is therefore not the technique of choice for use with the elderly, infirm, osteoporotic, or when a hip prosthesis is on the side to be treated. Some measure of trunk stabilization is obtained if the patient flexes the knee on the unaffected side and braces the foot on the treatment table foot rest (see Fig. 8.8.5a). With long lever techniques, there is a greater margin of patient safety if high velocity with minimum depth of thrust is used.

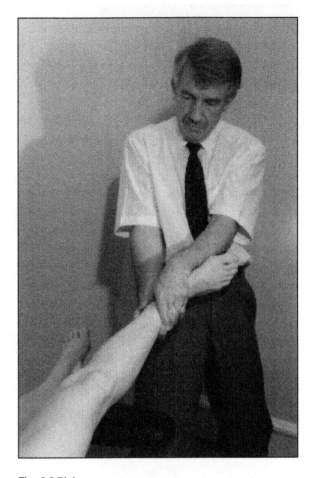

Fig. 8.8.5(a)

The right foot is forward and the chiropractor's back is held erect

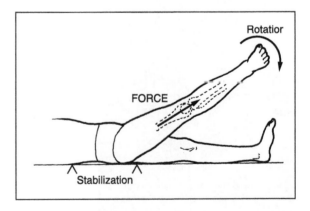

Fig. 8.8.5(b)

The directions of the adjustive forces applied to the knee joint

8.8.6 Supine modified tibio-femoral joint external to internal or internal to external traction/leverage rotation technique

Application
Rotational joint play glide loss of the tibia on the femur from external to internal.

Patient's position
The patient is placed supine or sitting with the affected knee flexed and the lower leg placed hanging down over the side of the treatment table. The treatment table is elevated horizontally to its highest setting. To increase the patient's comfort, a cushion or folded towel may be placed under the patient's leg just proximal to the knee joint.

Chiropractor's stance
Kneeling, facing cephalad, directly adjacent to the patient's affected knee.

Contact
Both hands are placed around the patient's lower leg just proximal to the ankle joint and the fingers are laced together at the posterior. The chiropractor's right forearm is placed against the lateral border of the patient's right foot, rotating the leg and ankle into internal rotation until tissue tension is felt.

Procedure
A rapid downward impulse is made whilst simultaneously adding further internal rotation. By flexing the patient's knee and allowing it to rest on the treatment table, the lever arm is effectively shortened, providing an additional safety factor when treating the elderly or infirm.

Note
This technique may also be applied if the joint play glide loss of the tibia on the femur is internal to external rotation. The patient's position, the chiropractor's stance and the contacts are all similar to those described. The procedure differs only in that the adjustive thrust is made in the direction from internal to external.

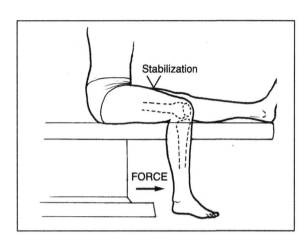

Fig. 8.8.6

The directions of the adjustive forces applied to the knee joint

8.8.7 Supine tibio-femoral joint external to internal or internal to external rotation/flexion/extension straddle technique

Application

Anterior to posterior and/or posterior to anterior joint play glide loss of the tibia on the femur. By adding a rotational component to the adjustive impulse, this technique may also be adapted to correct internal or external rotational joint play loss.

Patient's position

The patient is placed supine with the leg on the affected side abducted to approximately 25–35° with the affected knee held slightly flexed.

Chiropractor's stance

Standing facing cephalad straddling the patient's lower leg and holding it tightly between, or just proximal to, the knees.

Contact

a) The left hand is placed loosely around the lateral aspect of the tibia with the thenar eminence placed over the lateral part of the tibial plateau, the thumb pointing cephalad and the fingers curling to the posterior.
b) The right hand is similarly placed loosely around the medial side of the proximal tibia.

Procedure

The chiropractor leans backwards exerting traction on the knee joint to distract it. Using the fingers of both hands, the patient's knee is gently tapped upwards several times, which flexes it a little, to ensure that it is relaxed before the adjustment is performed. Whilst maintaining the traction with the legs, the adjustment is made by very rapidly and firmly tapping the posterior distal tibia, which again flexes the knee further. This is followed immediately by striking the knee on the tibial condyles with both thenar eminences on the anterior tibia directly distal to the joint, pushing it rapidly towards extension. Immediately after the strike, both hands are removed from their contacts so that there is no pressure on the knee as it fully extends into the screw home position. If joint play glide loss in rotation is also present, the adjustment is adapted to accommodate this factor by emphasizing the thrust in an internal or external direction.

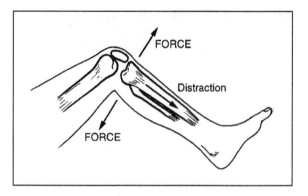

Fig. 8.8.7(a)

The direction of the adjustive forces applied to the tibio-femoral joint

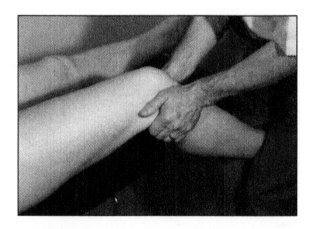

Fig. 8.8.7(b)

Phase I – the knee is flexed rapidly with both hands pulling upwards

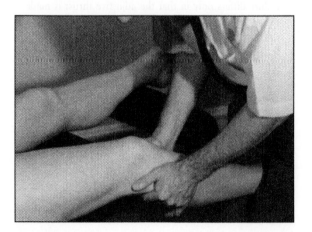

Fig. 8.8.7(c)

Phase II – the tibial condyles are struck very rapidly with both thenar eminences, taking the knee joint towards extension

8.8.8 Prone tibio-femoral joint flexion/rotation technique

Application
Rotational joint play glide loss of the tibia on the femur from external to internal.

Patient's position
The patient is placed prone with the affected knee flexed to approximately 90° with a cushion placed over the posterior lower thigh.

Chiropractor's stance
The chiropractor stands facing the patient's mid-line on the affected side adjacent to the patient's knee. A folded towel or small cushion is placed over the patient's thigh just proximal to the knee joint and the chiropractor places his right knee firmly but gently on it to anchor the patient's leg on to the treatment table.

Contact
Both hands, with all fingers laced together, grasp around the distal tibia and fibula just proximal to the ankle joint. Both elbows are held below the level of the contact and the forearms are held as near vertically as possible.

Procedure
The patient's lower leg is tractioned upwards until tissue slack is removed. Without releasing the tension, a swift upward impulse is made.

Note
If there is tibio-femoral joint play loss in rotation, this component may be adjusted by rotating the tibia in the appropriate direction while the upward impulse is being made.

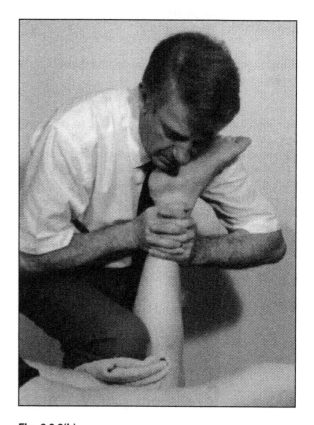

Fig. 8.8.8(b)

The contacts on the lower tibia. A towel may be wrapped around the leg to cushion the contact

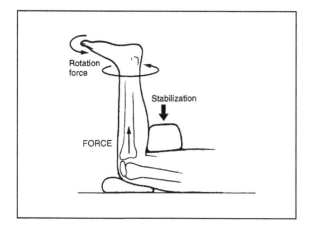

Fig. 8.8.8(a)

The direction of the adjustive forces applied to the tibio-femoral joint

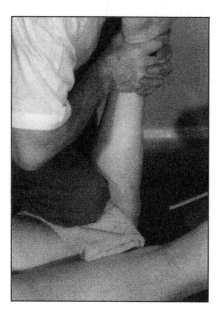

Fig. 8.8.8(c)

The final position for the adjustment. The trunk is flexed and the forearms held as close to the vertical as possible before the thrust is made

Tibio-femoral joint medial/lateral translation techniques

8.8.B Joint play evaluation of the knee – lateral translation

Procedure

1) Medial to lateral translation of the tibia on the femur: The patient is placed supine with the knee flexed several degrees to take it out of the 'screw home' position. The heel of the left hand is placed on the lateral epicondyle of the femur with the fingers along the lateral lower thigh. The heel of the right hand is placed against the medial condyle of the tibia with the fingers pointing medially over the anterior of the patella. Both hands press firmly towards the mid-line of the knee to elicit joint play.

2) Lateral to medial translation of the tibia on the femur:

The patient is supine with the affected knee slightly flexed. The hands are reversed so that the right hand contacts the medial epicondyle of the femur and the left hand contacts the lateral condyle of the tibia.

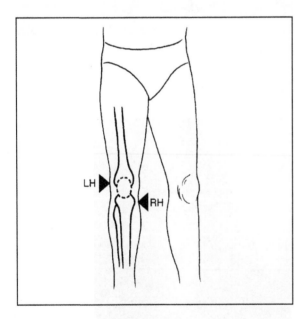

Fig. 8.8.B

The directions of the forces applied in medial to lateral joint play evaluation of the knee

8.8.9 Supine tibio-femoral joint lateral to medial distraction/straddle technique

Application
Joint play glide loss of lateral to medial translation of the tibia on the femur.

Patient's position
The patient is placed supine with the hip on the affected side abducted 30–40° from the mid-line with the knee extended and relaxed.

Chiropractor's stance
The chiropractor stands facing cephalad on the homolateral side straddling the patient's lower leg just proximal to the knees to stabilize the limb. The trunk is flexed forwards so that the arms fall vertically over the patient's knee. The left leg is placed ahead of the right, the right knee is flexed a little and the ankle is plantarflexed so that the right heel is lifted off the floor.

Contact
a) The left hand is placed around the lateral border of the tibia just distal to the knee joint with the fingers towards the posterior of the joint.

b) The right hand is placed on the medial side of the femur just proximal to the knee joint to act as a stabilizer.

Procedure
The patient's knee and hip are both flexed upwards approximately 30° and at the same time the chiropractor leans the flexed trunk backwards a little to distract the knee joint. Several rocking movements from lateral to medial and back to lateral are made, until the patient fully relaxes. A swift impulse is then initiated by the left arm, from lateral to medial, and the right arm continues to stabilize the patient's femur. Simultaneously, with equal speed, the right knee is fully extended, returning the heel down to the floor. The sudden lateral pressure of the chiropractor's calf against the patient's medial lower leg brings the patient's lower leg away from the mid-line, enhancing the thrust by the left arm.

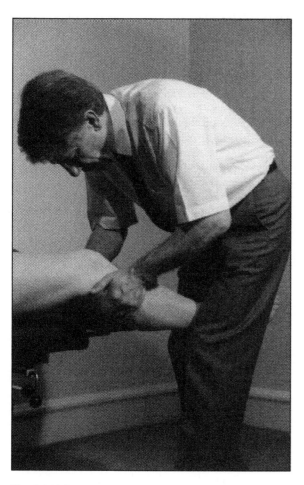

Fig. 8.8.9(a)

The initial position. The practitioner's right leg is flexed at the knee

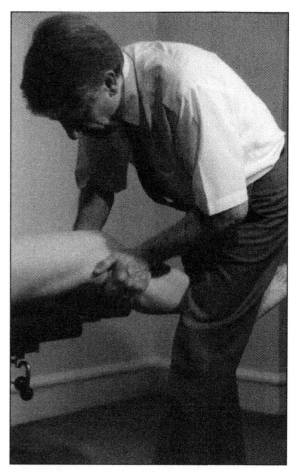

Fig. 8.8.9(b)

During the delivery of the thrust, the right knee is brought rapidly back into full extension in synchrony with the lateral to medial thrust of the left hand

Fig. 8.8.9(c)

The direction of the forces applied and the stabilization points used in this adjustment

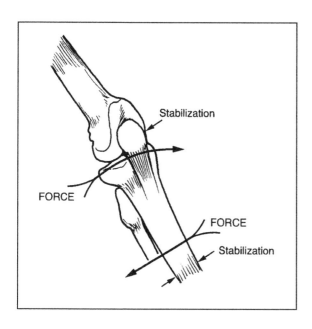

8.8.10 Supine tibio-femoral joint medial to lateral distraction/straddle technique

Application
Joint play glide loss of medial to lateral translation of the tibia on the femur.

Patient's position
The patient is placed supine with the hip on the affected side abducted to approximately 30° and the knee relaxed and extended.

Chiropractor's stance
The chiropractor stands alongside the patient on the homolateral side facing cephalad, straddling and holding the patient's mid lower leg to stabilize it. The right leg is placed ahead of the left. The left knee is flexed a little and the ankle is plantarflexed resulting in the left heel rising off the floor. The chiropractor flexes the trunk forward so that the arms fall vertically over the patient's knee.

Contact
a) The heel of the left hand is placed on the lateral side of the distal femur immediately proximal to the knee joint with the fingers contacting around towards the posterior of the thigh.
b) The thenar eminence of the right hand is placed on the medial side of the tibia just distal to the knee joint, with the fingers wrapped around towards the posterior.

Procedure
The patient's knee and hip are both passively flexed upwards approximately 30° and at the same time the chiropractor, whilst maintaining trunk flexion, leans backwards a little to distract the knee joint. Several rhythmical movements of the knee joint are made from medial to lateral and back again to relax the patient's leg. A swift impulse is then applied with the right arm from medial to lateral. Simultaneously, as the thrust with the arm is applied, the chiropractor's left leg is swiftly and fully extended. The sudden medial pressure on the patient's lateral lower leg enhances the lateral thrust from the chiropractor's right arm.

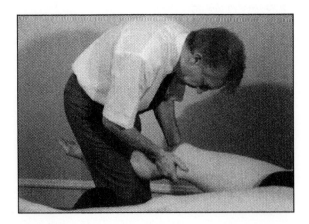

Fig. 8.8.10

The chiropractor flexes the trunk forward so that the arms fall vertically over the patient's knee

8.8.C Joint play evaluation of the tibio-femoral joint

Procedure
1) Valgus stress:
With the patient supine, the knee is flexed a little, sufficiently to take it out of the 'screw home' position, and the lower leg is straddled and held by the chiropractor's knees. The femur is stabilized on the medial side with the **right hand**. As the chiropractor's knees take the lower leg into lateral flexion, the **left hand** first stabilizes the lateral condyle of the patient's tibia then presses in a medial direction firmly into joint play. This has a dual purpose in that the integrity of the medial collateral ligament is also tested. 'The medial collateral ligament is critical to [knee] stability' (Hoppenfeld, 1976).
2) Varus stress:
The patient is placed supine, with the lower leg straddled and held by the chiropractor's knees. The patient's knee is slightly flexed. The left hand contacts the medial epicondyle of the femur to stabilize it and the knees take the patient's lower leg into medial flexion. The right hand first stabilizes the medial condyle then presses firmly in a lateral direction into joint play. This has a dual purpose in that the integrity of the lateral collateral ligament is also tested.

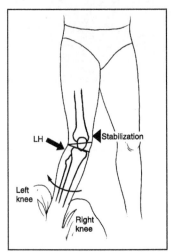

Fig. 8.8.C(a)

Right knee, anterior to posterior view: valgus stress

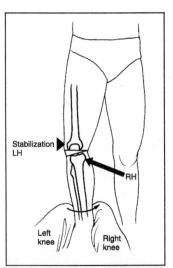

Fig. 8.8.C(b)

Right knee, anterior to posterior view: varus stress

8.8.11 Side-reclining tibio-femoral joint lateral to medial recoil technique

Application
Joint play glide loss of lateral to medial translation of the tibia on the femur.

Patient's position
The patient is placed in a side-reclining position with the affected side uppermost and semi-flexed at the knee and hip. A high-density foam-filled cushion is placed under the medial side of the lower thigh, just proximal to the knee joint. The other leg remains extended.

Chiropractor's stance
The chiropractor stands facing cephalad adjacent to the knee with the episternal notch directly above the contact.

Contact
a) The pisiform of the left hand is placed over the left 'anatomical snuff box' with the fingers and thumb wrapped around the left wrist.
b) The pisiform of the right hand is placed over the lateral aspect of the patient's right tibia just distal to the knee joint and by using a low arch (see Glossary of Terms, p. 285) the contact is broadened to include the whole of the heel of the hand.

Procedure
A rapid recoil thrust (see Chapter 2) of shallow depth using the pectoralis, triceps and anconius muscles is applied in a smooth synchronous harmony of movement.

8.8.12 Side-reclining tibio-femoral joint medial to lateral recoil technique.

Application
Joint play glide loss of medial to lateral translation of the tibia on the femur.

Patient's position
The patient is side-reclined with the affected knee down, semi-flexed and placed so that the tibia, just distal to the knee joint, is supported on the pelvic section of the treatment table. The upper leg remains extended and behind the right knee. The pelvic section drop mechanism of the treatment table is set for the patient's weight and cocked.

Chiropractor's stance
The chiropractor stands in front of the patient facing cephalad, opposite the patient's affected knee.

Contact
a) The pisiform of the left hand is placed over the medial aspect of the patient's right tibia, just distal to the knee joint and by using a low arch (see Glossary of Terms, p. 285) the contact is broadened and softened by including the heel of the hand.
b) The right hand is placed broadly over the posterior of the right hand and the fingers and thumb are extended.

Procedure
A rapid recoil thrust (see Chapter 2) of shallow depth is made with the pectoralis, triceps and anconius muscles in a smooth synchronous harmony of movement.

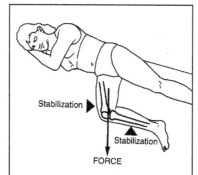

Fig. 8.8.12(a)

The direction of the adjustive forces and points of stabilization

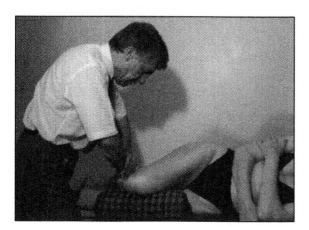

Fig. 8.8.11

The placement of a high density foam-filled cushion under the lower thigh, just proximal to the knee joint, provides the necessary height and support

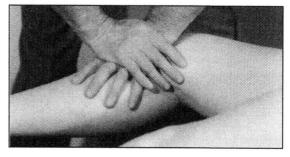

Fig. 8.8.12(b)

The final position for the adjustment. The episternal notch is directly above the point of contact

8.8.13   Supine tibio-femoral joint lateral to medial leg extension technique

Application
Joint play glide loss from lateral to medial translation of the tibia on the femur.

Patient's position
The patient is placed supine with the hip on the affected side abducted to approximately 20–30° and the knee held in semi-flexion by placing it over a soft cushion.

Chiropractor's stance
The chiropractor stands on the homolateral side facing the patient's mid-line, adjacent to the affected knee.

Contact
a)   The left hand is placed over the lateral side of the tibia immediately distal to the knee joint with the fingers over the anterior.
b)   The right hand holds the lower end of the tibia with the thumb over the anterior to clasp the medial side and the fingers wrapped around the posterior of the lower leg just proximal to the ankle joint.

Procedure
Joint pre-load tension is achieved by bracing the patient's knee with the left hand and by pulling the lower leg laterally with the right hand. Without releasing the tension, the adjustment is made with the left arm by a quick, deft, shallow thrust from lateral to medial.

Note
Even though the cushion under the knee has some stabilizing effect on the distal end of the femur, care must be taken with the delivery of the thrust to safeguard the joint by using minimal depth of thrust.

8.8.14   Supine tibio-femoral joint medial to lateral leg extension technique

Procedure
The previous technique can be adapted for joint play glide loss from medial to lateral of the tibia on the femur. The chiropractor stands on the medial side of the patient's leg and makes the thrust from medial to lateral with the right hand, which is placed over the medial tibial condyle. The left hand is placed over the lateral aspect of the lower tibia and acts as a stabilizer.

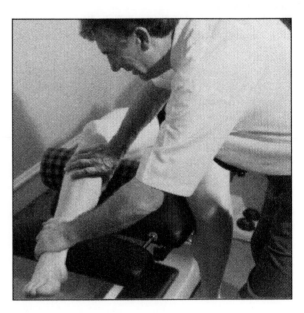

Fig. 8.8.14

Joint play glide loss from medial to lateral of the tibia on the femur. The chiropractor stands on the opposite side of the treatment table and makes the thrust from medial to lateral with the right hand

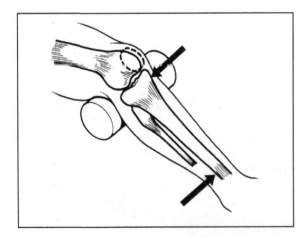

Fig. 8.8.13

The placement of a small soft cushion both flexes the knee and adds a stabilizing effect on the femur when the thrust is delivered

Tibio-femoral joint anterior to posterior techniques

8.8.D Joint play evaluation of the tibio-femoral joint anterior to posterior and posterior to anterior

Procedure
1) Anterior to posterior glide of the tibia on the femur:
The chiropractor's right foot is placed on the treatment table with the knee and hip each flexed to 90°. The right knee is placed under the posterior of the patient's mid-calf to stabilize the lower leg and act as a fulcrum. With both hands, posterior to anterior pressure is applied on the tibial tuberosity with both hands. Firm pressure is required to move the joint through anterior to posterior motion before joint play can be assessed.
2) Posterior to anterior glide of the tibia on the femur:
The patient is placed supine. The chiropractor's left knee is placed against the popliteal fossa. The left hand is placed over the distal end of the tibia to prevent movement. The right hand palpates for movement of the tibia from posterior to anterior. By plantarflexing the left foot and ankle, the patient's tibia is pushed upwards, allowing joint play to be assessed in that plane.

An alternative method is to adopt the **draw sign position** (see Glossary of Terms, p. 285). The patient's knee is flexed to approximately 90° with the foot flat on the examination table. The foot is anchored by sitting on the patient's toes and both hands are laced together at the posterior proximal tibia in the popliteal fossa. First all joint slack is removed by pulling posterior to anterior, then further firm anterior pressure is exerted to detect joint play integrity.

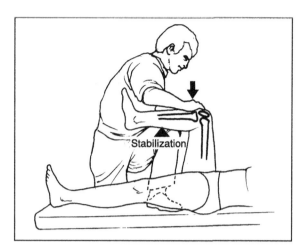

Fig. 8.8.D(a)

Anterior to posterior glide of the tibia on the femur

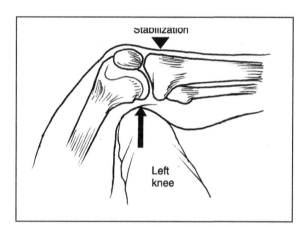

Fig. 8.8.D(b)

Posterior to anterior glide of the tibia on the femur

8.8.15 Supine tibio-femoral joint anterior to posterior flexion/extension straddle technique

See technique 8.8.9 on p. 203.

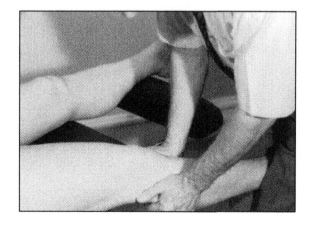

Fig. 8.8.15

Using the thenar eminences on the tibial condyles, the thrust is made from anterior to posterior whilst maintaining the knee in slight flexion

8.8.16 Supine tibio-femoral joint anterior to posterior recoil technique – Variations I, II and III

Application
Joint play glide loss from anterior to posterior of the tibia on the femur.

Patient's position
The patient either sits or lies supine with a small, high density cushion placed under the lower thigh just proximal to the affected knee joint. The knee is placed directly above the appropriate drop section on the treatment table, which is then set for the weight of the patient's limb, and cocked.

Chiropractor's stance
The chiropractor stands on the ipsilateral side facing cephalad adjacent to the affected knee and leans forward until the episternal notch is directly above the contact. The neck is flexed forwards.

Contact
The hands are placed on each side of the tibial condyles using the thenar eminences as the contact points. The fingers are wrapped around to the posterior of the knee and the thumbs remain on the anterior, pointing cephalad.

Procedure
Joint pre-load tension is achieved by leaning the trunk forwards a little on to the contacts. The elbows remain semi-flexed. A high velocity recoil adjustment (see Chapter 2) is then delivered using a smooth pectoralis, triceps, anconius thrust from anterior to posterior. The cushion supporting the patient's knee in flexion will absorb a proportion of the energy from the thrust, so it is necessary to increase the amplitude accordingly.

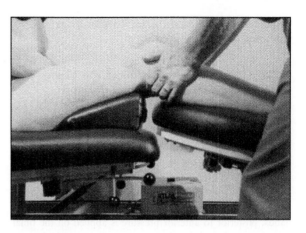

Fig. 8.8.16(a)

The placement of a medium density cushion or firm covered wedge-shaped block. When using the latter, the pelvic drop section is cocked with less resistance. The patient is shown lying supine

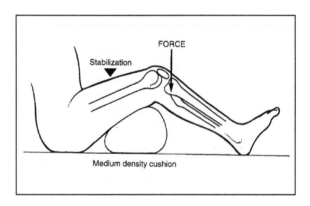

Fig. 8.8.16(b)

A medium density cushion is placed under the lower end of the femur to maintain knee flexion

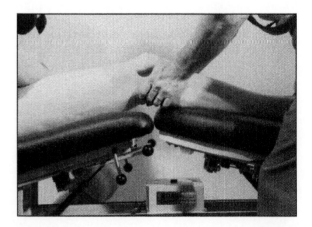

Fig. 8.8.16(c)

The patient is shown sitting with the table-angle increased to increase knee flexion

8.8.17 Supine tibio-femoral joint anterior to posterior flexion technique

Application
Joint play glide loss from anterior to posterior of the tibia on the femur.

Patient's position
The patient is placed supine with the affected leg flexed to approximately 90° at the hip and the knee.

Chiropractor's stance
The chiropractor stands facing cephalad on the homolateral side. The patient's leg is placed over the chiropractor's shoulder to about mid-way along the patient's calf. This position may vary depending on the length of the patient's lower leg and the length of the chiropractor's arms. It may also be advisable to place a small cushion on the chiropractor's shoulder to reduce the pressure discomfort on the patient's calf.

Contact
Approaching from the posterior, both hands are wrapped around the patient's knee just distal to the joint and the fingers are laced together over the anterior aspect.

Procedure
Joint pre-load tension is achieved by exerting considerable downward pressure and, without slackening, an impulse is made in a downward direction.

Note
This technique may be adapted to correct fixations with external or internal rotation components by altering the angle of the adjustive thrust accordingly (see Fig. 8.8.17b).

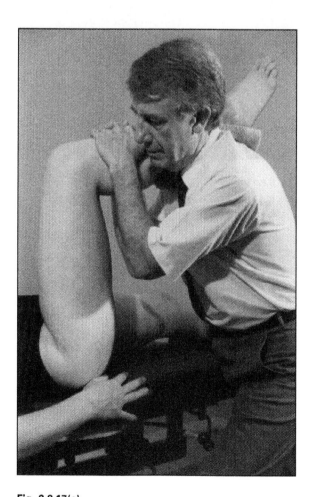

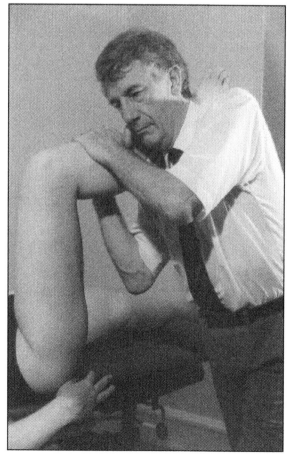

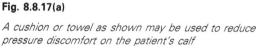

Fig. 8.8.17(a)

A cushion or towel as shown may be used to reduce pressure discomfort on the patient's calf

Fig. 8.8.17(b)

This technique may be adapted for additional external or internal fixation components by introducing the appropriate rotation with the downward thrust

Tibio-femoral joint posterior to anterior techniques

8.8.18   Supine tibio-femoral joint posterior to anterior flexion technique – Method I

Application
Joint play glide loss from posterior to anterior of the tibia on the femur.

Patient's position
The patient is placed supine with the affected leg fully flexed at the hip and the knee.

Chiropractor's stance
The chiropractor stands on the homolateral side facing cephalad, adjacent to the patient's knee.

Contact
The fingers of both hands are laced together at the posterior of the patient's tibia just distal to the joint. The chiropractor's right forearm, close to the elbow, is placed along the anterior of the patient's right lower tibia.

Procedure
Joint pre-load tension is achieved by the chiropractor pressing the forearm gently downwards on the patient's distal tibia and tractioning the proximal tibia upwards. Without releasing the tension, a rapid impulse is made in a posterior to anterior direction.

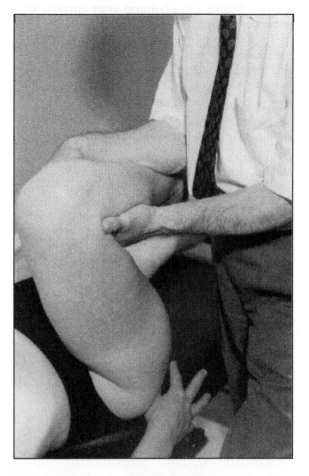

Fig. 8.8.18(a)

The leg on the affected side is fully flexed at the hip and knee

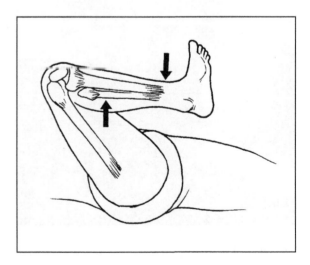

Fig. 8.8.18(b)

The directions of adjustive forces

8.8.19 Supine tibio-femoral joint posterior to anterior flexion technique – Method II

Application
Joint play glide loss from posterior to anterior of the tibia on the femur.

Patient's position
The patient is placed supine with the leg on the affected side flexed so that the foot can rest flat on the adjusting table.

Chiropractor's stance
The chiropractor sits facing caudad on the ipsilateral side, anchoring the patient's foot by sitting lightly on its lateral border.

Contact
Using both hands, the right hand from the medial side, the left hand from the lateral side, the fingers are wrapped around to the posterior of the tibia, just distal to the knee joint.

Procedure
Joint pre-load tension is produced by drawing the contact anteriorwards. With a firm contact and without slackening the tension, a swift impulse of medium depth is given from posterior to anterior.

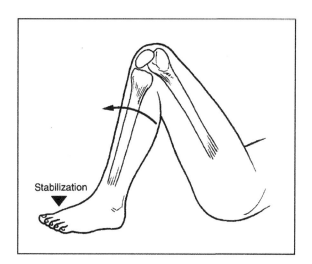

Fig. 8.8.19(a)

The adjustive forces applied to the knee

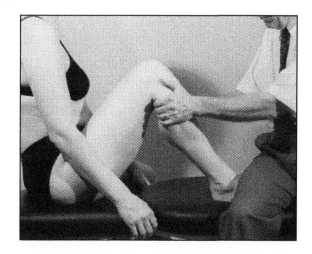

Fig. 8.8.19(b)

The patient's knee is flexed to approximately 45°. The practitioner's fingers are laced together at the posterior just distal to the knee joint

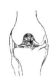

8.8.20 Prone tibio-femoral joint posterior to anterior flexion technique

Application
Joint play glide loss of the tibia on the femur from posterior to anterior.

Patient's position
The patient is placed prone with the knee on the affected side flexed to about 40–50° and the hip abducted to approximately 30°.

Chiropractor's stance
The chiropractor faces cephalad on the affected side and kneels down. The right foot is placed ahead of the left, adjacent to the patient's knee. The chiropractor then sits back on the left heel and patient's foot is rested over the chiropractor's left shoulder.

Contact
Both hands are laced around the posterior of the patient's knee holding the tibia just distal to the joint.

Procedure
Joint pre-load tension is achieved by tractioning with both arms. The chiropractor continues to pull, elevating the trunk until the patient's left thigh is almost vertical and the knee is flexed to approximately 90°. Without releasing the tension, a swift impulse is delivered in the same direction. The weight of the patient's thigh against the treatment table acts as a stabilizer to protect the joints proximal to the knee.

Note
Should joint play loss be found in either external or internal rotation as well as posterior to anterior motion, these factors may be corrected accordingly by suitable alteration in the vector of the thrust.

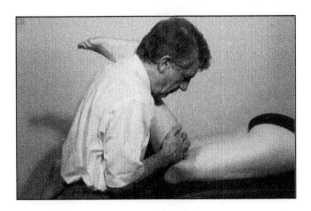

Fig. 8.8.20(b)

The joint is tractioned footwards and the patient's knee is flexed

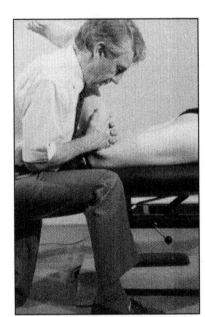

Fig. 8.8.20(c)

The dorsum of the patient's foot is rested against the practitioner's left shoulder. The right foot is placed level with the patient's knee. The thrust is made footwards

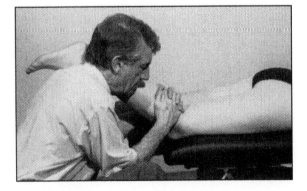

Fig. 8.8.20(a)

Starting position

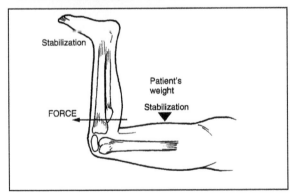

Fig. 8.8.20(d)

The direction of the adjustive forces applied. The patient's weight assists in stabilizing the thigh on the treatment table

Tibio-femoral joint long axis extension techniques

8.8.E Joint play evaluation of the tibio-femoral joint in long axis distraction

Procedure

The patient is either sitting or placed supine. When sitting, the lower leg is distracted downwards with one hand while the other palpates for gapping at the lateral or medial sides of the knee joint.

As an alternative, the patient may be placed supine, with the knee on the affected side flexed. The lower leg is straddled and held firmly between the chiropractor's legs. The hands hold the lateral and medial condyles and the first fingers are pressed along the knee joint to palpate for gapping. The chiropractor leans back, distracting the tibia in long axis, with the hands helping to stabilize the lower leg.

8.8.21 Supine tibio-femoral joint traction leverage/flexion technique

Application

Joint play glide loss of the tibio-femoral articulation in long axis extension and/or lateral translation.

Patient's position

The patient is placed supine with the affected leg abducted approximately 20–30° and the knee flexed to approximately 40–45°.

Chiropractor's stance

The chiropractor stands on the affected side facing cephalad and straddles the patient's lower leg just proximal to the ankle.

Contact

Both hands clasp around the head of the tibia from the anterior and hold the patient's relaxed knee in flexion at about 25° from full extension.

Procedure

Whilst maintaining the contact and keeping the knee flexed, the chiropractor leans back to distract the joint, until tissue tension is felt. The joint is then gently rocked several times into lateral and medial flexion to ensure that the patient's knee is relaxed and to help prevent the patient from anticipating when the thrust will be made. The thrust is then made swiftly in an upward direction and, at the same time, the chiropractor leans swiftly backwards to distract the joint.

Note

1) For lateral translation fixations, this technique may be varied as follows: Whilst maintaining the traction, a rapid and controlled-depth thrust from lateral to medial and back is initiated by the arms and assisted by a similar lateral to medial movement of the trunk. Rapidity is necessary because much of the energy is absorbed by the laxity of the patient's hip joint.

2) For medial to lateral joint play glide loss, the manipulation is performed as described above by reversing the initial direction of the thrust from medial to lateral.

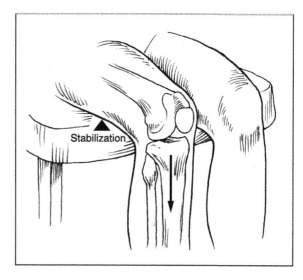

Fig. 8.8.E

Joint play evaluation of the knee. Long axis distraction

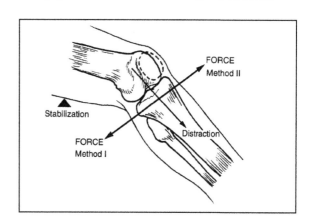

Fig. 8.8.21(a)

The adjustive force applied to the knee using this technique

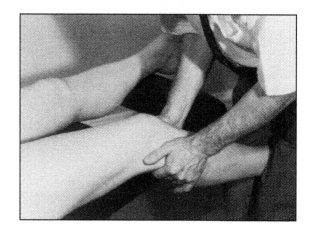

Fig. 8.8.21(b)

The joint is distracted until tissue tension is felt

Tibio-femoral joint mobilization techniques

Application

Mobilization methods are used to gently stretch tight ligaments and generally stimulate the soft tissues, by putting the patient's knee through gentle passive movements in all directions in which the joint is normally capable of functioning. If joint fixation is chronic, it is wise to use mobilization methods first, before manipulative procedures are undertaken. If degenerative joint changes are severe, osseous release methods may be precluded and treatment of a joint may be limited to gentle mobilization methods only.

8.8.22   Prone tibio-femoral joint flexion/distraction technique – Method I

Patient's position
The patient is placed prone with the affected knee flexed.

Procedure
A cylindrical shaped medium density foam cushion is placed tightly into the right popliteal space and held there. The right knee is then flexed over the cushion to the patient's tolerance. This is repeated as necessary in a rhythmical oscillating fashion.

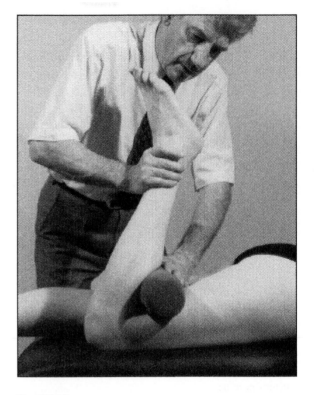

Fig. 8.8.22

Prone flexion/distraction technique – Method I

8.8.23   Prone tibio-femoral joint flexion/distraction technique – Method II

Patient's position
The patient is placed prone with the affected knee flexed.

Procedure
A modification of the method is to place a forearm into the patient's popliteus and then flex the patient's knee over it to the point of tension. The action is repeated as necessary in an oscillating fashion.

Note
Caution must be used with this method not to exceed the patient's tolerance.

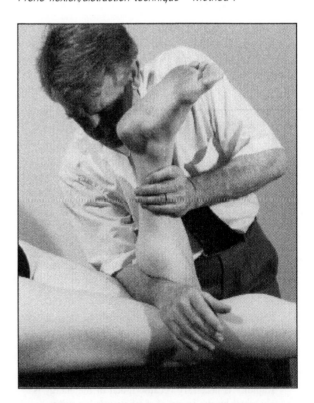

Fig. 8.8.23

Prone flexion/distraction technique – Method II

8.8.24   Supine tibio-femoral joint circumduction technique – Method I

Patient's position
The patient is placed supine with the knee flexed and held at 25–30° from full extension.

Procedure
The chiropractor straddles the patient's lower leg, holds it between the knees and leans back a little to distract the joint. The tibia is held with both hands just distal to the knee joint. The hands are placed over the tibial condyles. The joint is then gently moved in circumduction whilst continuing to maintain joint pre-load tension with the traction.

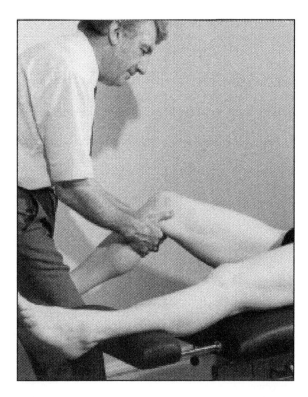

Fig. 8.8.24

Supine circumduction mobilization – Method I

8.8.25   Supine tibio-femoral joint circumduction technique – Method II

Patient's position
The patient is placed supine with the knee flexed and held at 25–30° from full extension.

Procedure
This is a modification of the foregoing procedure. The patient is placed supine with the hip and knee each flexed to approximately 90°. By supporting the patient's ankle under the arm and clasping the proximal tibia just distal to the knee joint, the chiropractor attempts to move the tibia in circumduction, working to the patient's tolerance.

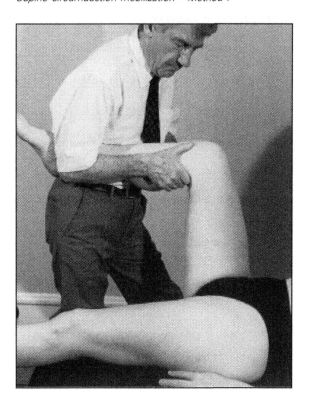

Fig. 8.8.25

Supine circumduction mobilization – Method II

8.8.26 Supine tibio-femoral joint circumduction technique – Method III

Procedure
With the patient supine and the affected leg flexed at the hip and knee to 90°, the chiropractor stabilizes the patient's knee with the right hand. The left hand holds the patient's right foot and describes a clockwise circle with it. As this is being carried out, the patient's foot is alternately placed into external and internal rotation, thus rotating the tibia on the femur.

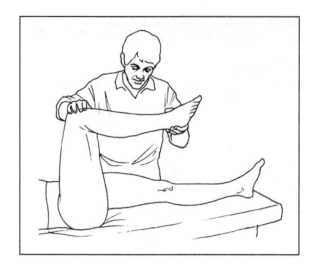

Fig. 8.8.26

Supine circumduction mobilization – Method III

Patellar mobilization techniques

8.8.27 Supine patellar superior to inferior technique

Procedure
With the patient placed supine, the chiropractor places the webs of the hands at the superior and inferior aspects of the patella and gently but firmly the patella is moved to the full extent of its normal excursion proximally and distally in a rhythmical way. When restriction is present, this should always be done to the patient's tolerance, gradually increasing the range of movement.

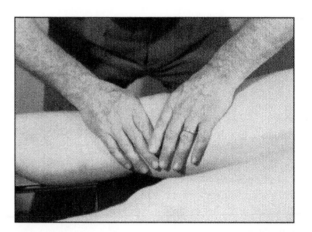

Fig. 8.8.27

Supine patellar superior to inferior mobilization technique

8.8.28 Supine patellar oblique technique

Procedure
This is performed as described in technique 8.8.27, but with oblique pressure on the patella from the superior medial aspect to the inferior lateral aspect and vice versa. The mobilization is carried out by using gentle, rhythmical, repetitive stretching movements.

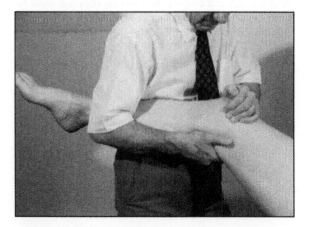

Fig. 8.8.28

The patella is pressed rhythmically from side to side, gradually increasing the range of movement, to patient tolerance

8.8.29 Supine lateral to medial patellar techniques

Procedure
Method I: With the patient placed supine, a double thumb contact is placed at the lateral border of the patella. The fingers of each hand are wrapped around the medial aspect of the leg for support. Pressure is then applied rhythmically with both thumbs, to move the patella medially. When restriction is present, this must be done to patient tolerance.

Note
As a precaution, the Patellar Apprehension Test (see Glossary of Terms, p. 285) should be carried out before this technique is used.

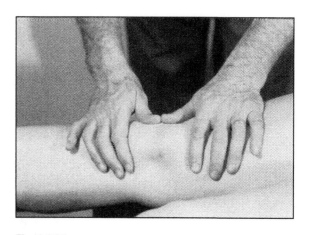

Fig. 8.8.29

Contact for lateral to medial patellar mobilization – Method I

Method II: The patient is placed supine with the leg flexed at the hip. The chiropractor stands facing cephalad, lateral to the patient's leg. The leg is held with approximately 30–40° of hip flexion by pressing the lower leg against the lateral aspect of the lower part of the chiropractor's rib cage with the right elbow. The right hand supports the patient's knee from the posterior. The left hand is placed against the lateral aspect of the patella and pressure is exerted medially in a rhythmical, repetitive way, gradually increasing the extent of patellar travel, to the patient's tolerance.

8.8.30 Supine medial to lateral techniques

Procedure
Method I: The procedure is similar to that described in technique 8.8.29 lateral to medial Method I except that the thumbs are placed on the medial aspect of the patella and the other fingers are wrapped around the lateral aspect of the patient's leg. The thumbs exert a lateral pressure.

Method II: The patient is placed supine with the affected leg abducted approximately 30–40° and flexed at the hip, also to approximately 30–40°. The chiropractor faces cephalad, standing between the patient's legs. The affected leg is held in flexion by firmly pressing it against the chiropractor's left lateral rib cage with the left elbow. The left hand supports the patient's knee by holding it from the posterior. The right hand is placed against the medial border of the patella and heel of hand pressure is exerted laterally, using a firm rhythmical, repetitive thrust, gradually increasing the extent of patellar travel. The technique is performed to the patient's tolerance.

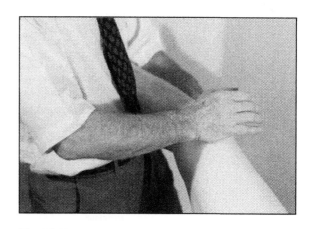

Fig. 8.8.30

Alternative contact for medial to lateral patellar mobilization. The heel of hand exerts a lateral pressure – Method II

REFERENCES

Hoppenfeld, S. (1976) *Physical Examination of the Spine and Extremities*. New York, Appleton–Century–Crofts.

Kapandji, L.A. (1983) *The Physiology of the Joints*, Vol. 2, Lower Limb. Edinburgh, Churchill Livingstone.

Segal, P. and Jacob, M. (1984) *The Knee*. London, Wolf Medical Publications.

The proximal and distal tibio-fibular joints

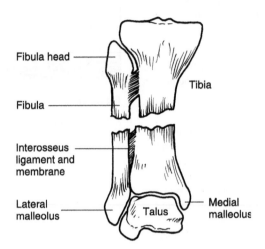

Proximal tibio-fibular joint play evaluation

8.9.A   Anterior to posterior and posterior to anterior glide

8.9.B   Inferior to superior glide with external rotation

8.9.C   Superior to inferior glide

Distal tibio-fibular joint play evaluation

8.9.D   Inferior to superior glide with external rotation

Proximal tibio-fibular joint techniques

8.9.1   Prone proximal tibio-fibular joint posterior to anterior traction/leverage flexion technique

8.9.2   Prone proximal tibio-fibular joint posterior to anterior flexion technique

8.9.3   Prone proximal tibio-fibular joint anterior to posterior flexion technique

8.9.4   Supine proximal tibio-fibular joint anterior to posterior recoil technique

8.9.5   Prone proximal tibio-fibular joint posterior to inferior technique

8.9.6   Side-reclining proximal tibio-fibular joint superior to inferior technique

8.9.7   Prone proximal tibio-fibular joint inferior to superior flexion technique

Distal tibio-fibular joint techniques

8.9.8   Side reclining distal tibio-fibular joint inferior to superior technique

8.9.9   Supine distal tibio-fibular joint superior to inferior traction/leverage technique

8.9.10   Supine distal tibio-fibular joint anterior to posterior direct thrust technique

8.9.11   Prone distal tibio-fibular joint posterior to anterior direct thrust technique

Proximal tibio-fibular joint play evaluation

8.9.A   Anterior to posterior and posterior to anterior glide

Procedure
The patient may be either sitting, reclining or lying supine. One hand stabilizes the proximal tibia while the anterior aspect of the 1st distal phalanx of the index finger presses the fibula until all joint slack is taken up. Then further pressure is applied to assess the joint play, which is perceived as an elasticity or soft end-feel.

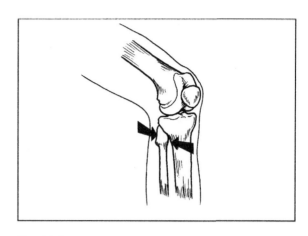

Fig. 8.9.A

Proximal tibio-fibular, anterior to posterior glide

8.9.B   Inferior to superior glide with external rotation

Procedure
The foot and ankle are passively dorsiflexed with one hand, as for the distal tibio-fibular joint (see 8.9.D). Normally, as the foot is fully dorsiflexed, the palpating fingers of the other hand feel the proximal tibio-fibular joint rise and externally rotate. It is wise to test both the distal and proximal joints whenever the fibula is examined for fixations.

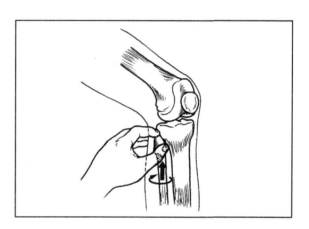

Fig. 8.9.B

Proximal tibio-fibular, inferior to superior glide and external rotation

8.9.C   Superior to inferior glide

Procedure
For the examination of the superior to inferior joint play glide of the proximal tibio-fibular joint, the patient is placed supine or side-reclining with the affected side up. The foot, ankle and lower leg must be kept relaxed and flexed at the knee. With one hand, the foot is gently held in plantar flexion. A thumb and first finger contact is made over the superior border of the head of the tibia and firm pressure is exerted from superior to inferior.

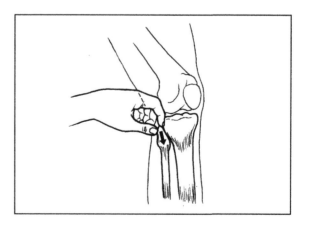

Fig. 8.9.C

Proximal tibio-fibular, superior to inferior glide

Distal tibio-fibular joint play evaluation

8.9.D   Distal tibio-fibular joint inferior to superior glide with external rotation

Procedure

The patient reclines supine with the affected foot relaxed. The right hand contacts the plantar surface of the foot and fully dorsiflexes the foot and ankle. As ligamentous resistance begins to be felt, further upward pressure is applied. With dorsiflexion, the widest part of the wedge-shaped superior surface of the talus is presented in the ankle mortice causing the fibula to rise superiorly (Cailliet). Also on dorsiflexion the triangular articular facet on the lateral border of the talus and the concave lateral articular surface of the lower extremity of the tibia cause the fibula to rotate a little externally. These joint play movements are palpated with the left hand using a first finger and thumb contact placed over the inferior tip of the distal fibula. The other movement of the fibula on dorsiflexion is a palpable widening of the articulation between the fibula and the tibia. This can be detected using a three-finger contact along the anterior border of the tibia and fibula (see Fig. 8.9.D(b)). This movement also tests for the laxity of the interosseous ligament. Loss of integrity of the interosseous ligament necessarily causes ankle joint instability.

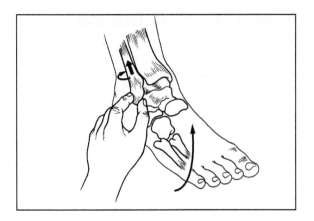

Fig. 8.9.D(a)

Distal tibio-fibular, inferior to superior glide with external rotation

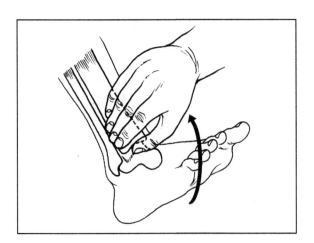

Fig. 8.9.D(b)

Palpation of the tibio-fibular articulation which normally opens on dorsiflexion

Proximal tibio-fibular joint techniques

8.9.1 Prone proximal tibio-fibular joint posterior to anterior traction/leverage flexion technique

Application
Joint play glide loss from posterior to anterior of tibio-fibular articulation.

Patient's position
The patient is placed prone with the knee on the affected side flexed to approximately 90°.

Chiropractor's stance
The chiropractor crouches down facing cephalad on the affected side with the right foot forward and placed opposite the patient's right knee. The trunk is rotated to the right, bringing the left shoulder forward. The patient's right lower leg is placed against the chiropractor's trunk and the patient's foot rests over the shoulder.

Contact
a) The anterior surface of the middle finger of the right hand, just proximal to the middle phalanx, is placed at the posterior lateral aspect of the proximal fibula.
b) The left hand is placed around the posterior of the knee from the medial side, to interlace with the fingers of the right hand.

Procedure
The patient's knee is tractioned towards the chiropractor until joint pre-load tension is felt. While maintaining the traction, the impulse is made in the same direction, mainly with the right hand, with the left hand used to maintain the traction and stabilize the knee.

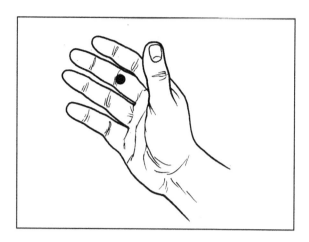

Fig. 8.9.1(a)

The contact point is the anterior head of the 1st phalanx of the middle finger

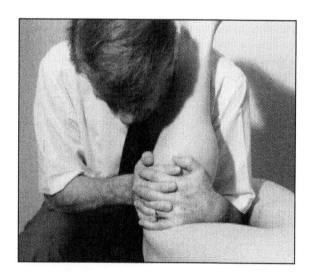

Fig. 8.9.1(b)

The chiropractor crouches down with the left foot placed opposite the patient's affected knee. The trunk is rotated, with both elbows held close to the sides

8.9.2   Prone proximal tibio-fibular joint posterior to anterior flexion technique

Application
Joint play glide loss from posterior to anterior of the fibula on the tibia.

Patient's position
The patient is placed prone with the knee on the affected side flexed to approximately 90°.

Chiropractor's stance
The chiropractor stands on the contralateral side facing the patient's mid-line, directly opposite the affected knee. The trunk is flexed forwards and rotated caudad.

Contact
a)   The heel of the left hand is placed at the posterior aspect of the proximal end of the fibula.

b)   The right hand is placed over the lateral border of the hind foot with the fingers wrapped around the lateral border of the patient's ankle.

Procedure
By externally rotating the patient's hip with the right hand, the patient's foot is pulled towards the chiropractor's trunk and the heel is wedged against the lower lateral chest wall. Joint pre-load tension is achieved by internally rotating the patient's foot. The impulse is made using a direct thrust and utilizing a body drop technique (see Chapter 2).

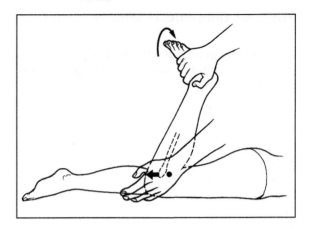

Fig. 8.9.2

The patient's hip is externally rotated and the right foot is braced against the chiropractor's chest

8.9.3 Prone proximal tibio-fibular joint anterior to posterior flexion technique

Application
Joint play glide loss from anterior to posterior of the fibula on the tibia.

Patient's position
The patient is placed prone with the knee on the affected side flexed to about 120° or until tissue tension is reached. On an older patient, less flexion may be required.

Chiropractor's stance
The chiropractor stands on the contralateral side, facing the patient's mid-line just distal to the knee on the affected side.

Contact
a) The left hand grasps the patient's right ankle on the lateral side and firmly holds the right knee in flexion. The patient's lower leg is pulled towards the mid-line by externally rotating the hip until tissue tension is felt.
b) The heel of the right hand is placed at the anterior aspect of the proximal fibula head.

Procedure
Whilst holding the contacts firmly, the chiropractor rotates the trunk cephalad, further increasing tissue tension. The right arm presses downwards against the contact to remove tissue slack and to move the joint through to pre-load tension. The impulse is made with a direct thrust and rapid body drop (see Chapter 2) initiated from the right shoulder in an anterior to posterior direction across the contact on the fibula head.

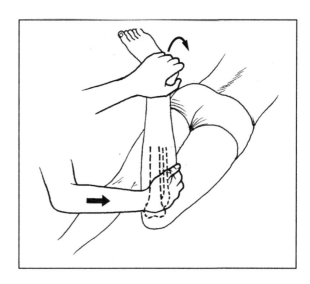

Fig. 8.9.3(a)

In order to achieve joint tension, the knee must be fully flexed. The hip is also slightly externally rotated

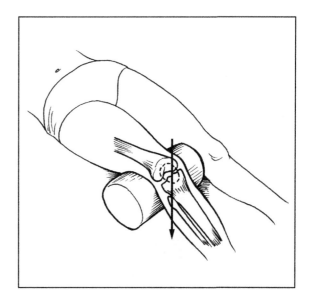

Fig. 8.9.3(b)

An alternative method is to place a firm cushion under the knee joint. The arrow shows the angle of the adjustive force

8.9.4 Supine proximal tibio-fibular joint anterior to posterior recoil technique

Application
Joint play glide loss from anterior to posterior of the fibula on the tibia.

Patient's position
The patient is placed supine with the leg on the affected side fully extended. The drop mechanism (see Glossary of Terms, p. 285) of the pelvic section on the treatment table is set for the patient's weight and cocked.

Chiropractor's stance
The chiropractor stands on the homolateral side facing the patient's midline opposite the right tibio-fibular articulation.

Contact
a) The pisiform of the right hand is placed over the anterior aspect of the joint and the wrist and hand are held in a high arch (see Glossary of Terms, p. 285) position.
b) The pisiform of the left hand is placed over the left 'anatomical snuff box' with the fingers wrapped around the lateral aspect of the left wrist. The thumb is wrapped around the medial aspect of the wrist to reach the posterior.

Procedure
A rapid shallow recoil adjustment (see p. 8) is applied utilizing a smooth pectoralis triceps anconius thrust.

8.9.5 Prone proximal tibio-fibular joint posterior to anterior recoil technique

Application
Joint play glide loss from posterior to anterior of the fibula on the tibia.

Patient's position
The patient is placed prone with the legs extended.

Chiropractor's stance
The chiropractor stands on the contralateral side facing the patient's mid-line and adjacent to the affected knee.

Contact
a) The pisiform of the left hand is placed over the left 'anatomical snuff box' with the fingers wrapped around the lateral aspect of the left wrist. The thumb is wrapped around the medial aspect of the wrist to reach the posterior.
b) The pisiform of the right hand contacts the posterior aspect of the proximal fibula and the hand is held in a low arch position (see Glossary of Terms, p. 285).

Procedure
A rapid, shallow recoil adjustment (see Chapter 2) is applied.

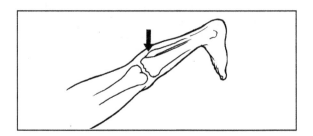

Fig. 8.9.5(a)

The arrow shows the contact point on the fibula

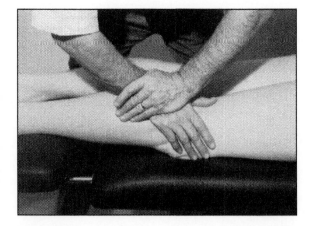

Fig. 8.9.5(b)

The patient is prone with the knee fully extended. The chiropractor stands on the contralateral side

Fig. 8.9.4

The patient is placed with the pelvic section cushion giving support under the posterior of the proximal tibia

8.9.6 Side-reclining proximal tibio-fibular joint superior to inferior technique

Application
Joint play glide loss from superior to inferior of the proximal fibula on the tibia.

Patient's position
The patient is placed in the side reclining position on the unaffected side, with the pelvis rotated well forwards and the affected leg flexed, allowing the medial side of it to rest flat against the pelvic section cushion of the adjusting table.

Chiropractor's stance
The chiropractor stands facing caudad, in front of the patient and adjacent to the knee on the affected side.

Contact
a) The left hand is placed over the lateral aspect of the patient's right ankle, holding it firmly against the adjusting table, in plantarflexion.
b) The heel of the right hand is placed over the superior border of the fibular head, with the fingers extended and held flat against the fibula, pointing caudad.

Procedure
With the patient's ankle held in plantarflexion and against the treatment table, an impulse is made with the right hand from superior to inferior on the fibular head.

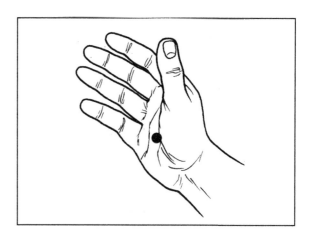

Fig. 8.9.6(a)

The contact is point is the heel of the hand

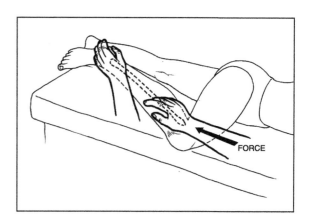

Fig. 8.9.6(b)

The patient's ankle is held in plantarflexion, thus slackening the distal fibula joint while the proximal fibula joint is being treated

8.9.7 Prone proximal tibio-fibular joint inferior to superior flexion technique

Application
Joint play glide loss from inferior to superior of the proximal fibula on the tibia.

Patient's position
The patient is placed prone with the affected leg flexed to approximately 90°. The hip is rotated externally, allowing the foot to cross the patient's mid-line.

Chiropractor's stance
The chiropractor stands at the contralateral side facing the patient's mid-line, directly opposite the patient's knees. The trunk is then rotated caudad.

Contact
a) The heel of the left hand is placed over the inferior aspect of the fibular head. The fingers remain extended and are held firmly against the lateral border of the patient's knee. The left arm remains rigid, with slight elbow flexion.

b) The right hand is placed over the lateral border of the foot with the fingers curled around the dorsum of the mid-foot. The patient's right foot is then pulled against the chiropractor's lower right chest wall to stabilize the lower leg and held there firmly. The patient's foot is then passively dorsiflexed.

Procedure
As the right hand stabilizes the patient's right leg, the chiropractor leans forwards to contact the patient's right foot to further dorsiflex it. The thrust is then applied using a rapid impulse from the left shoulder down to the rigidly held left arm.

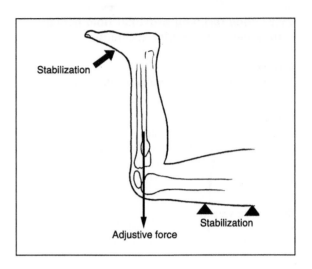

Fig. 8.9.7(a)

The contact on the fibula head is the heel of the left hand

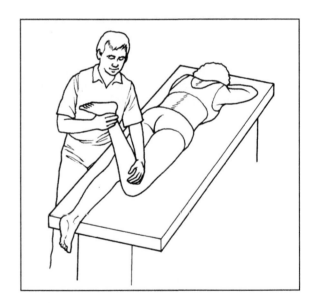

Fig. 8.9.7(b)

The patient's hip is externally rotated sufficiently to allow the foot to be braced against the chiropractor's chest to stabilize the lower leg. The depth of the adjustive thrust must be increased if the treatment table cushion is soft

Distal tibio-fibular joint techniques

8.9.8 Side-reclining distal tibio-fibular joint inferior to superior technique

Application
Joint play glide loss from inferior to superior of the medial convex margin of the distal end of the fibula and the lateral concave margin of the distal end of the tibia.

Patient's position
The patient is placed in a side-reclining position on the unaffected side. The knee and hip on the affected side are flexed to allow the medial side of the foot to be comfortably placed against the surface of the treatment table.

Chiropractor's stance
The chiropractor stands behind the patient at the foot end of the treatment table facing cephalad.

Contact
a) The web of the right hand is placed firmly against the inferior aspect of the distal tip of the fibula with the thumb wrapped around to the posterior of the ankle and the fingers curled around the medial inferior border of the hind/midfoot.

b) With the wrist flexed back, the pisiform of the left hand is placed against the proximal aspect of the first right metacarpal. The fingers are wrapped around the lateral border of the ulna on the right hand.

Procedure
a) Using both arms, a short, quick impulse is made as close to the direction of the plane line of the joint as possible, without allowing the patient's foot to slide along the cushion. Inevitably, some of the thrust force is dissipated into the supporting cushion.

b) An alternative to the above procedure is to position the patient's foot over the treatment table pelvic drop section, which is cocked and set for the patient's weight. A drop technique (see Chapter 2) with a recoil-type thrust is then used.

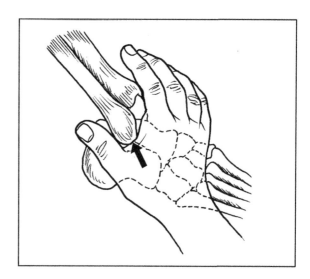

Fig. 8.9.8(a)

The contact uses the web of the thumb against the inferior tip of the fibula

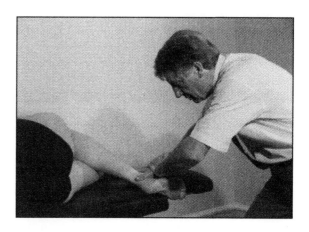

Fig. 8.9.8(b)

The medial malleolus is held firmly against the treatment table cushion to prevent the patient's foot from slipping

8.9.9 Supine distal tibio-fibular joint superior to inferior traction/leverage technique

Application
Joint play glide loss from superior to inferior of the medial convex margin of the distal end of the fibula and the lateral concave margin of the distal end of the tibia.

Patient's position
The patient is placed supine and requested to hold on to the sides of the treatment table with both hands. The leg on the affected side is held relaxed and extended. The non-affected leg is slightly flexed to allow the foot to brace against the foot rest, if available. If not, the leg is allowed to remain extended.

Chiropractor's stance
The chiropractor stands at the foot end of the table, facing cephalad, favouring the side of the affected leg.

Contact
a) The anterior of the joint between the first and second phalanges of the middle finger of the right hand is placed around the dorsal surface of the ankle to contact the lateral border of the distal fibula just proximal to the joint. Backed up by the other fingers, a firm contact is made.

b) The left hand is placed over the right hand as support.

Procedure
The patient's affected leg is allowed to remain on the treatment table and a quick impulse of minimum depth is made towards the chiropractor. The disadvantage of this technique, in common with other long lever techniques, is that the thrust stresses the joints of the leg, pelvis and low back. High speed with minimal depth of thrust is advised when using this technique.

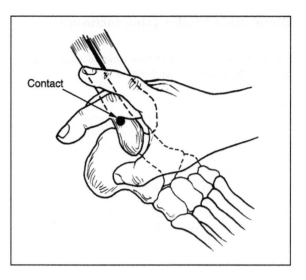

Fig. 8.9.9(a)

The contact is the anterior aspect of the 2nd–3rd phalanx of the middle finger

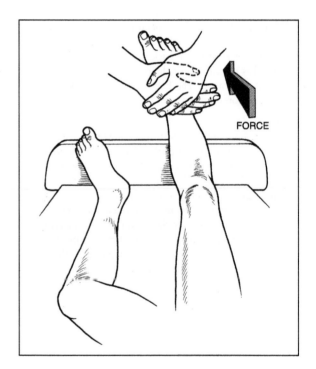

Fig. 8.9.9(b)

The unaffected leg is braced against the footrest of the treatment table. The affected leg remains resting on the cushion to stabilize the ankle and reduce the force affecting the leg

8.9.10 Supine distal tibio-fibular joint anterior to posterior direct thrust technique

Application
Joint play glide loss from anterior to posterior of the fibula on the tibia at the distal articulation.

Patient's position
The patient is placed supine with the legs extended.

Chiropractor's stance
The chiropractor stands at the foot end of the treatment table facing cephalad, favouring the affected side.

Contact
a)   The thenar eminence and thumb of the left hand are placed along the anterior border of the distal fibula. The fingers are wrapped around the lateral border to grasp the distal fibula from the posterior.
b)   The anterior of the 1st metacarpal of the right hand is placed on the anterior of the distal tibia and all the fingers are wrapped around the medial border to hold it at the posterior.

Procedure
The chiropractor bends forwards at the waist until the arms are almost vertical. The elbows are slightly flexed. The height of the treatment table should be raised or lowered to accommodate this position. The adjustment is made by swiftly snapping the elbows into full extension, making a minimal downward thrust on to the fibula with the left hand whilst simultaneously pulling the right shoulder girdle up and back producing an additional upward thrust on the tibia.

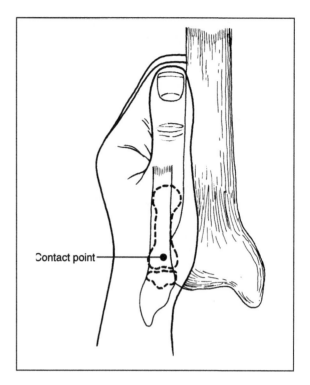

Fig. 8.9.10(a)

The medial aspect of the base of the 1st metacarpal is used as the contact point and is placed over the anterior of the lateral malleolus

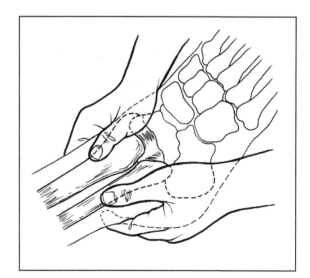

Fig. 8.9.10(b)

The arms are held in a near vertical position to deliver the thrust

8.9.11 Prone distal tibio-fibular joint posterior to anterior direct thrust technique

Application
Joint play glide loss of the distal fibula articulation from posterior to anterior on the tibia.

Patient's position
The patient is placed prone on the treatment table with both legs extended.

Chiropractor's stance
The chiropractor stands at the foot end of the treatment table facing cephalad, favouring the side of involvement.

Contact
a)   The left hand is placed around the medial side of the ankle to contact the anterior of the distal end of the tibia. The thenar eminence is placed over the posterior aspect of the tibia and the fingers are wrapped around the medial aspect of the ankle to stabilize the contact.
b)   The thenar eminence and thumb of the right hand are placed firmly along the distal end of the fibula at the posterior with the fingers wrapped around to the anterior to support the thumb.

Procedure
a)   The trunk is flexed forward at the waist so that the arms are nearly vertical, with the elbows slightly bent. The height of the treatment table should be raised or lowered to allow for this posture. The adjustment is made by swiftly extending the elbows to full extension, simultaneously producing a rapid minimal downward thrust on the fibula and, by drawing the right shoulder upwards and backwards, a corresponding counter thrust is effected upwards on the tibia with the right hand.
b)   As an alternative, the use of a drop mechanism section on the treatment table may be employed, using similar hand positions as described.

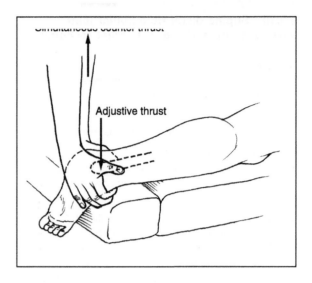

Fig. 8.9.11

The arms are held nearly vertical for this adjustment. Only minimal depth of adjustive and counter-thrust is required

REFERENCE

Caillet, R. (1968) *Foot and Ankle Pain*. Philadelphia, F.A. davis Company.

8.10

The joints of the foot and ankle

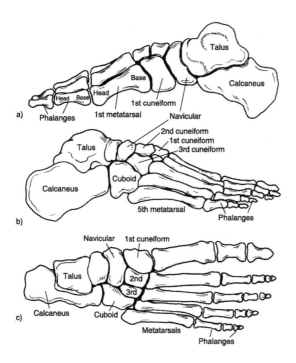

Interphalangeal techniques
8.10.A Joint play evaluation of the interphalangeal joints
8.10.1 Supine and prone interphalangeal direct thrust and distraction techniques

Metatarso-phalangeal techniques
8.10.B Joint play evaluation of the metatarso-phalangeal joints
8.10.2 Supine 1st metatarso-phalangeal joint inferior to superior and superior to inferior short lever pull techniques
8.10.3 Supine 1st metatarso-phalangeal long axis distraction technique – Method I
8.10.4 Supine 1st metatarso-phalangeal long axis distraction technique – Method II
8.10.5 Supine 1st metatarso-phalangeal long axis distraction technique – Method III
8.10.6 Prone 2nd to 5th metatarso-phalangeal inferior to superior direct thrust technique
8.10.7 Supine 2nd to 5th metatarso-phalangeal flexion/distraction technique

Intermetatarsal techniques
8.10.8 Supine intermetatarsal clasp mobilization technique
8.10.9 Prone intermetatarsal clasp mobilization technique
8.10.10 Supine and prone intermetatarsal shuttle mobilization technique

---

continued overleaf

Metatarso-tarsal techniques
8.10.C Joint play evaluation of the tarsals and metatarsals on the medial side of the foot
8.10.D Joint play evaluation of the 1st metatarsal on the 1st cuneiform
8.10.E Joint play evaluation of the tarsals and metatarsals on the lateral side of the foot
8.10.11 Supine 1st metatarsal on the 1st cuneiform superior to inferior traction/leverage distraction technique
8.10.12 Supine 2nd or 3rd metatarsal/2nd or 3rd cuneiform traction leverage technique
8.10.13 Supine 1st metatarsal/1st cuneiform inferior to superior short lever pull technique
8.10.14 Supine 1st metatarsal/1st cuneiform superior to inferior short lever pull technique
8.10.15 Prone 1st metatarsal/1st cuneiform superior to inferior short lever pull technique
8.10.16 Prone 1st metatarsal/1st cuneiform inferior to superior short lever pull technique
8.10.17 Prone 2nd metatarsal/1st cuneiform superior to inferior short lever pull technique
8.10.18 Supine 2nd metatarsal/1st cuneiform superior to inferior short lever pull technique
8.10.19 Prone 3rd metatarsal/2nd cuneiform superior to inferior short lever pull technique
8.10.20 Prone 1st, 2nd or 3rd metatarso-tarsal and intertarsal inferior to superior pectoralis/triceps thrust technique
8.10.21 Prone metatarso-tarsal and intertarsal superior to inferior pectoralis/triceps thrust and check technique
8.10.22 Standing metatarso-tarsal and intertarsal inferior to superior pectoralis/triceps thrust technique
8.10.23 Supine figure-of-eight metatarso-tarsal mobilization technique
8.10.24 Supine 4th or 5th metatarso-cuboid superior to inferior short lever pull technique
8.10.25 Supine 4th or 5th metatarso-cuboid inferior to superior short lever pull technique
8.10.26 Supine 4th or 5th metatarso-cuboid superior to inferior recoil technique
8.10.27 Supine 4th or 5th metatarso-cuboid superior to inferior body drop thrust technique
8.10.28 Prone 4th or 5th metatarso-cuboid superior to inferior short lever pull technique

Intertarsal techniques
8.10.29 Supine navicular/1st cuneiform inferior to superior short lever pull technique
8.10.30 Supine navicular/1st cuneiform superior to inferior short lever pull technique
8.10.31 Prone talo-navicular inferior to superior short lever pull technique

8.10.32 Supine 1st and 2nd or 2nd and 3rd intercuneiform superior to inferior compression technique
8.10.33 Supine 1st or 2nd cuneiform–navicular superior to inferior traction leverage technique
8.10.34 Supine 3rd cuneiform–cuboid superior to inferior traction/leverage technique
8.10.35 Supine calcaneo-cuboid superior to inferior traction/leverage technique
8.10.36 Prone calcaneo-cuboid inferior to superior short lever technique
8.10.37 Supine calcaneo-cuboid inferior to superior short lever technique
8.10.38 Prone calcaneo-cuboid inferior to superior thrust technique
8.10.F Joint play evaluation of the talus on the calcaneus
8.10.39 Prone talo-calcaneal lateral to medial short lever technique
8.10.40 Prone talo-calcaneal medial to lateral short lever technique
8.10.41 Supine talo-calcaneal lateral to medial traction/leverage technique
8.10.42 Supine talo-calcaneal medial to lateral traction/leverage technique
8.10.43 Supine talo-calcaneal lateral to medial strike technique
8.10.44 Supine talo-calcaneal medial to lateral strike technique
8.10.G Joint play evaluation of the talo-calcaneal joint
8.10.45 Prone talo-calcaneal anterior to posterior short lever technique
8.10.46 Prone talo-calcaneal posterior to anterior short lever technique
8.10.47 Supine or prone intertarsal circumduction mobilization technique

The talo-crural (ankle) joint
8.10.H Joint play evaluation of the talo-crural joint
8.10.48 Supine talo-crural long axis distraction technique
8.10.49 Supine talo-crural lateral to medial short lever technique
8.10.50 Supine talo-crural medial to lateral short lever technique
8.10.51 Prone talo-crural lateral to medial short lever technique
8.10.52 Prone talo-crural medial to lateral short lever technique
8.10.53 Supine talo-crural lateral to medial distraction technique
8.10.54 Supine talo-crural medial to lateral distraction technique
8.10.55 Supine talo-crural lateral to medial modified distraction technique
8.10.56 Supine talo-crural medial to lateral modified distraction technique
8.10.I Anterior to posterior and posterior to anterior joint play evaluation of the talo-crural joint
8.10.57 Prone talo-crural anterior to posterior short lever technique
8.10.58 Prone talo-crural posterior to anterior short lever technique
8.10.59 Supine talo-crural anterior to posterior and posterior to anterior thrust technique

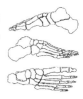

Interphalangeal techniques

8.10.A   Joint play evaluation of the interphalangeal joints

Procedure
Adjacent phalanges are held each in turn with a first finger and thumb contact as illustrated in Fig. 8.10.A(a). Using a firm pressure, each joint is examined for joint play in flexion, extension, lateral flexion, lateral translation, rotation, superior to inferior glide and long axis extension. To reach joint play, the joint is first put through its normal range of movement. At the point of ligamentous resistance at the end of the range, momentary further firm pressure is exerted in the same direction. Joint play loss is perceived as resistance with a hard end-feel.

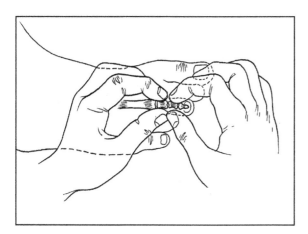

Fig. 8.10.A(a)

Each phalanx is taken through the ranges of movement to end-play

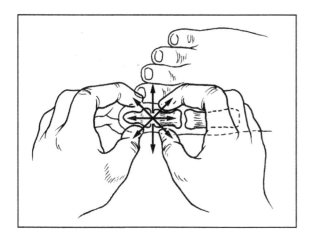

Fig. 8.10.A(b)

Close up view illustrating the directions of the joint movements

8.10.1   Supine and prone interphalangeal joint direct thrust and distraction techniques

Application
Joint play glide loss of the inter-phalangeal joints in lateral flexion, rotation, dorsiflexion, plantarflexion or distraction.

Patient's position
The patient may be placed supine or prone.

Chiropractor's stance
a) Patient supine: the chiropractor stands at the foot end of the treatment table, facing cephalad.
b) Patient prone: the chiropractor stands at the foot end of the treatment table on the homolateral side facing medially, with the patient knee flexed.

Contact
While one hand stabilizes the proximal phalanx to be adjusted, the other grasps the distal one between the thumb and lateral border of the 2nd phalanx of the index finger.

Procedure
Short, swift, shallow thrusts are made in the direction or directions in which joint play glide is restricted. Distraction is used if joint play in long axis extension is restricted.

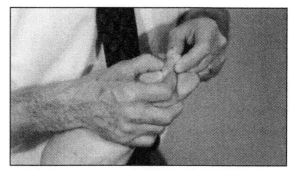

Fig. 8.10.1(a)

The patient is prone. It is a matter of clinical preference whether the technique is performed prone or supine

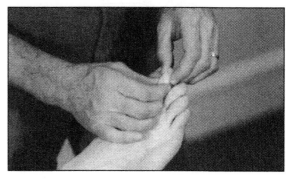

Fig. 8.10.1(b)

The patient is supine. Short, swift, shallow thrusts are used

Metatarso-phalangeal techniques

8.10.B Joint play evaluation of the metatarso-phalangeal joints

Procedure

One hand firmly holds the distal metacarpals, allowing the proximal phalanges to be moved in all planes of motion, through to the limit of joint play in lateral flexion, flexion and extension, rotation, long axis extension, lateral and medial translation. Clinically, the great toe is frequently found to have gross passive mobility loss on plantarflexion while in contrast maintaining greater dorsiflexion. The normal gross range of movement of the toes is 70–90° in dorsiflexion and 45° in plantar flexion (Hoppenfeld, 1976). Joint play glide loss of the 1st metatarso-phalangeal joint from superior to inferior and inferior to superior planes is clinically seen most frequently and is tested by using opposing thumb pressures along the plane line of the joint.

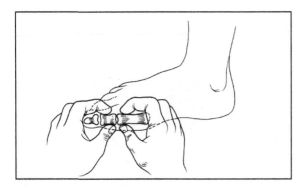

Fig. 8.10.B(a)

Joint play evaluation of the metatarso-phalangeal joint

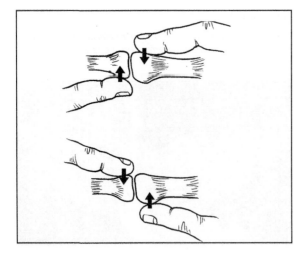

Fig. 8.10B(b)

Opposing thumb pressures are used along the plane line of the 1st metatarso-phalangeal joint

8.10.2 Supine 1st metatarso-phalangeal joint inferior to superior and superior to inferior short lever pull techniques

Inferior to superior technique

Application

Joint play glide loss of the 1st metatarsal from inferior to superior on the 1st phalanx. This fixation is commonly found when examining patients for gross passive movements of the great toe.

Patient's position

The patient is placed supine with the leg on the affected side fully extended.

Chiropractor's stance

The chiropractor may either sit or stand on the affected side, facing the patient's mid-line at the foot end of the treatment table. The lateral border of the patient's right foot is held nearly vertically along the mid-line of the chiropractor's sternum.

Contact

a) The anterior of the first finger of the left hand at the junction of the 1st and 2nd phalanges is wrapped around the medial border of the foot from the dorsum to contact the inferior surface of the head of the first metatarsal, supported closely by the other fingers.

b) The right hand is wrapped around the medial border of the foot from the plantar surface and an anterior middle finger contact, using the junction of the 1st and 2nd phalanges, is made on the dorsal surface of the base of the 1st phalanx of the great toe. This contact is held firmly, with the rest of the fingers closing up to support the contact.

Procedure

By rotating the trunk several degrees caudad and flexing it forwards a little, the chiropractor increases the joint pre-load tension. The impulse is made rapidly in equal and opposite directions along the plane line of the joint, combined with moderate distraction in long axis. Little depth of thrust is needed to achieve a joint release.

Superior to inferior technique:

Application

Joint play glide loss of the 1st metatarsal from superior to inferior on the 1st phalanx.

Patient's position

As for inferior to superior technique

Chiropractor's stance

As for inferior to superior technique.

Contact

The hands are reversed.

a) The middle finger of the left hand contacts the inferior surface of the base of the first phalanx and is supported closely by the remaining fingers.

b) The first finger of the right hand contacts the dorsal surface of the 1st metatarsal head and is supported closely by the remaining fingers.

Procedure

As for inferior to superior technique.

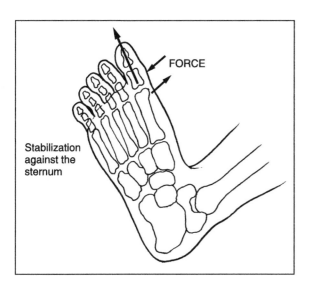

Fig. 8.10.2(a)

The arrows show the directions of the adjustive forces. The lateral border of the foot is stabilized against the chiropractor's sternum

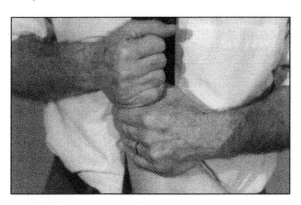

Fig. 8.10.2(b)

To enhance the joint pre-load tension, the chiropractor's trunk is rotated several degrees caudad and then flexed forwards a little

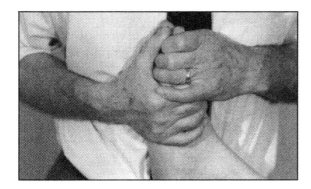

Fig. 8.10.2(c)

Superior to inferior. This technique is similar to the previous technique but with the hand positions reversed

8.10.3 Supine 1st metatarso-phalangeal long axis distraction technique – Method I

Application
Joint play loss of the 1st metatarsal and the 1st phalanx on long axis extension.

Patient's position
The patient is placed supine with the leg on the affected side fully extended.

Chiropractor's stance
The chiropractor sits at the foot end of the treatment table on the affected side, facing the mid-line of the patient, with the trunk rotated slightly cephalad.

Contact
a) The left hand is turned palm upwards. The 1st phalanx of the great toe is held firmly between the chiropractor's first and middle fingers.
b) The right hand firmly holds the distal end of the 1st metatarsal, the fingers wrapped over the dorsum of the foot, the thumb placed under the plantar surface of the foot.

Procedure
The right hand stabilizes the first metatarsal and the rest of the foot. The left hand tractions until tissue tension is felt. Without slackening the tension, an impulse with rapid minimum depth is made along the long axis of the joint.

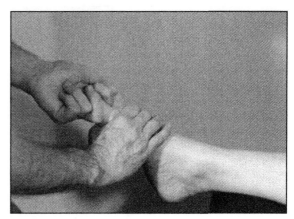

Fig. 8.10.3

To support the two fingers contacting the proximal phalanx, the web of the right hand is pressed against them

8.10.4 Supine 1st metatarso-phalangeal long axis distraction technique – Method II

Application
Joint play glide loss of the 1st metatarsal on the 1st phalanx in long axis extension.

Patient's position
The patient is placed supine with the affected leg extended and the hip flexed about 45°.

Chiropractor's stance
The chiropractor stands at the foot end of the treatment table on the affected side, facing caudad. The patient's extended affected leg is lifted to about 45° and held at the region of the mid-calf, under the left upper arm.

Contact
a) The right hand is held palm upwards. The patient's great toe is held firmly between the index and middle fingers around the first phalanx. These two fingers are curled back towards the palm of the hand. The right elbow is held high.

b) The web of the left hand is placed palm downwards over the dorsum of the foot to contact the right index and middle fingers to support them.

Procedure
Without flexing the great toe, a rapid impulse is made directly away from the contact.

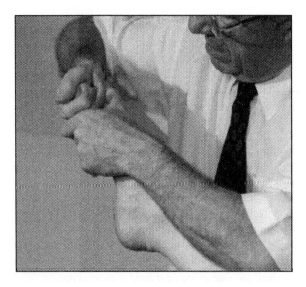

Fig. 8.10.4

The patient's heel is placed on the chiropractor's knee for support. The elbow is held very high to avoid toe flexion on extension

8.10.5 Supine 1st metatarso-phalangeal long axis distraction technique – Method III

Application
Joint play glide loss of the 1st metatarsal and 1st phalanx on long axis extension.

Patient's position
The patient is placed supine with the leg on the affected side fully extended and raised to about 45° by flexing the hip.

Contact
a) The index and middle fingers of the right hand grasp around the proximal phalanx from the inferior, with the elbow held high and the fingers pointing upwards.

b) The web of the supporting left hand is placed around the fingers of the right hand, with the palm against the dorsum of the patient's foot. For added support, the forearm may be held low and pressed against the patient's lower leg and ankle.

Procedure
A rapid impulse is made with the right arm directly away from the contact. If mobility restriction is found in other planes, for example rotation or plantarflexion loss, the impulse may be directed to include this additional direction component.

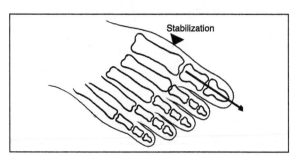

Fig. 8.10.5(a)

The directions of the adjustive forces and stabilization of the metatarsals

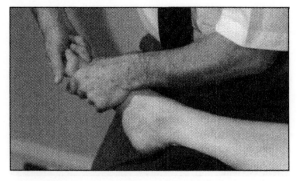

Fig. 8.10.5(b)

The left hand firmly supports the distal metatarsals and presses the patient's heel downwards

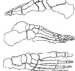

8.10.6 Prone 2nd to 5th metatarso-phalangeal inferior to superior direct thrust technique

Application
Joint play glide loss of the metatarsal from inferior to superior on the proximal phalanx.

Patient's position
The patient is placed prone with the affected leg flexed at the knee.

Chiropractor's stance
The chiropractor stands on the affected side facing caudad and with the left foot placed well ahead of the right.

Contact
a) The left hand is placed palm upwards under the dorsal surface of the patient's foot from the lateral side. The hand is placed so that the palm is directly beneath the line of metatarso-phalangeal joints.
b) The thumb of the right hand is placed directly over the inferior surface of the metatarso-phalangeal joint to be treated, the thenar eminence resting on the plantar surface of the foot.

Procedure
The chiropractor leans forwards on to the left leg. This movement extends the patient's knee, plantarflexing the ankle and the toes. Joint pre-load tension should now be felt. Continuing in a smooth motion, the chiropractor's right thumb impulses towards the palm of the right hand. Little depth of thrust is needed to effect a joint release.

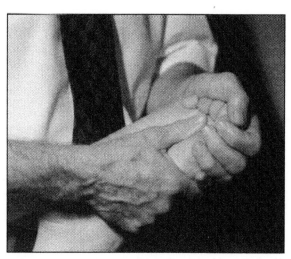

Fig. 8.10.6(a)

The right thumb contacts the inferior of the metatarsal. The heel of the left hand supports the dorsum of the foot and the fingers plantarflex the toes as the knee is extended and the ankle plantarflexed

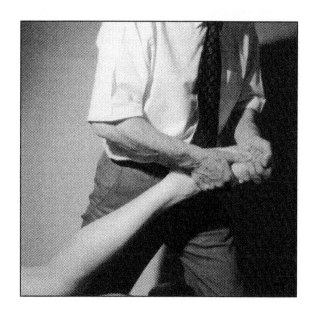

Fig. 8.10.6(b)

The chiropractor leans forward to produce joint pre-load tension before the thrust is given

8.10.7 Supine 2nd to 5th metatarso-phalangeal flexion/distraction technique

Application
Joint play glide loss of long axis extension and plantarflexion of the 2nd to 5th phalanges on the adjacent metacarpals.

Patient's position
The patient is placed supine with the leg on the affected side extended.

Chiropractor's stance
The chiropractor stands or sits on the affected side at the foot end of the treatment table facing cephalad.

Contact
The fingers of both hands are flexed and laced together with the right index finger on top. The laced fingers are then placed under the plantar surface of the base of the phalanx to be adjusted. The thumbs are placed on top of each other over the dorsal surface just distal to the joint.

Procedure
The patient's toe is plantarflexed and distracted in long axis extension until joint tension is reached. This is carried out to the patient's tolerance. Without slackening the tension, the chiropractor lifts his hands, to slightly dorsiflex the ankle and further distract the joint to produce the pre-load tension. The impulse is made towards the chiropractor with rapidity and with little depth of thrust.

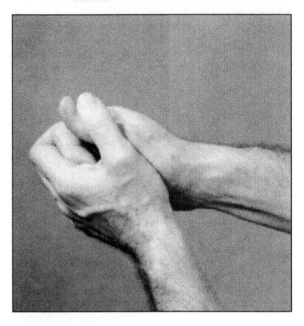

Fig. 8.10.7(a)

The position of the hands. The fingers are laced together making a stable platform under the proximal phalanx. The double thumb contact is placed over the anterior proximal phalanx, close up to the joint

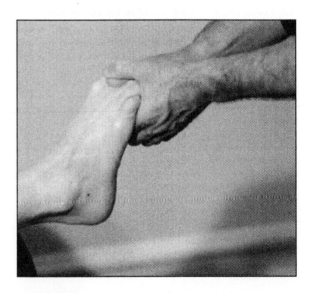

Fig. 8.10.7(b)

The final position for the technique. Before the adjustive thrust is employed, the toe is first plantarflexed to tolerance and distracted a little to produce joint pre-load tension

Intermetatarsal techniques

8.10.8   Supine intermetatarsal clasp mobilization technique

Application
Stiffness and restriction of movement between adjacent metatarsals.

Patient's position
The patient is placed supine with the legs fully extended.

Chiropractor's stance
The chiropractor stands at the foot end of the treatment table, facing cephalad.

Contact
The fingers of both hands are laced together, palms facing towards each other.
a)   The left hand is placed over the dorsum of the foot from the lateral side, with the fingers pointing towards the medial side.
b)   The right hand is placed under the plantar surface of the foot.

Procedure
The medial of the two adjacent metatarsals affected is placed against the heel of the left (upper) hand. The heel of the right hand is placed against the lateral of the two metatarsals. The chiropractor's hands are first separated a little, then brought very rapidly and forcefully together, the heel of the right hand striking towards the palm of the left. This has the effect of moving the lateral metatarsal into dorsiflexion and the medial one into plantarflexion. This procedure may be repeated several times as necessary. The strike bias may be reversed if restrictions are found in the opposite direction to those described above.

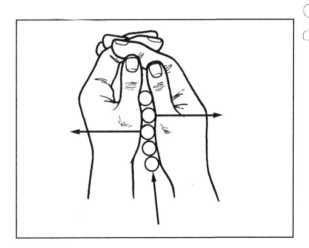

Fig. 8.10.8(a)

The strike bias shown here can be reversed

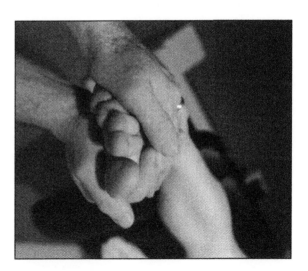

Fig. 8.10.8(b)

Supine metatarsal clasp technique

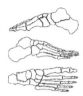

8.10.9 Prone intermetatarsal clasp mobilization technique

Application
Stiffness and restriction of movement between adjacent metatarsals.

Patient's position
The patient is placed prone with the leg on the affected side flexed to 45–55°.

Chiropractor's stance
The chiropractor stands on the homolateral side facing caudad.

Contact
The fingers of both hands are laced together, with the palms facing each other.
a) The left hand is placed around the dorsum of the foot from the lateral side.
b) The right hand is placed over the plantar surface of the foot from the medial side.

Procedure
The heel of the left hand is placed against the lateral of the two adjacent metatarsals affected and the heel of the right hand is placed against the medial of the two. The heels of the hands are first separated and then brought very rapidly together again, so that the heel of the left hand strikes towards the palm of the right hand. This has the effect of moving the medial metatarsal into dorsiflexion and the lateral one into plantarflexion. This procedure may be repeated several times as necessary. The strike bias may also be reversed if required.

Note
This mobilization method can also be employed as an intermetacarpal and carpal mobilization technique.

8.10.10 Supine and prone intermetatarsal shuttle mobilization technique

Application
Stiffness and restriction of movement between adjacent metatarsals.

Patient's position
The patient is placed supine with the affected leg extended or prone with the knee on the affected side flexed.

Chiropractor's stance
The chiropractor stands at the foot end of the treatment table facing cephalad favouring the side of involvement.

Contact
With the palms facing each other and the fingers close together and parallel to the tibia, the hands are placed one on each side of the affected foot.

Procedure
Maintaining a firm contact on the lateral and medial borders of the foot, the hands are moved up and down in a see-saw motion (see shuttle mobilization technique, Chapter 2) bringing the foot repeatedly into inversion and evertion.

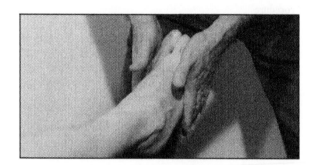

Fig. 8.10.10(a)

The patient is supine. With the palms facing each other and the fingers pointing downwards, the hands are moved repeatedly in opposite directions, bringing the foot into inversion followed by eversion

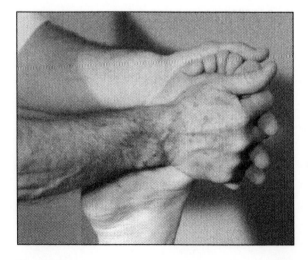

Fig. 8.10.9

Prone intermetatarsal mobilization technique

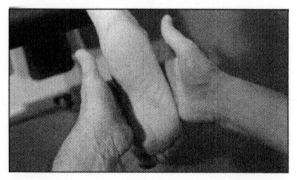

Fig. 8.10.10(b)

The patient is prone. The hands, palms facing, contact the medial and lateral borders of the foot, working in a see-saw movement

Metatarso-tarsal techniques

8.10.C Joint play evaluation of the tarsals and metatarsals on the medial side of the foot: inferior to superior and superior to inferior glide

Procedure

1) The patient lies supine with the foot relaxed. The left hand is placed over the dorsum of the mid- and fore-foot. The fingers of the right hand hold around the patient's heel to stabilize the hind foot. The anterior tip of the right thumb is first placed against the inferior border of the navicular and is pressed firmly upwards. As the right thumb presses a tarsal upward in passive movement, the left hand presses the foot downwards into plantarflexion, enhancing the pressure exerted by the right thumb. If no resistance is detected, the right thumb presses next against the inferior of the 1st cuneiform and on to the inferior of the first metatarsal in succession. The 2nd and 3rd cuneiforms are similarly tested as are the 2nd and 3rd metatarsals in succession.

   If resistance is detected by the right thumb against any of the joints in the complex, it is then necessary to isolate which articulation or articulations are fixated. For example, if fixation is met to upward pressure under the navicular, it is essential to test which one, or more, of its five articulations is involved before treatment can accurately be applied. This can be done quite rapidly.

2) **Isolating fixations in the intertarsal and metatarso-tarsal joint complex**

   When joint mobility restriction of a tarsal or metatarsal is found by the procedure described above, the particular articulation involved may be isolated as follows:

   - While still maintaining the thumb pressure from the inferior, the other thumb presses firmly downwards from the superior border of each of the neighbouring articulating bones in turn, along the plane lines of the joints. This challenges the function of each of the individual joints.
   - Resistance will be felt as a hard end-feel on the articulation which is fixated.
   - The appropriate adjustment can then be selected and applied with contacts on the adjacent bones, and the force applied in the direction in which joint play glide is lost.
   - Not infrequently in chronic cases, fixation of a joint will be detected in more than one direction. This is determined by reversing the thumbs and applying the pressure in the opposite directions. This type of fixation may require a separate adjustment in each direction of mobility loss in order to correct it. In some cases, however, it is seen clinically that the correction of a fixation in one plane will mobilize the joint in other planes as well.
   - Faye also points out, 'It is not unusual for joint play to be restricted in some planes and not others' (Schafer and Faye, 1990).

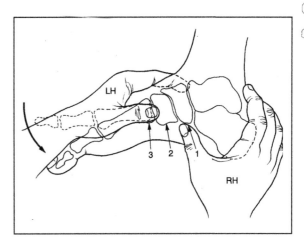

Fig. 8.10.C(a)

Medial view of the right foot. Inferior to superior glide. The thumb presses superior on 1 the navicular, 2 the 1st cuneiform, and 3 the 1st metatarsal. The left hand blocks movement of the remaining joints and plantarflexes the foot

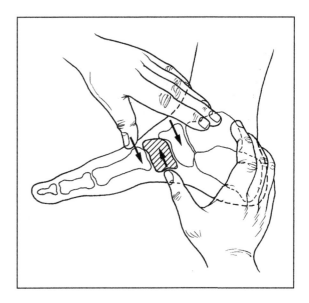

Fig. 8.10.C(b)

Medial view of the right foot. Isolating the fixation. Pressure is maintained by the right thumb while the left thumb, pressing downwards, assesses the joint play of 1 the navicular and 2 the 1st metatarsal in succession

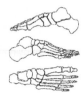

8.10.D   Joint play evaluation of the 1st metatarsal on the 1st cuneiform: inferior to superior and superior to inferior glide

Procedure

1) Example: Joint play glide loss of the 1st metatarsal from superior to inferior on the 1st cuneiform is detected as a hard resistance to opposing pressures by the thumbs. The adjustive correction is made in the direction in which joint play is lost.
2) If joint play glide loss is detected, the joint should also be examined for motion integrity in all other planes in which it normally moves. In this example, joint play is tested from superior to inferior, then the thumbs are reversed as illustrated. Opposing thumb pressure is then used to test whether joint play glide loss is also present from inferior to superior.

8.10.E   Joint play evaluation of the tarsals and metatarsals on the lateral side of the foot: inferior to superior and superior to inferior glide

Procedure

The tarsals and metatarsals on the lateral side of the foot are also examined using the same method as on the medial side. First the presence of fixation is detected by thumb pressure on the underside of the tarsal or metatarsal using the left hand. The foot is put into plantar flexion with the right hand over the dorsum of the mid- and forefoot, enhancing the pressure of the left thumb on the calcaneus, cuboid and 4th and 5th metatarsals successively. If a fixation is detected, shearing stress is used by applying pressure with the right thumb from the superior border on the adjacent bones to isolate the articulations involved.

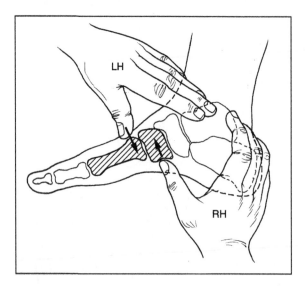

Fig. 8.10.D(a)

Medial view of the right foot. Joint play glide loss from superior to inferior of the 1st metatarsal on the 1st cuneiform

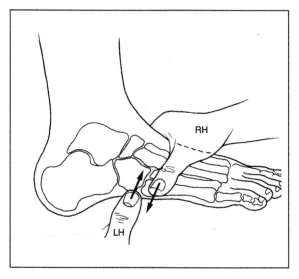

Fig. 8.10.E

Lateral view of the right foot. With the left thumb maintaining a firm pressure from under the cuboid, by pressing inferiorly on the bases of the metatarsals in turn, joint restriction can be isolated. Shown here is an inferior pressure on the fifth metatarsal

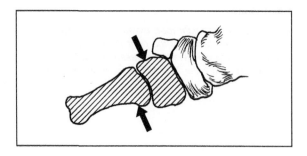

Fig. 8.10.D(b)

Medial view of the right foot. The thumbs are reversed to test for joint play glide loss from inferior to superior

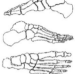

8.10.11 Supine 1st metatarsal on the 1st cuneiform superior to inferior traction/leverage distraction technique

Application
Joint play glide loss from superior to inferior of the 1st metatarsal on the 1st cuneiform.

Patient's position
The patient is placed supine with the affected extended and relaxed. The patient's leg is elevated and the foot is dorsiflexed.

Chiropractor's stance
The chiropractor stands on the affected side at the foot end of the treatment table facing cephalad, with the left foot ahead of the right.

Contact
a) The anterior surface of the joint between the 1st and 2nd phalanges of the right hand is placed over the dorsal surface of the 1st metatarsal just distal to the joint. The hand wraps around the patient's foot with the thumb placed under the distal end of the metatarsal.
b) The left hand supports the right hand by interlacing the fingers. The left thumb wraps around the lateral border of the foot and is placed over the right thumb to form a double thumb contact under the distal end of the 1st metatarsal.

Procedure
The patient's foot is further dorsiflexed until joint tension is felt. The leg is tractioned by the chiropractor leaning backwards without bending the trunk. The foot is medially rotated to provide some protection to the patient's hip. Without slackening the traction, a fast minimal depth impulse is made straight towards the chiropractor.

Note
Due to the long leverage employed in this technique, it should be used with caution, especially with the elderly or infirm. It should be avoided with osteoporotic patients or where joint surgery has been performed on the limb proximal to the contact.

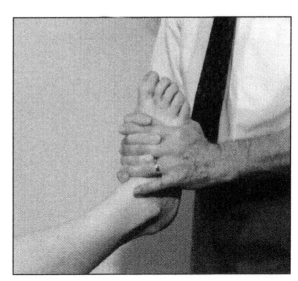

Fig. 8.10.11(a)

The contact is held firmly by interlacing the fingers

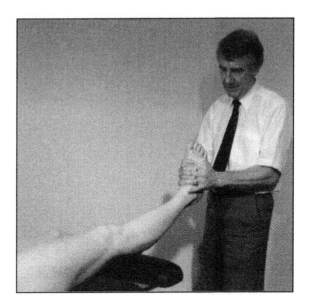

Fig. 8.10.11(b)

By leaning back and keeping the trunk straight, the chiropractor's body weight assists in achieving joint distraction

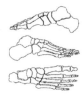

8.10.12   Supine 2nd or 3rd metatarsal/2nd or 3rd cuneiform traction leverage technique

Application
Joint play glide loss of the 2nd or 3rd metatarsal from superior to inferior on either the 2nd or 3rd cuneiform, as applicable following joint play analysis.

Patient's position
The patient is placed supine with the leg on the affected side held relaxed and fully extended, and elevated to 30–40°.

Chiropractor's stance
The chiropractor stands at the foot end of the treatment table, with the right leg ahead of the left, facing cephalad and favouring the side of involvement. The right leg is held straight and the left leg is kept slightly flexed.

Contact
The anterior second phalanx of the middle finger of either hand is used as the contact. The fingers of both hands are laced together over the dorsum of the patient's foot to reinforce the contact on the superior border of the second or third metatarsal base. A double thumb contact under the distal end of the same metatarsal enhances the leverage on the joint being adjusted.

Procedure
The elbows are held to the sides and flexed to about 90°. The trunk and the right leg are held stiff and erect and the weight placed back over the left, slightly flexed leg. Joint pre-load tension is obtained by rotating the trunk several degrees to the left, which has the effect of inverting the patient's foot. By dorsiflexing the foot there is a dual effect of enhancing the joint tension for the adjustment and stabilizing the ankle joint. Without releasing the tension, a quick minimal depth impulse is made in a caudad direction.

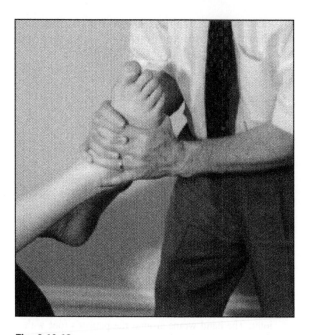

Fig. 8.10.12

Joint pre-load tension is achieved both by rotating the trunk to the left thus inverting the foot, and by dorsiflexing the patient's ankle

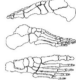

8.10.13   Supine 1st metatarsal/1st cuneiform inferior to superior short lever pull technique

Application
Joint play glide loss of the 1st metatarsal from inferior to superior on the 1st cuneiform.

Patient's position
The patient is placed supine with the leg on the affected side fully extended.

Chiropractor's stance
The chiropractor either sits or stands on the homolateral side, level with the patient's affected foot, facing the patient's mid-line.

Contact
a)   The left hand wraps over the dorsum of the foot from the lateral side. The middle finger contacts the inferior surface of the 1st metatarsal, supported closely by the remaining fingers.
b)   The right hand wraps under the plantar surface of the foot from the medial side. The index finger contacts the superior surface of the 1st cuneiform supported closely by the remaining fingers.

Procedure
Joint tension is achieved in the following stages:
1)   *The lateral border of the patient's foot is placed vertically along the chiropractor's mid-sternum.*
2)   *The chiropractor's trunk is then rotated several degrees caudad.*
3)   *The chiropractor's elbows are kept at approximately 90°, are relaxed and drawn into the sides.*
4)   *The chiropractor's trunk is flexed several degrees forwards and joint pre-load tension will then be felt.*
Typical short lever pull technique (see Chapter 2) is applied by swiftly approximating the scapulae, producing a thrust in equal and opposite directions across the joint.

Note
This is one of the most common foot fixations which the author has encountered in clinical practice.

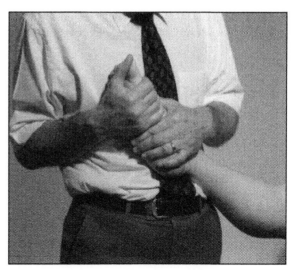

Fig. 8.10.13(a)

The chiropractor is standing, with the trunk rotated caudad and flexed forwards to obtain joint pre-load tension

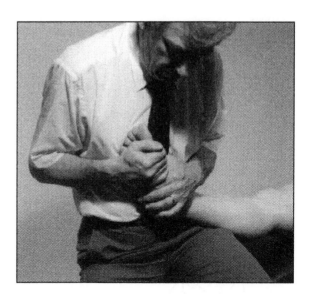

Fig. 8.10.13(b)

The chiropractor is sitting, with the patient's lower leg and ankle resting on the left thigh. The foot is held against the sternum

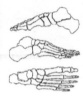

8.10.14 Supine 1st metatarsal/1st cuneiform superior to inferior short lever pull technique

Application
Joint play glide loss from superior to inferior of the 1st metatarsal on the 1st cuneiform.

Patient's position
The patient is placed supine with the leg on the affected side fully extended and abducted approximately 20–30°.

Chiropractor's stance
The chiropractor may sit or stand facing the patient's midline at the foot end of the treatment table, opposite the patient's affected foot.

Contact
a) The left hand is wrapped over the dorsum of the foot towards the medial border. The index finger contacts the 1st cuneiform on the inferior surface. The remaining fingers support it closely.

b) The right hand is passed under the plantar surface of the foot and reaches around so that the middle finger contacts the superior surface of the 1st metatarsal. The remaining fingers support it closely.

Procedure
1) The lateral border of the patient's foot is placed against the chiropractor's mid-sternum.
2) The chiropractor flexes the trunk forward and rotates caudad.
3) The elbows are brought to the sides.

The adjustive impulse is produced by rapidly contracting the rhomboids, thus approximating the scapulae, and bringing both shoulders posterior. Little depth of thrust is required and joint release is easily obtained. The thrust is made by both arms in equal and opposite directions, along the plane line of the joint.

This fixation may also be corrected using SLPT, with the patient prone (see technique 8.10.15).

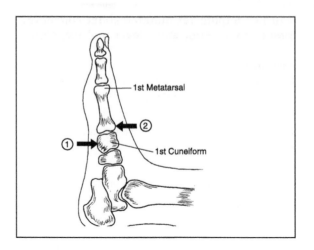

Fig. 8.10.14(b)

The lateral border of the foot is placed vertically along the sternum. Arrow 1 shows where the left index finger contacts the inferior surface of the 1st cuneiform. The right hand approaches from the opposite side and arrow 2 shows where the middle finger contacts the superior surface of the 1st cuneiform

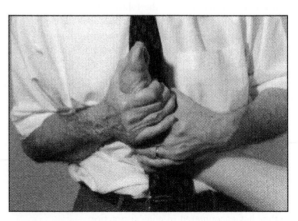

Fig. 8.10.14(c)

The trunk is rotated a few degrees in a caudad direction and then flexed forwards until joint pre-load tension is felt. Alternatively, the chiropractor may sit lateral to the foot, facing the patient's mid-line with the lower leg and ankle rested across the chiropractor's knee

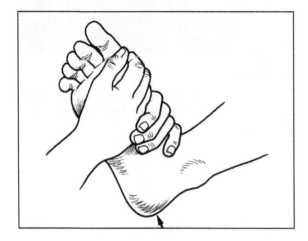

Fig. 8.10.14(a)

The position of the hands

8.10.15   Prone 1st metatarsal/1st cuneiform superior to inferior short lever pull technique

Application
Joint play glide loss of the 1st metatarsal from superior to inferior on the 1st cuneiform.

Patient's position
The patient is placed prone with the knee on the affected side flexed to approximately 90°. The affected foot is plantarflexed.

Chiropractor's stance
The chiropractor stands on the affected side facing caudad and bends forward to place the lateral border of the patient's right foot along the sternum.

Contact
a)   The left hand reaches around the dorsum of the foot to the medial side and the index finger contacts the inferior surface of the 1st cuneiform.
b)   The right hand is wrapped around the medial border of the foot and the middle finger contacts the superior surface of the 1st metatarsal base just distal to the joint.

Procedure
The chiropractor turns further caudad, which slightly increases the plantarflexion of the patient's foot, and by flexing the trunk forwards and bringing the elbows to the sides, joint pre-load tension will be felt. The impulse is achieved by rapidly approximating the scapulae (see short lever technique, Chapter 2).

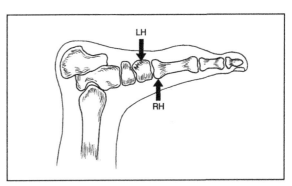

Fig. 8.10.15(a)

Medial view of the inverted right foot. The arrows show the direction of joint play glide loss of the 1st metatarsal from superior to inferior on the 1st cuneiform

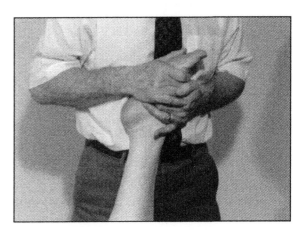

Fig. 8.10.15(b)

The lateral border of the foot is stabilized against the chiropractor's mid-sternal area

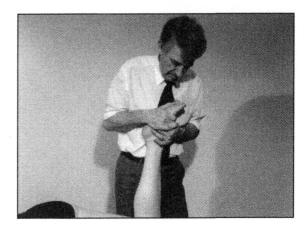

Fig. 8.10.15(c)

The chiropractor stands adjacent to the affected foot, with the elbows flexed to approximately 90° and drawn down and relaxed to the sides. The height of the treatment table should be adjusted to allow for this

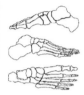

8.10.16 Prone 1st metatarsal/1st cuneiform inferior to superior short lever pull technique

Application
Joint play glide loss of the 1st metatarsal from inferior to superior on the 1st cuneiform.

Patient's position
The patient is placed prone with the knee on the affected side flexed to approximately 90°. The affected foot is plantarflexed.

Chiropractor's stance
The chiropractor stands on the affected side facing caudad and bends forwards to place the lateral border of the patient's right foot along the sternum.

Contact
a) The middle finger of the left hand contacts the inferior surface of the base of the 1st metatarsal. The contact is made secure by support from the remaining fingers held tightly up against it.
b) The index finger of the right hand wraps around the medial border of the foot and contacts the superior surface of the 1st cuneiform, supported closely by the remaining fingers.

Procedure
The chiropractor turns further caudad, which slightly increases the plantarflexion of the patient's foot, and by flexing the trunk forwards and bringing the elbows to the sides, joint pre-load tension will be felt. The impulse is achieved by rapidly approximating the scapulae (see short lever technique, Chapter 2).

8.10.17 Prone 2nd metatarsal/1st cuneiform superior to inferior short lever pull technique

Application
Joint play glide loss of the 2nd metatarsal from superior to inferior on the 1st cuneiform.

Patient's position
The patient is placed prone with the knee on the affected side flexed to approximately 90° and the affected foot is plantarflexed.

Chiropractor's stance
The chiropractor stands on the affected side facing caudad and bends forwards to place the lateral border of the patient's right foot along the sternum.

Contact
a) The middle finger of the left hand reaches medially around the foot to contact the inferior of the 2nd metatarsal, supported by the remaining fingers. To make the best contact, the middle and distal digits must be flexed, and held flexed throughout the procedure.

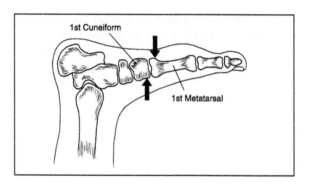

Fig. 8.10.16(a)

Medial view of the inverted right foot. The arrows show the direction of joint play glide loss of the 1st metatarsal from inferior to superior on the 1st cuneiform

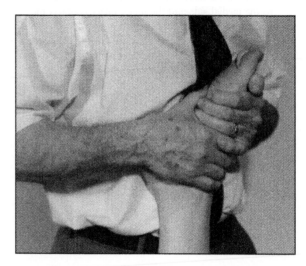

Fig. 8.10.16(b)

Inferior to superior short lever pull technique. The left middle finger contacts the inferior surface of the 1st cuneiform. The right index finger contacts the superior surface of the 1st cuneiform. Both contacts are supported closely by the other fingers

b)   The index finger of the right hand contacts the superior surface of the 1st cuneiform, supported by the remaining fingers.

Procedure

The chiropractor turns further caudad, which slightly increases the plantarflexion of the patient's foot, and by flexing the trunk forwards and bringing the elbows to the sides, joint pre-load tension will be felt. The impulse is achieved by rapidly approximating the scapulae (see short lever technique, Chapter 2).

8.10.18   Supine 2nd metatarsal/1st cuneiform superior to inferior short lever pull technique

Application

Joint play glide loss from superior to inferior of the 2nd metatarsal on the 1st cuneiform.

Patient's position

The patient is placed prone with the knee on the affected side flexed to approximately 90°. The affected foot is plantarflexed.

Chiropractor's stance

The chiropractor stands on the affected side facing caudad and bends forward to place the lateral border of the patient's right foot along the sternum.

Contact

a)   The index finger of the left hand contacts the inferior surface of the 1st cuneiform, supported by the remaining fingers.

b)   The middle finger of the right hand contacts the superior border of the 2nd metatarsal, closely supported by the remaining fingers. The index and the middle fingers are held straight at the middle and distal phalanges.

Procedure

The chiropractor turns further caudad, which slightly increases the plantarflexion of the patient's foot, and by flexing the trunk forwards and bringing the elbows to the sides, joint pre-load tension will be felt. The impulse is achieved by rapidly approximating the scapulae (see short lever pull technique, Chapter 2).

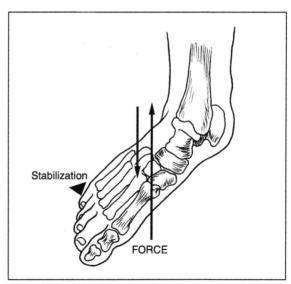

Fig. 8.10.18(a)

The direction of the adjustive forces on the joints

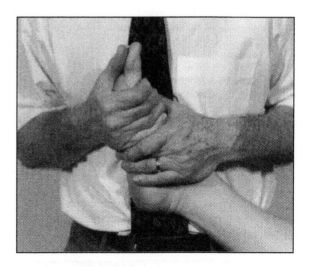

Fig. 8.10.18(b)

To make a firm contact, the index and middle fingers of the right hand are held as straight as possible at the middle and distal phalanges

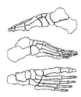

8.10.19 Prone 3rd metatarsal/2nd cuneiform superior to inferior short lever pull technique

Application
Joint play glide loss of the 3rd metatarsal from superior to inferior on the 2nd cuneiform.

Patient's position
The patient is placed prone with the knee on the affected side flexed to approximately 90° and the affected foot is plantarflexed.

Chiropractor's stance
The chiropractor stands on the affected side facing the patient's mid-line and bends forward to place the lateral border of the patient's right foot along the sternum.

Contact
a) The tips of the index finger and middle fingers of the left hand contact both the 1st and 2nd cuneiforms from the inferior. This is achieved by flexing the index and middle fingers and closing all the fingers together to support the contact.
b) The middle finger of the right hand stretches under the dorsum of the foot from the medial side, to contact the superior proximal base of the 3rd metatarsal. The proximal phalanx is flexed, the middle and distal phalanges are kept extended.

Procedure
The chiropractor turns further caudad, which slightly increases the plantarflexion of the patient's foot and by flexing the trunk forwards and bringing the elbows to the sides, joint pre-load tension will be felt. The impulse is achieved by rapidly approximating the scapulae (see short lever pull technique, Chapter 2) producing a force in equal and opposite directions across the contacts.

Note
If there is difficulty in holding the contact on the 3rd metatarsal, a piece of sticking plaster attached to the patient's skin prevents the contact from slipping.

8.10.20 Prone 1st, 2nd or 3rd metatarso-tarsal and intertarsal inferior to superior pectoralis/triceps thrust technique

Application
Joint play glide loss from inferior to superior of adjacent tarsals and 1st to 3rd metatarso-tarsal joints.

Patient's position
The patient is placed prone in a position which allows the leg on the affected side to hang freely over the side of the treatment table. Both the knee and hip are flexed to approximately 90°. The lower leg is kept parallel to the surface of the treatment table and the ankle is held in a neutral position.

Chiropractor's stance
The chiropractor crouches at the foot end of the treatment table on the affected side, facing cephalad and flexing the trunk forwards.

Contact
A double thumb contact is placed on the plantar surface of the tarsal or metatarsal to be adjusted. The fingers of both hands are wrapped around the sides of the foot and laced together over the dorsum, firmly contacting the adjacent tarsal or metatarsal.

Procedure
To relax the patient, the foot is pushed rhythmically headwards and footwards several times. The ankle is kept in a neutral position and the lower leg kept parallel to the surface of the treatment table throughout the procedure. As the patient's foot is being pushed headwards, the thrust is given by rapidly snapping the elbows into full extension. The travel is immediately restrained by the fingers laced over the dorsum of the foot, which contact the adjacent tarsal or metatarsal, thus reducing the amplitude of the thrust. See Fig. 8.10.20(a and b).

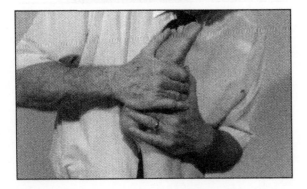

Fig. 8.10.19

The lateral border of the foot is held closely against the chiropractor's sternum. The elbows are held as close to 90° as possible

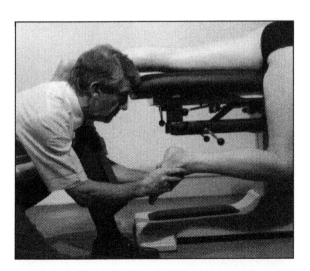

Fig. 8.10.20(a)

The final position for the set up. The patient's foot is placed in a neutral position and the lower leg kept parallel to the surface of the treatment table

8.10.21   Prone metatarso-tarsal and intertarsal superior to inferior pectoralis/triceps thrust and check technique

This is an adaptation of technique 8.10.20; to correct superior to inferior joint play glide loss of inter-tarsal or metatarso-tarsal joints.

Application
Joint play glide loss from inferior to superior of adjacent tarsals and 1st to 3rd metatarso-tarsal joints.

Patient's position
The patient is placed prone in a position which allows the leg on the affected side to hang freely over the side of the treatment table. Both the knee and hip are flexed to approximately 90°. The lower leg is kept parallel to the surface of the treatment table and the ankle is held in a neutral position.

Chiropractor's stance
The chiropractor crouches at the foot end of the treatment table on the affected side, facing cephalad and flexing the trunk forwards.

Contact
The laced fingers become the contact on the dorsum of the foot and the double thumb contact on the plantar surface is the stabilizer.

Procedure
The same rhythmical movement of the patient's leg is used to produce relaxation. As the foot is being pushed away, the thrust is made and immediately followed by a rapid snatch back towards the foot end of the table, to achieve the adjustment.

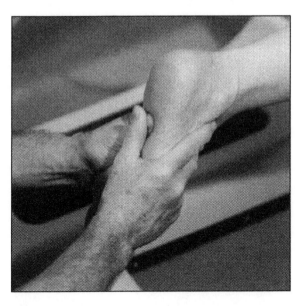

Fig. 8.10.20(b)

The thumbs are on the proximal contact and the crooked, laced index fingers are on the distal contact

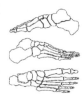

8.10.22 Standing metatarso-tarsal and intertarsal inferior to superior pectoralis/triceps thrust technique (sometimes inaccurately referred to as the 'Black Snake Whip')

Application
Joint play glide loss from inferior to superior of adjacent mid-tarsals and the 1st to 3rd metatarso-tarsal joints.

Patient's position
The patient stands facing away from the chiropractor, holding on to a support. The leg on the affected side is flexed at the hip and knee and remains so during the entire procedure.

Chiropractor's stance
The chiropractor crouches down behind the patient, favouring the affected side.

Contact
A double thumb contact is placed on to the plantar surface of the tarsal to be adjusted. The fingers of both hands are wrapped around the sides of the foot and laced together, grasping firmly around the dorsum, contacting the adjacent fixated tarsal or metatarsal, whichever is relevant.

Procedure

1) The affected foot is pushed forwards and upwards until it is adjacent to the opposite knee.
2) The foot is made to describe a large circle, starting towards the patient's mid-line, then downwards towards the opposite ankle.
3) As the foot approaches the mid-line, it is taken into eversion and the joint contacted is held in pre-load tension.
4) As the circle continues smoothly downwards, the pre-load tension is maintained on the foot by incorporating some plantarflexion in addition to the eversion.
5) At the bottom of the circle, the pre-load tension is still maintained by starting to invert the foot. At this point a fast impulse, with minimal depth, is made along the plane line of the joint to be adjusted. This is achieved by rapidly snapping the elbows into full extension using a pectoralis triceps thrust.

Caution
In order to avoid stress on the ligaments of the dorsum of the foot, great care must be taken not to increase the plantarflexion as the adjustive thrust is made.

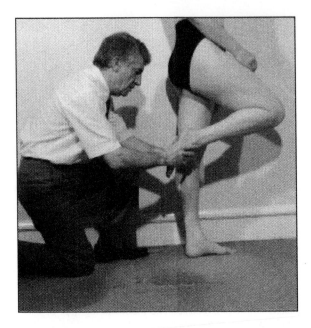

Fig. 8.10.22(a)

The patient's hip is held in a flexed position and the affected foot is held adjacent to the opposite knee. Minimal plantarflexion is made. A common error made when using this technique is to extend the hip and reduce the joint pre-load tension before the adjustive thrust is made

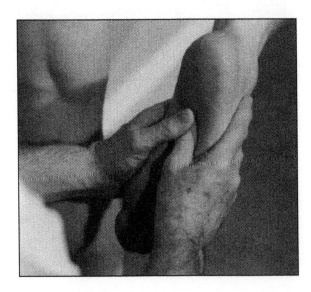

Fig. 8.10.22(b)

A double thumb contact is made on the plantar surface of the relevant metatarsal or tarsal and the foot describes a circle in a medial direction

8.10.23 Supine figure-of-eight metatarso-tarsal mobilization technique

Application
Mobility restriction and stiffness of the tarsals and metatarsals.

Patient's position
The patient is placed supine with the leg on the affected side fully extended.

Chiropractor's stance
The chiropractor stands at the foot end of the treatment table facing cephalad, favouring the affected side.

Contact
a) The left hand wraps over the dorsum of the distal end of the foot from the lateral side, covering the metatarsals. The thumb is placed against the plantar surface.
b) The right hand wraps over the proximal end of the dorsum of the foot from the medial side, covering the tarsals. The thumb is placed against the plantar surface proximal to the left thumb.

Procedure

1) (a) The left hand first plantarflexes the forefoot, inverts it and medially flexes it.
   (b) As the left hand inverts the forefoot, the right hand attempts to evert the hindfoot.
2) (a) Whilst holding the forefoot in inversion, the left hand then dorsiflexes and laterally flexes it. The right hand opposes this movement.
   (b) When the foot is fully dorsiflexed, the left hand everts the forefoot and the right hand attempts to invert the hindfoot.

This procedure is carried out smoothly and repeated to requirement and patient tolerance.

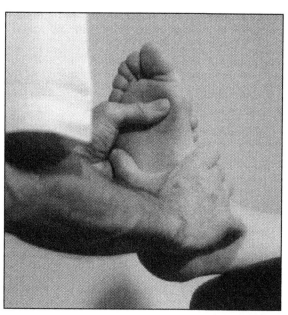

Fig. 8.10.23(a)

Stage 1: the left hand dorsiflexes the forefoot, inverts it and medially flexes it. The right hand resists the movement and everts the mid-foot

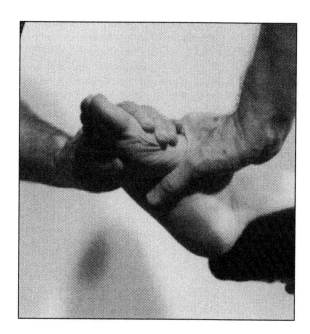

Fig. 8.10.23(b)

Stage 2: the forefoot is plantarflexed, laterally flexed and everted with the left hand. The right hand resists and attempts to dorsiflex and invert the tarsals

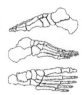

8.10.24 Supine 4th or 5th metatarso-cuboid superior to inferior short lever pull technique

Application
Joint play glide loss of the 4th or 5th metatarsal from superior to inferior on the cuboid.

Patient's position
The patient is placed supine with the leg on the affected side fully extended and abducted 20–30°.

Chiropractor's stance
The chiropractor sits or stands between the patient's legs, adjacent to the affected foot, facing laterally. The medial side of the patient's foot is placed against the mid-sternum.

Contact
a) The left hand reaches under the foot to the lateral side. The anterior middle phalanx of the middle finger is placed firmly over the superior aspect of the affected 4th or 5th metatarsal, as close to the joint as possible. The remaining fingers close up against it as support.

b) The right hand reaches over the dorsum of the mid-foot to the lateral side. The anterior of the middle phalanx of the middle finger is placed firmly under the inferior surface of the cuboid, as close to the joint as possible, with the remaining fingers closed up against it as support.

Procedure
To achieve joint tension, the chiropractor partially rotates the trunk caudad and draws the elbows gently to the sides. Standard short lever technique (see Chapter 2) is applied using a swift bilateral 'scissor-type' (see Glossary of Terms, p. 285) thrust. The impulse is made in equal and opposite directions across the joint.

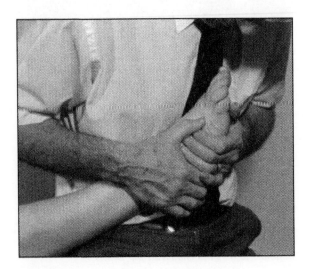

Fig. 8.10.24

The adjustment may be made either sitting as shown, or in the standing position

8.10.25 Supine 4th or 5th metatarso-cuboid inferior to superior short lever pull technique

Application
Joint play glide loss of the 4th or 5th metatarsal from inferior to superior on the cuboid.

Patient's position
The patient is placed supine with the leg on the affected side fully extended and abducted 20–30°.

Chiropractor's stance
The chiropractor sits or stands between the patient's legs, adjacent to the affected foot, facing laterally. The medial side of the patient's foot is raised and placed against the mid-sternum.

Contact
a) The middle finger of the left hand contacts the superior border of the cuboid, supported by the remaining fingers.

b) The middle finger of the right hand contacts the inferior border of the distal 4th or 5th metatarsal, supported by the remaining fingers.

Procedure
To achieve joint tension, the chiropractor partially rotates the trunk cephalad and draws the elbows gently to the sides. Standard short lever pull technique (see Chapter 2) is applied using a swift bilateral 'scissor-type' (see Glossary of Terms, p. 285) thrust. The impulse is made in equal and opposite directions.

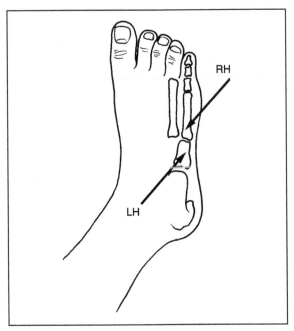

Fig. 8.10.25

The points of contact and the directions of the adjustive forces

8.10.26 Supine 4th or 5th metatarso-cuboid superior to inferior recoil technique

Application
Joint play glide loss from superior to inferior of either the 4th or 5th metatarsal on the middle or lateral cuneiform respectively.

Patient's position
The patient is placed supine with the affected leg flexed at the knee and the right foot placed flat on the treatment table, on a section with a drop mechanism. The patient's right hip is slightly medially rotated.

Chiropractor's stance
The chiropractor stands on the contralateral side, facing the patient's mid-line adjacent to the affected foot. The drop mechanism is set for the patient's weight and cocked.

Contact
The patient's right knee is gently pulled towards the chiropractor by adducting the hip, past the patient's mid-line and held there by pinning the patient's lower leg against the chiropractor's lower trunk with the medial border of the right upper arm.

a) The pisiform of the right hand contacts the relevant metatarsal base, the skin slack is taken downwards and a low arch (see Glossary of Terms, p. 285) position of the wrist is assumed.
b) The left hand is placed over the right wrist for a recoil adjustment (see Chapter 2).

Procedure
A high velocity recoil thrust (see Glossary of Terms, p. 285) initiated by the pectoralis triceps and anconius muscles is used.

8.10.27 Supine 4th or 5th metatarso-cuboid superior to inferior body drop thrust technique

Application
Joint play glide loss from superior to inferior of either the 4th or 5th metatarsal on the middle or lateral (3rd) cuneiform respectively.

Patient's position
The patient is placed supine with the affected leg flexed at the knee and the right foot placed flat on the treatment table, on a section with a drop mechanism. The patient's right hip is slightly medially rotated.

Chiropractor's stance
The chiropractor stands on the contralateral side, facing the patient's mid-line adjacent to the affected foot. The drop mechanism is set for the patient's weight and cocked.

Contact
The patient's right knee is gently pulled towards the chiropractor by adducting the hip, past the patient's mid-line and held there by pinning the patient's lower leg against the chiropractor's lower trunk with the medial border of the right upper arm.

a) The pisiform of the right hand contacts the relevant metatarsal base, the skin slack is taken downwards and a low arch (see Glossary of Terms, p. 285) position of the wrist is assumed.
b) The left hand is placed over the right wrist for a recoil adjustment (see Chapter 2).

Procedure
A rapid body drop technique is employed (see Chapter 2).

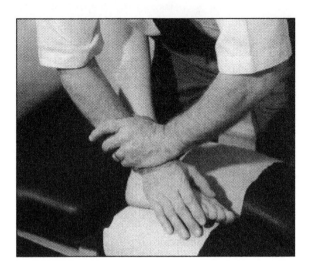

Fig. 8.10.26

The foot is placed flat on a drop section. Here the patient's foot is placed on the head piece of the treatment table. The knee is pulled over and held by the chiropractor's right arm and the skin slack is taken out downwards before the impulse is made

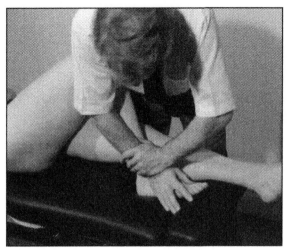

Fig. 8.10.27

An alternative method is the body drop thrust technique. The episternal notch is placed directly above the contact and a low arch hand position is used. Little depth of thrust is required

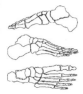

8.10.28   Prone 4th or 5th metatarso-cuboid superior to inferior short lever pull technique

Application
Joint play glide loss from superior to inferior of the 4th or 5th metatarsal on the cuboid.

Patient's position
The patient is placed prone with the leg on the affected side flexed to approximately 90° and the hip abducted approximately 30°.

Chiropractor's stance
The chiropractor stands or sits between the patient's legs facing laterally and adjacent to the patient's affected foot. The medial border of the patient's foot is placed along the chiropractor's sternum.

Contact
a) The middle finger of the left hand is placed over the lateral border of the foot and wrapped around to contact the superior surface of the relevant 4th or 5th metatarsal. The remaining fingers close around to support the contact. To increase the leverage, the left thumb is placed against the anterior distal end of the affected metatarsal.

b) The index finger of the right hand is placed right under the dorsum of the foot from the medial border to contact the inferior surface of the cuboid. The remaining fingers close around to support the contact.

Procedure
Standard short lever pull technique (see Chapter 2) is applied with the force applied in equal and opposite directions across the joint.

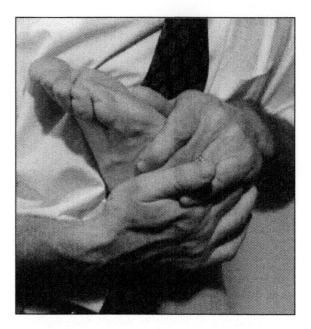

Fig. 8.10.28(b)

The index finger of the right hand contacts the inferior surface of the cuboid. The middle finger of the left hand contacts the superior surface of the relevant 4th or 5th metatarsal

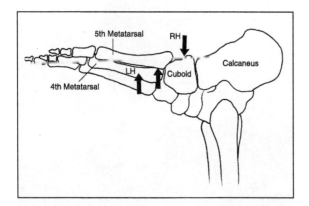

Fig. 8.10.28(a)

Lateral view of the right foot. The arrows show the direction of joint play glide loss from superior to inferior of either the 4th or 5th metatarsals on the cuboid

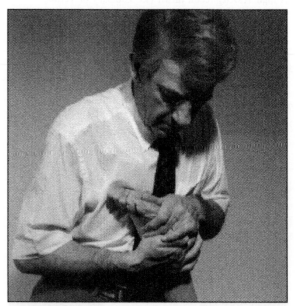

Fig. 8.10.28(c)

For this adjustment the chiropractor stands or sits between the patient's legs, facing laterally. The patient's knee is flexed to approximately 90°

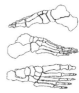

Intertarsal techniques

8.10.29 Supine navicular/1st cuneiform inferior to superior short lever pull technique

Application

Joint play glide loss from inferior to superior of the navicular on the 1st cuneiform.

Patient's position

The patient is placed supine with the limb on the affected side fully extended.

Chiropractor's stance

The chiropractor stands or sits facing the patient, lateral to and adjacent to the affected foot.

Contact

a) The left hand reaches over the dorsum of the foot from the lateral side and the anterior of the second phalanx of the index finger contacts the inferior surface of the navicular.

b) The right hand reaches under the plantar surface of the foot from the lateral side and the anterior of the second phalanx of the middle finger contacts over the superior surface of the 1st cuneiform.

Procedure

Joint pre-load tension is achieved as follows:

1) The lateral border of the foot is placed vertically along the chiropractor's sternum.

2) The trunk is then rotated several degrees caudad.

3) Whilst keeping the elbows flexed to about 90°, they are drawn in to the sides and kept relaxed.

4) The trunk is then flexed several degrees forwards until the joint tension is felt. Standard short lever pull technique (see Chapter 2) is then applied.

8.10.30 Supine navicular/1st cuneiform superior to inferior short lever pull technique

Application

Joint play glide loss from superior to inferior of the navicular on the 1st cuneiform.

Patient's position

The patient is placed supine with the limb on the affected side fully extended.

Chiropractor's stance

The chiropractor stands or sits facing the patient, lateral to and adjacent to the affected foot.

Contact

a) The left hand reaches under the plantar surface of the foot from the lateral side and the anterior of the second phalanx of the middle finger contacts over the superior surface of the 1st cuneiform.

b) The right hand reaches over the dorsum of the foot from the lateral side and the anterior of the second phalanx of the index finger contacts the inferior of the navicular.

Procedure

Joint pre-load tension is achieved as follows:

1) The lateral border of the foot is placed vertically along the chiropractor's sternum.

2) The trunk is then rotated several degrees caudad.

3) Whilst keeping the elbows flexed to about 90°, they are drawn in to the sides and kept relaxed.

4) The trunk is then flexed several degrees forwards until the joint tension is felt. Standard short lever pull technique (see Chapter 2) is then applied.

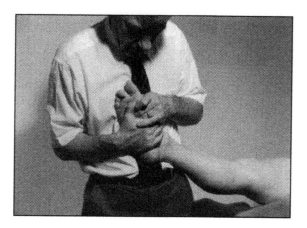

Fig. 8.10.29

The first finger of the left hand contacts the inferior of the navicular. The anterior of the middle finger of the right hand contacts the superior surface of the 1st cuneiform. The lateral border of the foot is held vertically against the sternum to stabilize the patient's lower leg

Fig. 8.10.30

The hands are reversed compared with technique 8.10.29. The middle finger of the left hand now contacts the inferior of the 1st cuneiform and the index finger of the right hand contacts the superior border of the navicular

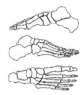

8.10.31 Prone talo-navicular inferior to superior short lever pull technique

Application
Joint play glide loss of the navicular from inferior to superior on the talus.

Patient's position
The patient is placed prone with the knee on the affected side flexed to 90°.

Chiropractor's stance
The chiropractor stands on the homolateral side, lateral to the patient's leg, facing medially and adjacent to the affected knee. The elbows are held flexed to approximately 90°.

Contact
a) The left hand reaches under the plantar surface of the foot from the lateral side. The anterior of the second phalanx of the middle finger reaches around to the medial border of the foot to contact the inferior surface of the navicular.
b) The right hand reaches over the plantar surface of the foot from the medial side. The anterior surface of the index finger contacts the superior border of the neck of the talus.

Procedure
The lateral border of the patient's foot is placed against the chiropractor's sternum. By rotating the trunk several degrees caudad and by flexing the trunk a little forwards, joint pre-load tension is achieved. Using standard short lever pull technique (see Chapter 2) the impulse is initiated by rapidly approximating the scapulae with the force exerted in equal and opposite directions at the contacts.

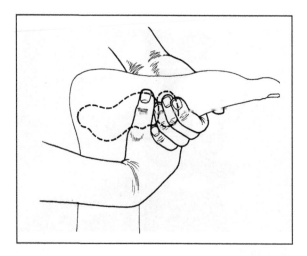

Fig. 8.10.31

The talus is stabilized by the right hand contacting the superior surface. The anterior surface of the middle finger of the left hand contacts the inferior surface of the navicular and is supported by the remaining fingers

8.10.32 Supine 1st and 2nd or 2nd and 3rd intercuneiform superior to inferior compression technique

Application
Joint play glide loss from superior to inferior of the 3rd cuneiform on the 2nd cuneiform.

Patient's position
The patient is placed supine or sitting, with the hip and knee on the affected side sufficiently flexed to allow the foot to rest flat on the treatment table.

Chiropractor's stance
The chiropractor stands on the homolateral side at the foot end of the treatment table facing cephalad, adjacent to the affected foot.

Contact
For the adjustment of the 2nd and 3rd cuneiforms:
a) The left hand is placed over the dorsum of the foot from the lateral side, using the pisiform low arch (see Glossary of Terms, p. 285) contact on the 3rd cuneiform.
b) The right hand is closed with the distal two phalanges of all fingers held straight and the thumb held to the side. The hand is then placed under the plantar surface of the foot so that the proximal end of the first phalanx of the middle finger (the knuckle) is beneath the 2nd cuneiform. The heel remains on the treatment table. If the cushion is soft, a stiffening board beneath the right hand may be necessary.

For the adjustment of the 1st and 2nd cuneiforms, the hands are reversed:
c) The left hand is closed, as described in (b) above, and placed under the plantar surface of the second cuneiform.
d) The right hand is placed over the dorsum of the foot, using a pisiform low arch contact on the 1st cuneiform.

Procedure
The chiropractor leans forwards over the contacts, using the body weight to achieve joint pre-load tension. Without releasing the tension, a shallow swift body drop technique (see Chapter 2) is employed with the pressure applied to the relevant cuneiform, compressing it downwards on its neighbour.

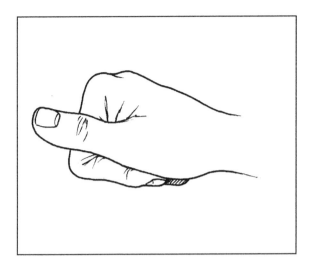

Fig. 8.10.32(a)

The right hand is closed with the distal digits of all fingers held flat. The knuckle of the 3rd metacarpal is used as the contact point

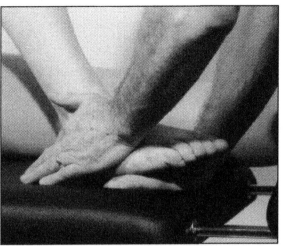

Fig. 8.10.32(b)

The right hand held closed is placed under the 2nd cuneiform. The patient's heel remains on the treatment table

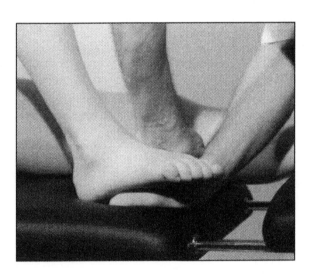

Fig. 8.10.32(c)

The hand positions are reversed when the 1st and 2nd cuneiforms are involved

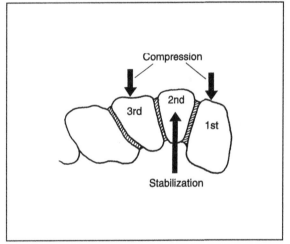

Fig. 8.10.32(d)

The 2nd cuneiform is stabilized on the plantar surface. Compression downwards, respecting the plane line of the joint, is directed on to the relevant 1st or 3rd cuneiform

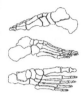

8.10.33 Supine 1st or 2nd cuneiform–navicular superior to inferior traction leverage technique

Application
Joint play glide loss of either the 1st or 2nd cuneiform from superior to inferior on the navicular.

Patient's position
The patient is placed supine with the leg on the affected side fully extended and with the hip abducted approximately 20° and flexed to approximately 30°. The other leg may be flexed a little and the foot placed on the foot rest to brace the patient if required.

Chiropractor's stance
The chiropractor stands at the foot end of the treatment table facing cephalad, favouring the side of the affected foot. The right leg is placed ahead of the left and fully extended. The hind left leg remains slightly flexed at the knee.

Contact
The fingers of both hands are laced together and placed over the dorsum of the foot so that the anterior of the middle phalanx of the left hand firmly contacts either the 1st or 2nd cuneiform, whichever is fixated. A double thumb contact is placed on the plantar surface of the foot.

Procedure
The chiropractor's elbows are held in semi-flexion. To achieve joint pre-load tension, the thumbs press the patient's foot into dorsiflexion and the laced fingers evert the foot. Traction on the joint is applied by pressing the trunk away from the contact with the leading right foot. Without slackening the tension, a quick impulse is made straight towards the chiropractor with minimal depth of thrust.

Note
Caution must be exercised whenever long lever techniques are employed.

8.10.34 Supine 3rd cuneiform–cuboid superior to inferior traction leverage technique

Application
Joint play glide loss of the 3rd cuneiform from superior to inferior on the cuboid.

Patient's position
The patient is placed supine with the leg on the affected side fully extended. The hip is abducted to approximately 20° and also flexed to between 20° and 30°. The other leg may be used as a brace by flexing the knee a little and placing the foot on the treatment table foot rest. The patient may also feel more secure if instructed to hold on to the sides of the treatment table.

Chiropractor's stance
The chiropractor stands at the foot end of the treatment table facing cephalad, favouring the side to be adjusted. The right foot, with the leg fully extended, is placed ahead of the left. The left knee remains flexed throughout the procedure.

Contact
The fingers of both hands are laced together and placed over the dorsum of the foot, ensuring that the anterior of the second phalanx of the middle finger of the left hand contacts the 3rd cuneiform on the superior border. Both thumbs are placed under the plantar surface of the foot.

Procedure
To achieve joint pre-load tension, both thumbs press the patient's foot up and into dorsiflexion, and into inversion by rotating the trunk to the left. Traction is then applied by pressing away from the contact with the leading right foot. Without slackening the tension, a rapid minimal depth impulse is made straight towards the chiropractor.

Note
Because the force is extended over several joints, great care must be taken when using traction leverage techniques.

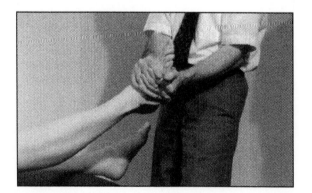

Fig. 8.10.33

The fingers are laced together and a middle finger, middle phalanx contact is used on the 1st or 2nd cuneiform

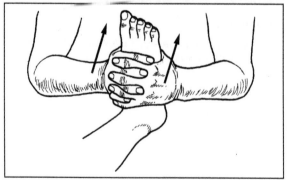

Fig. 8.10.34

The chiropractor dorsiflexes and inverts the foot as traction is applied

8.10.35 Supine calcaneo-cuboid superior to inferior traction/leverage technique

Application
Joint play glide loss of the cuboid from superior to inferior on the calcaneus.

Patient's position
The patient is placed supine with the affected limb extended and elevated to approximately 30°. The unaffected limb may be flexed at the knee and can be used to brace the patient by pressing the foot against the foot rest. The patient holds on to the sides of the treatment table to prevent sliding.

Chiropractor's stance
The chiropractor stands at the foot end of the treatment table facing cephalad with the right foot ahead of the left. The low back and thoracics are held erect.

Contact
Both hands are laced together. The anterior surface of the middle phalanx of the middle finger is placed over the superior surface of the cuboid. The arms are held out ahead with the elbows semi-flexed.

Procedure
To produce joint pre-load tension, the patient's foot is held in dorsiflexion throughout the procedure. The foot is rotated internally to afford protection to the ipsilateral coxal joint. While keeping the trunk erect, the chiropractor tractions the joint by pushing away from the contact with the leading foot. To apply the thrust, further traction is suddenly and rapidly applied towards the chiropractor with moderate depth of thrust.

Note
Because the force is applied over several joints, great care must be taken when using traction/leverage techniques. Speed of delivery and cautious control of thrust depth must be exercised. The use of traction/leverage techniques is not advised when treating the infirm, elderly or frail.

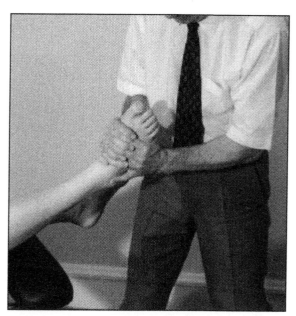

Fig. 8.10.35

Dorsiflexion of the foot helps to stabilize the ankle and the hip is medially rotated to aid stability

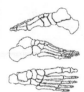

8.10.36   Prone calcaneo-cuboid inferior to superior short lever technique

Application
Joint play glide loss from inferior to superior of the cuboid on the calcaneus.

Patient's position
The patient is placed prone with the knee on the affected side flexed to approximately 40°.

Chiropractor's stance
The chiropractor sits between the patient's legs, facing laterally.

Contact
a)   The left hand is wrapped around the lateral border of the patient's foot from the posterior of the heel. The middle finger contacts the anterior aspect of the calcaneus as close to the cuboid as is practicable. The remaining fingers support the contact.

b)   The right hand reaches under the dorsum of the foot to the lateral side. The middle finger reaches around the lateral border to contact the inferior surface of the cuboid. The remaining fingers close up to produce a firm contact.

Procedure
The chiropractor rotates the trunk away from the contact approximately 30° caudad or until joint pre-load tension is felt. Trunk rotation also has the effect of plantarflexing the patient's mid-foot, opening the dorsal aspect of the calcaneo-cuboid joint. When joint tension has been achieved, a swift short lever (see Chapter 2) impulse is given in equal and opposite directions across the contacts.

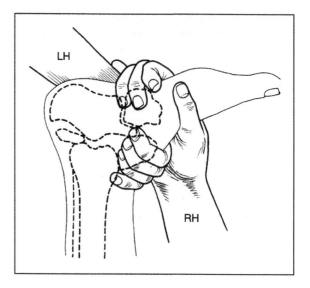

Fig. 8.10.36(a)

Medial view of the right foot, showing the contacts for the correction of joint play glide loss from inferior to superior of the calcaneus on the cuboid

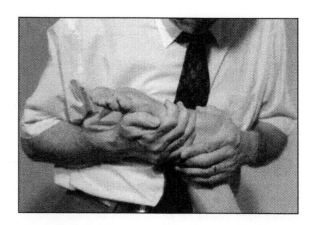

Fig. 8.10.36(b)

Lateral view of the right foot. The chiropractor's caudad trunk rotation assists in producing joint pre-load tension. To open the dorsal aspect of the calcaneo-cuboid joint, the foot is plantarflexed

8.10.37 Supine calcaneo-cuboid inferior to superior short lever technique

Application
Joint play glide loss from inferior to superior of the cuboid on the calcaneus.

Patient's position
The patient is placed supine in a relaxed position, with the legs spread apart.

Chiropractor's stance
The chiropractor either stands or sits between the patient's legs, facing laterally and adjacent to the affected foot.

Contact
a) The left hand is placed around the inferior medial aspect of the patient's foot to the lateral side. The lateral border of the hand (the knife edge) is then placed along the lateral border of the calcaneus with a firm contact.
b) The right hand is placed around the lateral border of the foot. A middle finger contact is made on the inferior aspect of the cuboid, as close to the joint with the calcaneus as possible, and the remaining fingers support the contact.

Procedure
To achieve joint pre-load tension, the chiropractor holds the medial border of the patient's affected foot vertically against the sternum and rotates the trunk several degrees in a caudad direction. The relaxed elbows are held close to the sides, bent at approximately 90°. Trunk rotation also plantarflexes the foot, opening the dorsal aspect of the calcaneo-cuboid joint. When joint tension has been achieved, a swift short lever (see Chapter 2) impulse is given with a force in equal and opposite directions across the contacts.

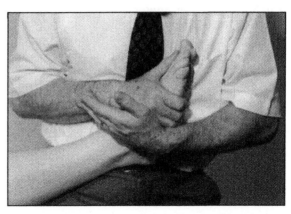

Fig. 8.10.37(a)

The knife-edge of the left hand is held firmly against the lateral border of the calcaneus to stabilize it

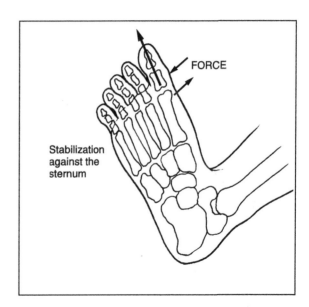

Fig. 8.10.37(b)

The contact on the calcaneus with the left hand is a broad one, using the lateral border of the hand to stabilize it. The arrows show the direction of the forces applied to the joint

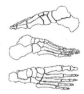
8.10.38 Prone calcaneo-cuboid inferior to superior thrust technique

Application
Joint play glide loss of the cuboid from inferior to superior on the calcaneus.

Patient's position
The patient is placed prone with the knee on the affected side flexed to 90°.

Chiropractor's stance
The chiropractor stands on the ipsilateral side facing caudad. It is necessary to have the patient on a low treatment table or to stand on a stool to achieve sufficient height above the patient to perform the adjustment.

Contact
a) The left hand slides under the dorsum of the foot from the lateral side to stabilize the cuboid and the other tarsals and prevents any movement of the patient's knee.

b) The right hand uses a low arch (see Glossary of Terms, p. 285) pisiform contact on the inferior ridge of the cuboid, just proximal to the peroneal sulcus. The fingers rest on the left wrist.

Procedure
The left hand plantarflexes and inverts the foot to produce joint tension and to stabilize it. The right hand then thrusts rapidly downwards and slightly laterally to respect the plane line of the joint. The patient's knee on the affected side must not be permitted to move during the procedure.

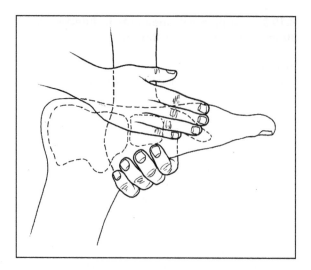

Fig. 8.10.38(a)

The chiropractor must be high enough above the patient to perform this technique efficiently. The patient's knee must not be permitted to move during the adjustment. The foot is first plantarflexed and inverted and the thrust with the right arm is from inferior to superior and slightly laterally to conform to the plane line of the joint

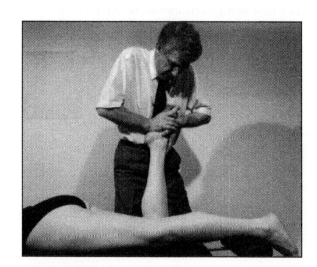

Fig. 8.10.38(b)

Joint pre-load tension is achieved by plantarflexing the foot

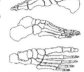

8.10.F   Joint play evaluation of the talus on the calcaneus

Procedure

The patient may be placed either prone or supine for this examination. When the patient is supine, the anterior aspect of the distal digit of the thumbs applies pressure across the joint. The thumb of the right hand contacts the posterior lateral side of the calcaneus and presses medially. The thumb of the left hand contacts the medial side of the talus and presses laterally. The pressure applied is in equal and opposite directions into joint play, which is felt as a perception of elasticity at the end of the movement induced by the pressure.

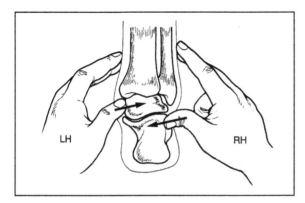

Fig. 8.10.G

Posterior view of the right foot. The patient is in the prone position

8.10.39   Prone talo-calcaneal lateral to medial short lever technique

Application

Joint play glide loss from lateral to medial of the calcaneus on the talus.

Patient's position

The patient is placed prone with the knee on the affected side flexed to 90° and the hip abducted.

Chiropractor's stance

Facing laterally, the chiropractor stands between the patient's legs, adjacent to the knee on the affected side.

Contact

a) The left hand is placed around the calcaneus from the lateral side with the fingers tightly grasping the medial side.

b) The index and middle fingers of the right hand contact the talus around the lateral side of the foot over the dorsum and contact the medial border. The remaining fingers support the contact.

Procedure

Using standard short lever technique (see Chapter 2), the elbows are drawn to the sides, the trunk is rotated a little to the right to achieve joint pre-load tension and the impulse is made with equal and opposite force across the contacts.

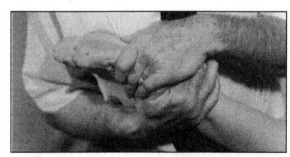

Fig. 8.10.39(a)

Facing cephalad, the chiropractor stands between the patient's knees. The medial border of the patient's foot is placed across the mid-sternal region for stabilization

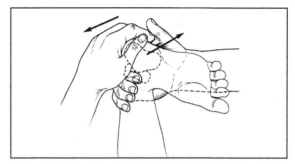

Fig. 8.10.39(b)

The contacts on the talus and calcaneus. The arrows show the direction of thrust

8.10.40 Prone talo-calcaneal medial to lateral short lever technique

Application
Joint play glide loss from medial to lateral of the calcaneus on the talus.

Patient's position
The patient is placed prone with the knee on the affected side flexed to 90°.

Chiropractor's stance
The chiropractor faces cephalad and stands lateral to the patient's affected leg.

Contact
a) The index finger of the left hand is placed around the posterior of the talus to contact the medial border. It is supported by the remaining fingers.
b) The right hand is placed around the calcaneus from the lateral side with the fingers tightly grasping the medial side.

Procedure
Using standard short lever technique (see Chapter 2) the elbows are drawn to the sides, the trunk is rotated a little to the right to achieve joint pre-load tension and the impulse is made with equal and opposite force across the contacts.

8.10.41 Supine talo-calcaneal lateral to medial traction/leverage technique

Application
Joint play glide loss from lateral to medial of the talus on the calcaneus.

Patient's position
The patient is placed supine with the affected leg fully extended and the hip on the affected side flexed to approximately 30°.

Chiropractor's stance
The chiropractor stands at the foot end of the treatment table facing cephalad and favouring the affected side.

Contact
a) The left hand wraps around the posterior of the calcaneus from the lateral side and all four fingers curl round to contact the medial side of the calcaneus.
b) The middle finger of the right hand, supported by the remaining fingers, reaches across the dorsum of the foot to contact the lateral side of the talus.

Procedure
To achieve joint pre-load tension, the chiropractor keeps both elbows slightly flexed and leans back with the back held straight to traction the joint. By lowering the right shoulder a little, the patient's foot is rotated internally. Without slackening the tension, the chiropractor then tractions swiftly backwards with equal force through both arms. The thrust is enhanced by simultaneously pressing the trunk rapidly backwards.

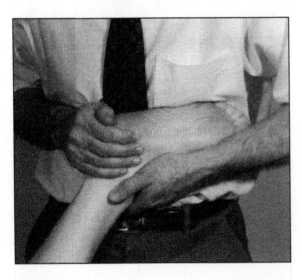

Fig. 8.10.40

The chiropractor stands lateral to the patient's affected leg, which is flexed to approximately 90°. The trunk is flexed forwards to bring it as close to the contact as possible

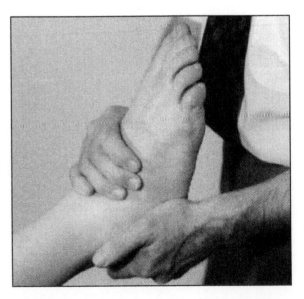

Fig. 8.10.41

Joint pre-load tension is achieved by internal rotation of the foot and by leaning backwards with the back straight

8.10.42 Supine talo-calcaneal medial to lateral traction/leverage technique

Application
Joint play glide loss of the talus from medial to lateral on the calcaneus.

Patient's position
The patient is placed supine with the affected leg fully extended and the hip on the affected side flexed to approximately 30°.

Chiropractor's stance
The chiropractor stands at the foot end of the treatment table facing cephalad and favouring the affected side.

Contact
a)   The left hand wraps around the dorsum of the foot from the lateral side to grasp the medial side of the talus with the middle finger, backed up closely by the remaining fingers.
b)   All four fingers of the right hand reach across the posterior of the foot to contact the lateral aspect of the calcaneus.

Procedure
To achieve joint pre-load tension, the chiropractor keeps both elbows slightly flexed and leans back with the back held straight to traction the joint. By lowering the left shoulder a little, the patient's foot is rotated externally. Without slackening the tension, the chiropractor then tractions swiftly backwards with equal force through both arms. The thrust is enhanced by simultaneously pressing the trunk rapidly backwards. The depth of thrust is minimal.

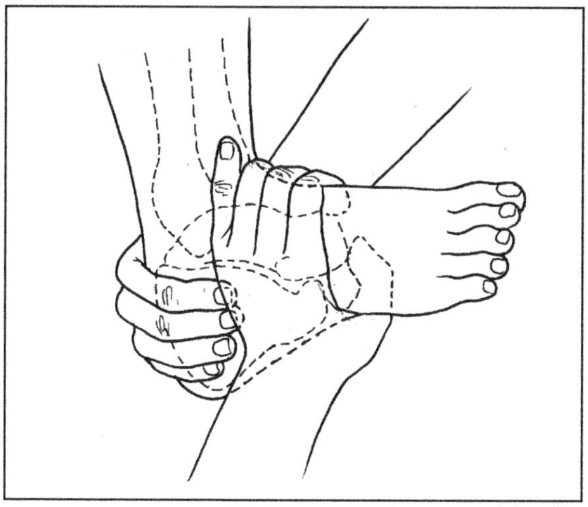

8.10.43 Supine talo-calcaneal lateral to medial strike technique

Application
Joint play glide loss of the calcaneus from lateral to medial on the talus.

Patient's position
The patient is placed supine with the affected leg extended and the hip flexed to approximately 30°.

Chiropractor's stance
The chiropractor stands at the foot end of the treatment table facing cephalad and favouring the affected side.

Contact
a)   The left hand is held away from the patient's ankle.
b)   The right hand is cupped around the calcaneus from the medial side with the thenar eminence against the talus to stabilize it. All four fingers hold closely together around the lateral aspect of the calcaneus ensuring that they remain distal to the talo-calcaneal joint.

Procedure
The right hand everts the ankle, gently tractions and dorsiflexes it as much as possible to prevent any ligamentous strain and to stabilize the talo-crural joint. The right arm remains fully extended. The adjustment is made by swiftly striking with the palm of the left hand precisely against the fingers of the right hand. Very little force is required.

Note
Caution must be exercized at all times when using this technique to avoid traumatizing the joint. It should not be used on the frail or the elderly.

Fig. 8.10.42

For this technique the contacts are reversed and the foot and ankle externally rotated

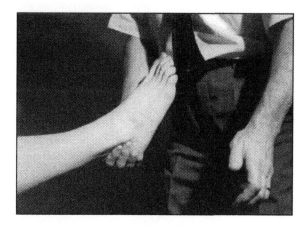

Fig. 8.10.43

The relaxed leg is held in extension and the ankle is everted. The right thenar eminence is placed against the medial border of the talus to stabilize it. All four fingers are wrapped around the posterior of the calcaneus to the lateral side

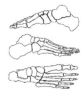

8.10.44   Supine talo-calcaneal medial to lateral strike technique

Application
Joint play glide loss of the calcaneus from medial to lateral on the talus.

Patient's position
The patient is placed supine with the affected leg extended and the hip flexed to approximately 30°.

Chiropractor's stance
The chiropractor stands at the foot end of the treatment table facing cephalad and favouring the affected side.

Contact
a)   The left hand is cupped around the posterior of the calcaneus. All four fingers grasp the medial side. The foot is then inverted to open the talo-crural joint on the lateral side. The foot is also dorsiflexed as much as possible to prevent movement in the talo-crural joint.
b)   The right hand is held away from the patient's ankle.

Procedure
The adjustment is made by swiftly striking the fingers of the left hand with the palm of the right hand. The right arm remains fully extended throughout the procedure. Very little force should be applied.

Note
Except for the direction of thrust, this technique employs a similar method to technique 8.10.43.

8.10.G   Joint play evaluation of the talo-calcaneal joint

Procedure
a)   Anterior to posterior glide of the talus on the calcaneus: The foot is plantarflexed allowing a better contact on the anterior of the talus. Opposing pressure from the posterior of the calcaneus is exerted along the plane line of the joint.
b)   Posterior to anterior glide of the talus on the calcaneus: The foot is plantarflexed to slacken the achilles tendon, allowing for a contact on the posterior of the talus.

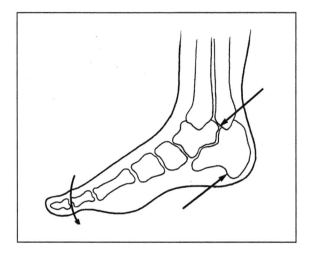

Fig. 8.10.H(a)

Right foot from the medial side. Posterior to anterior glide of the talus on the calcaneus

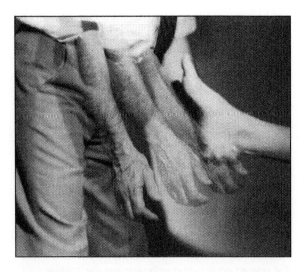

Fig. 8.10.44

For this technique the hands are reversed. The patient's relaxed leg is extended and the foot and ankle inverted

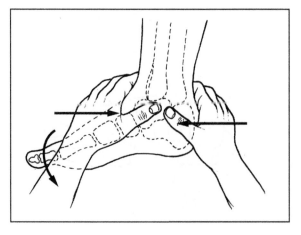

Fig. 8.10.H(b)

Anterior to posterior glide of the talus on the calcaneus. Right foot, medial view

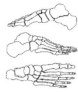

8.10.45   Prone talo-calcaneal anterior to posterior short lever technique

Application
Joint play glide loss of the talus from anterior to posterior on the calcaneus.

Patient's position
The patient is placed prone with the knee on the affected side flexed to 90°.

Chiropractor's stance
The chiropractor stands facing the mid-line of the patient, adjacent to the knee on the affected side. The lateral aspect of the patient's ankle is placed against the sternum.

Contact
a) The left hand contacts from the medial side around the posterior of the calcaneus and all four fingers, held closely together, grasp it.
b) the right hand approaches from the medial side around the anterior border of the talus. The anterior of the middle finger contacts the talus, backed up closely by the remaining fingers.

The chiropractor's forearms in the contact position must be horizontal, with the elbows flexed to approximately 90°. Depending on the relative heights of the patient and doctor, it may be necessary to use variable height equipment or, failing this, for the chiropractor to flex at the knees to reduce height and achieve the correct contact position.

Procedure
Joint pre-load tension is achieved by drawing the elbows to the sides. The tension may be enhanced by rotating the trunk moderately so that the patient's ankle is externally rotated. Standard short lever technique (see Chapter 2) is applied, with equal and opposite force applied across the contacts.

8.10.46   Prone talo-calcaneal posterior to anterior short lever technique

Application
Joint play glide loss of the talus from posterior to anterior on the calcaneus.

Patient's position
The patient is placed prone with the knee on the affected side flexed to 90°.

Chiropractor's stance
The chiropractor stands facing the mid-line of the patient, adjacent to the knee on the affected side. The medial aspect of the patient's ankle is placed against the sternum.

Contact
a) The middle finger of the left hand is flexed and the anterior of the joint between the proximal and middle phalanx reaches around the medial side of the foot to contact the posterior of the talus. The ankle is passively plantarflexed to slacken the overlying achilles tendon, allowing a small but firm contact. All the fingers close up to strengthen the contact.
b) The middle finger of the right hand from the medial side is placed transversely across the inferior process and is hooked against the lateral and medial processes of the calcaneal tuberosity. The contact is supported by the remaining fingers.

Procedure
The lateral border of the patient's foot is placed against the chiropractor's sternum to stabilize the contacts and to hold the foot in plantarflexion. Standard short lever pull technique (see Chapter 2) is applied, with the elbows held at approximately 90°. Joint pre-load tension is facilitated by drawing the elbows downwards to the sides and the shoulders slightly into extension. The force is applied in equal and opposite directions across the joint.

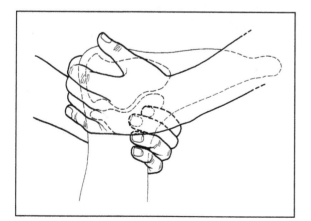

Fig. 8.10.45

The forearms in the contact position are horizontal. The lateral border of the patient's foot is placed against the chiropractor's sternum

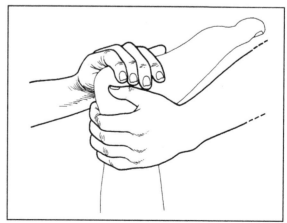

Fig. 8.10.46

The ankle is plantarflexed to slacken the achilles tendon and allow a firm contact on the talus

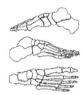

8.10.47   Supine or prone intertarsal circumduction mobilization technique

Application
Stiffness and general restriction of movement of the intertarsal joints.

Patient's position
The patient is placed either supine or prone. If supine, the leg is held fully extended and the hip abducted to approximately 20°.

Chiropractor's stance
The chiropractor stands at the foot end of the treatment table on the affected side, adjacent to the patient's foot, facing cephalad.

Contact
a)   The left hand is cupped firmly over the calcaneus.
b)   The right hand is placed around the dorsum of the mid-foot.

Procedure

1)   The left hand moves the calcaneus in a wide circular movement and the right hand blocks any movement of the mid- and forefoot. The procedure is repeated as necessary and to the patient's tolerance.
2)   The left hand holds the calcaneus still and the right hand moves the mid-foot in circular motion. This is performed gently at the joint mobility limits, and to the patient's tolerance.

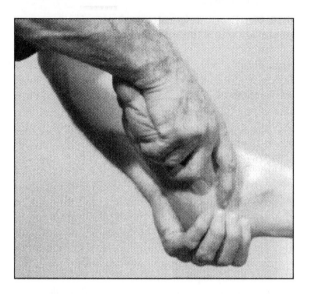

Fig. 8.10.47(a)

The right hand is placed over the dorsum of the foot to block any mid- and forefoot movement. The left hand moves the hind foot in a circular movement

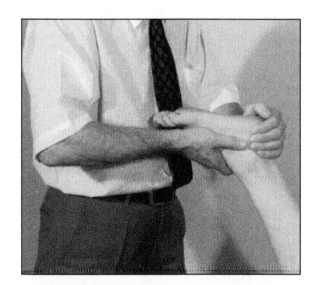

Fig. 8.10.47(b)

In the prone position, the patient's knee is flexed to 90°. The chiropractor stands lateral to the patient and facing cephalad. The right hand blocks the articulations of the mid-foot and the left hand moves the hind foot in a circular motion

The talo-crural (ankle) joint

8.10.H   Joint play evaluation of the talo-crural joint

Procedure

1) Lateral to medial glide
   The right hand contacts the dorsum of the foot just distal to the talo-navicular joint, laterally flexes the foot and slightly everts it, holding it firmly. This effectively blocks all joint movement distal to the talus. The fingers of the left hand wrap around the posterior of the calcaneus blocking talo-calcaneal movement. The thumb of the left hand is placed over the lateral border of the talus, superior to the anterior talo-fibular ligament. Without further movement of the mid- and forefoot, the talus is pressed steadily and firmly with the anterior distal pad of the left thumb into joint play glide from lateral to medial. Normally, a perception of elasticity should be felt by the palpating thumb at the end of the joint movement. A hard end-feel denotes the presence of fixation. Clinically, this is one of the most commonly encountered fixations in the foot and ankle.

2) Medial to lateral glide
   The left hand is placed over the dorsum of the foot so that the thumb and index finger contact the superior border of the navicular and the cuboid. The foot is then medially flexed and slightly inverted. This effectively prevents any foot movement distal to the talus. The fingers of the right hand are placed around the posterior of the calcaneus to block talo-calcaneal movement and the anterior distal pad of the thumb of the right hand is placed on the medial border of the talus. Care must be taken to ensure the contact is superior to the anterior talo-tibial part of the deltoid ligament. Without slackening the medial flexion of the foot, lateral pressure with the right thumb presses the talus laterally into joint play glide. Fixation of this movement is less commonly encountered in clinical practice.

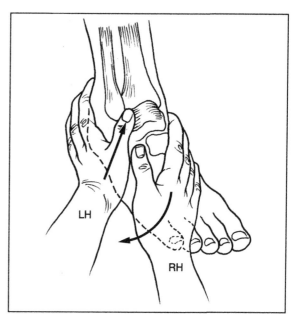

Fig. 8.10.J1

Right foot, lateral oblique view. While pressure is exerted with the left thumb from lateral to medial on the talus, all distal joints are effectively blocked by the right hand holding the mid-foot firmly and laterally flexing it. The left fingers wrapped around the heel block any movement of the calcaneus. The foot is held in plantar flexion to open the talo-crural joint

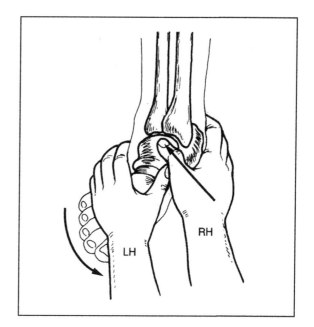

Fig. 8.10.J2

The left hand is placed over the dorsum of the foot so that the thumb and first finger contact the superior border of the navicular and the cuboid. The foot is plantar flexed to open the talo-crural joint

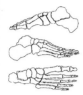

8.10.48 Supine talo-crural long axis distraction technique

Application
Joint play glide loss of the talo-crural joint in long axis extension.

Patient's position
The patient is placed supine, with the leg on the affected side fully extended.

Chiropractor's stance
The chiropractor stands at the foot end of the treatment table facing cephalad. The left leg is placed ahead of the right.

Contact
a)   All four fingers of the left hand are placed around the posterior of the calcaneus as close to the malleoli as possible.
b)   The right hand reaches over the foot and the fingers contact the superior surface of the talus, as close to the talo-crural joint as possible.

Procedure
Joint pre-load tension is achieved by leaning the body weight backwards with the trunk held erect and the elbows held in a semi-flexed position. Without slackening the tension, a rapid minimal depth impulse is made towards the chiropractor. Because of the potential stress over joints proximal to the ankle when using this technique, a high velocity shallow thrust provides a measure of protection.

Alternatively, the patient's lower leg may be placed over the side of the treatment table, with the thigh still supported and the knee flexed, with the same contacts as described above. The chiropractor, facing cephalad, crouches down and impulses downwards into long axis distraction. This latter method affords considerably more protection to the joints of the patient's leg and lower back.

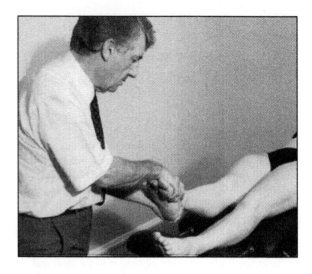

Fig. 8.10.48

The right hand contacts as close to the talocrural joint as possible

8.10.49   Supine talo-crural lateral to medial short lever technique

Application
Joint play glide loss from lateral to medial of the talus on the tibia and fibula.

Patient's position
The patient is placed supine with the hip on the affected side flexed to about 40°.

Chiropractor's stance
The chiropractor stands at the foot end of the treatment table with the left leg ahead of the right. Facing cephalad and favouring the affected side, the plantar surface of the affected foot is placed against the mid-sternal area.

Contact
a)   The left hand reaches across the dorsum of the foot from the lateral side and all four fingers contact the lower lateral border of the tibia.
b)   The right hand reaches across the dorsum of the foot from the medial side and the anterior of the middle phalanx of the middle finger contacts the lateral border of the neck of the talus. The remaining fingers close up to support the contact.

Procedure
From the waist, the chiropractor leans backwards several degrees. This has the effect of first further plantarflexing the foot and ankle and presenting the narrowest portion of the talus under the tibia and fibula, at which point the joint is at its least stable. Second, the ankle joint is modestly tractioned, further destabilizing the articulation. The trunk is then rotated slightly medially to tension the joint. Without releasing the traction, a standard short lever technique thrust (see Chapter 2) is employed.

Note
Because there is very little ligamentous stress when applying this technique, it may be employed even when the ankle is in a sub-acute state.

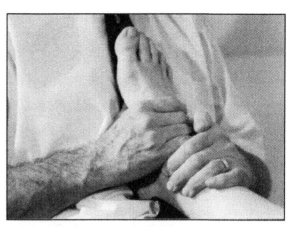

Fig. 8.10.49(a)

The patient's foot is pressed firmly against the chiropractor's sternum

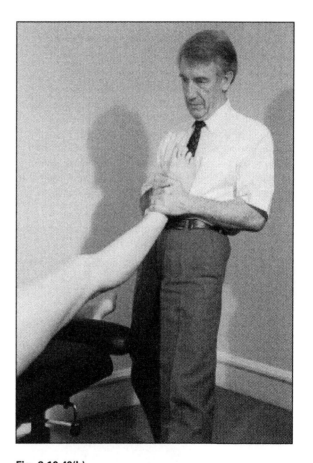

Fig. 8.10.49(b)

By leaning backwards, further plantarflexion is obtained and by turning the trunk several degrees medially, joint pre-load tension is achieved

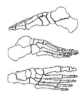

8.10.50 Supine talo-crural medial to lateral short lever technique

Application
Joint play glide loss from medial to lateral of the talus on the tibia and fibula.

Patient's position
The patient is placed supine with the hip on the affected side flexed to 30–40°.

Chiropractor's stance
The chiropractor stands at the foot end of the treatment table with the right leg ahead of the left. Facing cephalad and favouring the affected side, the plantar surface of the patient's foot is placed against the mid-sternal area.

Contact
a) The left hand reaches over the dorsum of the foot with a middle finger contact on the medial side of the talus. The remaining fingers close up to support the contact.
b) The right hand reaches across the dorsum of the foot with all four fingers contacting the lateral lower border of the fibula.

Procedure
The chiropractor leans several degrees backwards from the waist. With this stance and by rotating the trunk several degrees laterally, the joint is tractioned and pre-load tension is produced. By bringing the foot further into plantarflexion, the talo-crural joint is less stable. Without releasing the traction, a swift standard short lever pull technique (see Chapter 2) is employed. The force exerted is in equal and opposite directions across the contacts.

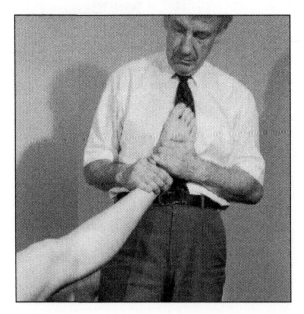

Fig. 8.10.50
The chiropractor rotates the trunk several degrees caudally

8.10.51 Prone talo-crural lateral to medial short lever technique

Application
Joint play glide loss from lateral to medial of the talus on the tibia and fibula.

Patient's position
The patient is placed prone. The knee on the affected side is flexed to 90°.

Chiropractor's stance
The chiropractor stands lateral to the patient adjacent to the affected foot facing the patient's mid-line. The lateral border of the foot is placed against the mid-sternum.

Contact
a) The left hand reaches beneath the dorsum of the foot and around the ankle to the medial side. All four fingers contact the lower tibia as close to the medial malleolus as possible.
b) The right hand reaches around the dorsum of the foot from the medial side. The middle phalanx of the middle finger contacts the lateral border of the neck of the talus, supported closely by the remaining fingers. The thumb reaches around the medial side to contact the plantar surface of the 1st cuneiform. The index finger, still held closely against the middle finger, is placed over the dorsal surface of the navicular and, if possible, also over the row of cuneiforms. This will depend upon the size of the chiropractor's hand and of the patient's foot. The index finger and the web of the hand are used to plantarflex the foot and ankle.

Procedure
To achieve joint pre-load tension, the foot and ankle are first plantarflexed with the right hand. Whilst pressing the lateral border of the foot against the mid-sternum, the chiropractor rotates the trunk several degrees caudad, then flexes forwards until the tension is felt. The elbows are flexed to approximately 90° and drawn relaxed to the sides, and without releasing the joint tension, standard short lever technique (see Chapter 2) is applied in equal and opposite directions across the plane line of the joint.

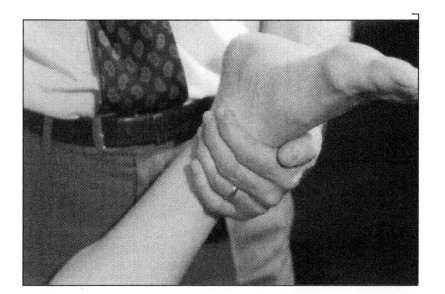

Fig. 8.10.51(a)

The fingers of the left hand contact the medial malleolus

Fig. 8.10.51(b)

The right middle finger contacts the lateral border of the talus

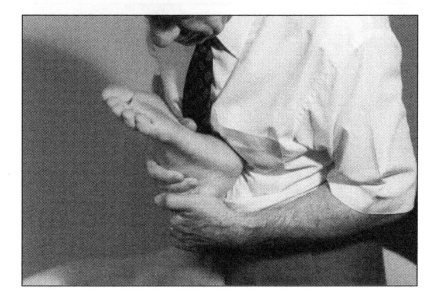

Fig. 8.10.51(c)

The right hand plantarflexes the foot and ankle. The trunk is rotated caudad and flexed forwards to produce joint pre-load tension. This ankle fixation is frequently found following inversion sprain/strain injuries and is one of the most common foot fixations encountered in clinical practice

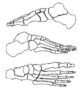

8.10.52 Prone talo-crural medial to lateral short lever technique

Application
Joint play glide loss from medial to lateral of the talus in the talo-crural joint.

Patient's position
The patient is placed prone with the knee on the affected side flexed to approximately 90°.

Chiropractor's stance
The chiropractor stands on the homolateral side facing the patient's mid-line adjacent to the patient's knee.

Contact
a) The left hand wraps around under the dorsum of the foot from the lateral side and the anterior of the second phalanx of the middle finger contacts the medial border of the talus. The remaining fingers close around the middle finger to support it.
b) The right hand wraps around the patient's ankle from the medial side to contact the lateral distal aspect of the fibula with all fingers.

Procedure
The patient's right lower leg is held vertically against the chiropractor's sternum. The right hand, whilst maintaining the contact on the talus, plantarflexes the foot with the lateral border of the index finger and web of the hand. Joint pre-load tension is achieved by drawing the elbows to the sides and extending the upper arms. Standard short lever technique (see Chapter 2) is then applied, with the force pulling in equal and opposite directions across the joint.

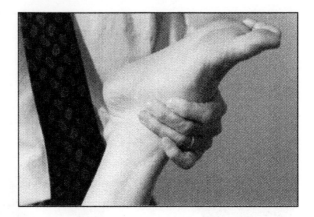

Fig. 8.10.52(b)

The left middle finger contacts the medial border of the talus

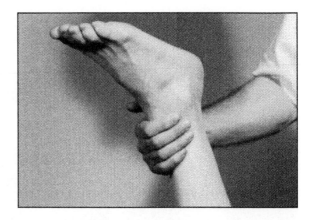

Fig. 8.10.52(c)

The right fingers contact the lateral border of the distal fibula

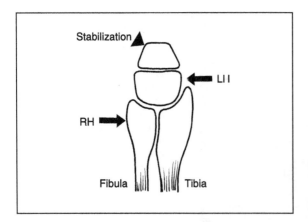

Fig. 8.10.52(a)

Schematic posterior view of the right inverted ankle

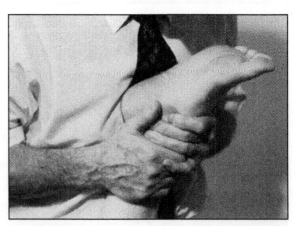

Fig. 8.10.52(d)

The lower leg and foot are pressed against the chiropractor's mid-sternum for stability. The foot is plantarflexed with the web of the left hand

8.10.53 Supine talo-crural lateral to medial distraction technique

Application
Joint play glide loss from lateral to medial of the talus on the tibia and fibula.

Patient's position
The patient is placed supine with the leg on the affected side fully extended and relaxed. The hip is flexed by a few degrees.

Chiropractor's stance
The chiropractor stands at the foot end of the treatment table facing cephalad, favouring the affected side.

Contact
a) The left hand is placed over the lateral side of the hind foot. The thenar eminence contacts the lateral border of the talus with the thumb pointing upwards. The fingers contact around the posterior of the calcaneus to reach the medial side, to block joint movement of the talo-calcaneal joint.

b) The right hand is placed over the dorsum of the foot from the lateral side. The index finger contacts over the talo-navicular joint with the remaining fingers holding the mid-foot. This effectively blocks all joint movement distal to the talus.

Procedure
To achieve joint pre-load tension, the foot and ankle are rotated medially and the hip is abducted approximately 20°. The foot is then plantarflexed and the foot and ankle are distracted in long axis. The elbows are held slightly flexed. Without slackening the tension, the leg is rapidly adducted. As the foot passes across the patient's mid-line, the chiropractor's elbows are snapped into full extension, giving a lateral to medial thrust against the talus.

8.10.54 Supine talo-crural medial to lateral distraction technique

Application
Joint play glide loss from medial to lateral of the talus on the tibia and fibula.

Patient's position
The patient is placed supine with the leg on the affected side fully extended and relaxed. The hip is flexed by a few degrees.

Chiropractor's stance
The chiropractor stands at the foot end of the treatment table facing cephalad, favouring the affected side.

Contact
a) The left hand stabilizes the mid-foot. The index finger approaches from the medial side and contacts the dorsal surface of the cuboid and the navicular on the medial side. The remaining fingers support it closely.

b) The thenar eminence of the right hand contacts the medial neck of the talus, with the thumb pointing upwards. The remaining fingers contact around the posterior of the calcaneus.

Procedure
The foot and ankle are plantarflexed, externally rotated and slightly inverted. Whilst maintaining the traction, the adjustment is given in a smooth swing from medial to lateral, bringing the hip into abduction. As the foot crosses the patient's mid-line, the impulse thrust is generated by snapping the slightly flexed elbows into full extension.

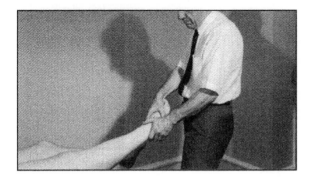

Fig. 8.10.53

The leg is held with the knee straight and the hip flexed 30° and abducted. The foot and ankle are plantar flexed and internally rotated. The chiropractor's elbows are flexed a little. The adjustment is given with a lateral to medial swing of the patient's leg into adduction while maintaining traction. As the foot crosses the mid-line, the impulse is generated by swiftly snapping the elbows into full extension

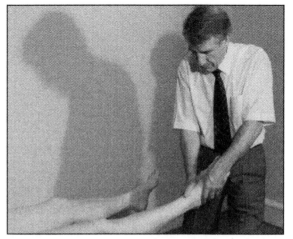

Fig. 8.10.54

Supine talo-crural medial to lateral distraction technique. This procedure is similar to technique 8.10.53 but with the hands reversed

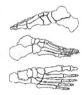

8.10.55 Supine talo-crural lateral to medial modified distraction technique

This technique provides a shorter lever compared to technique 8.10.53.

Application
Joint play glide loss from lateral to medial of the talus on the tibia and fibula.

Patient's position
The patient is placed supine with the hip on the affected side abducted 20–30° and the knee flexed to 90°, with the lower leg hanging freely over the side of the treatment table.

Chiropractor's stance
The chiropractor crouches at the foot end of the treatment table on the affected side and facing cephalad.

Contact
a) The thenar eminence of the left hand contacts the lateral border of the talus, with the thumb pointing upwards. The remaining fingers contact around the posterior of the calcaneus.
b) The right hand is placed over the dorsum of the foot from the lateral side so that the index finger contacts the talo-navicular joint and the cuboid. The thumb curls under the plantar surface on the lateral side.

Procedure
With the patient's knee relaxed and flexed to almost 90°, the foot is moved laterally away from the treatment table by internally rotating the patient's hip. The foot is plantarflexed, laterally flexed and everted, and tractioned downwards. The adjustment is given in a smooth swing of the foot from lateral to medial and downwards. As the lower leg approaches the vertical, the thrust is initiated by snapping the partly flexed elbows into full extension, producing a rapid thrust of minimal depth.

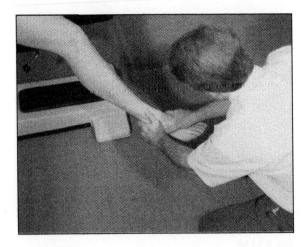

Fig. 8.10.55

This technique provides a shorter lever than that described for the distraction technique 8.10.53

8.10.56 Supine talo-crural medial to lateral modified distraction technique

Application
Joint play glide loss of the talus from medial to lateral on the tibia and fibula.

This technique is similar in all respects to that described in technique 8.10.55 except that the thrust is from medial to lateral, whilst maintaining plantarflexion, inversion and long axis distraction.

8.10.I Anterior to posterior and posterior to anterior joint play evaluation of the talo-crural joint

Procedure

1) Anterior to posterior glide of the tibia and fibula on the talus
The patient is placed supine and the web of the left hand is placed over the malleoli. The ankle is allowed to passively plantarflex in order to slacken the achilles tendon, allowing for the web of the right hand to contact the small available area at the posterior of the talus. Plantarflexion also presents the narrowest part of the trochlea of the talus under the tibia, allowing freer movement of the joint. As the left hand presses posterior, the right hand opposes this and presses anterior to elicit anterior to posterior joint play.
2) Posterior to anterior glide of the tibia and fibula on the talus
The patient is placed supine and the foot is plantarflexed. The web of the left hand contacts the anterior of the talus and the web of the right hand contacts the posterior of the malleoli. The left hand presses anterior to posterior, and the right hand opposes this and presses posterior to anterior into joint play.

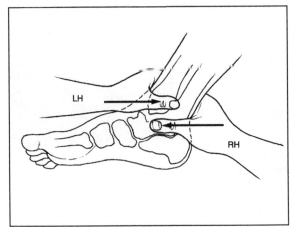

Fig. 8.10.K

Joint play evaluation of the anterior to posterior glide of the tibia and fibular on the talus

8.10.57 Prone talo-crural anterior to posterior short lever technique

Application
Joint play glide loss of the tibia and fibula from anterior to posterior on the talus.

Patient's position
The patient is placed prone and the knee is flexed to 90°. The ankle is plantarflexed to slacken the achilles tendon.

Chiropractor's stance
The chiropractor stands on the contralateral side, adjacent to the patient's foot, facing the patient's mid-line. The medial border of the patient's foot is pressed against the mid-sternum to stabilize it.

Contact
a) The left hand reaches around the lateral side of the ankle to the anterior of the foot and all the fingers contact the anterior of the tibia and fibula as close to the talo-crural joint as possible.
b) The right hand reaches under the dorsum of the foot from the medial side. The fingers curl around the posterior of the ankle so that the anterior of the second phalanx of the index finger contacts the posterior of the talus and the anterior of the second phalanx of the middle finger contacts the posterior of the calcaneus on the lateral side. The thumb rests on the inferior aspect of the calcaneus.

Procedure
The foot is held in plantarflexion and standard short lever technique (see Chapter 2) is applied. The elbows are drawn down to the sides and the shoulders extended a little to produce the joint pre-load tension. The thrust is applied in equal and opposite direction across the joint.

8.10.58 Prone talo-crural posterior to anterior short lever technique

Application
Joint play glide loss of the tibia and fibula from posterior to anterior on the talus.

Patient's position
The patient is placed prone with the knee on the affected side flexed to approximately 90°.

Chiropractor's stance
The chiropractor stands on the contralateral side facing the patient's mid-line adjacent to the affected foot. The medial side of the foot is placed against the sternum.

Contact
a) The left hand reaches around the lateral side of the foot so that the second phalanx of the index finger contacts the anterior of the talus. All the remaining fingers close up to support the contact. To facilitate this contact, the left wrist bears upwards to plantarflex the patient's foot which in turn slackens the achilles tendon and makes the joint less stable.
b) The right hand reaches around the lateral side of the foot to enable all four fingers to contact the posterior of the distal tibia and fibula.

Procedure
The lateral border of the patient's foot is placed against the chiropractor's sternum to stabilize it and to hold the foot in plantarflexion. Joint pre-load tension is achieved by drawing the elbows to the sides and extending the shoulders. The impulse is generated using short lever pull technique (see Chapter 2) with the force applied in equal and opposite directions across the contacts.

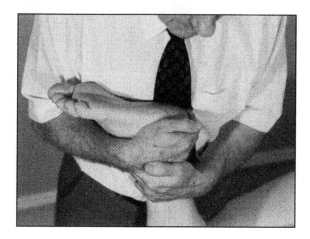

Fig. 8.10.57

For stability, the medial border of patient's foot is pressed against the chiropractor's mid-sternum. The adjustive thrust is made in equal and opposite directions

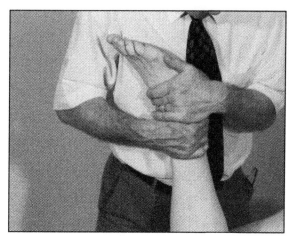

Fig. 8.10.58

The foot is plantarflexed with the left hand before the adjustive impulse is delivered

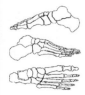

8.10.59 Supine talo-crural anterior to posterior and posterior to anterior thrust technique

Procedure

As an alternative to the short lever technique described in 8.10.57, the patient is placed supine with the ankle supported on the foot rest of the treatment table. A rapid shallow anterior to posterior thrust is made using a double thenar (see Glossary of Terms, p. 285) contact. If the joint play glide loss of the tibia and fibula is from posterior to anterior, the patient is placed prone with the ankle resting on the foot rest of the treatment table. A double thenar contact is made on the posterior of the malleoli and the thrust is from posterior to anterior.

REFERENCES

Hoppenfeld, S. (1976) *Physical Examination of the Spine and Extremities*. New York, Appleton–Century–Crofts.

Schafer, R.C. and Faye, L.J. (1990) *Motion Palpation and Chiropractic Technique – Principles of Dynamic Chiropractic*. 2nd edn. Huntington Beach, CA, Motion Palpation Institute.

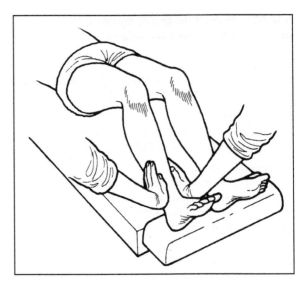

Fig. 8.10.59(a)

The patient is placed supine and the heel is supported by a high density cushion. The thrust is delivered along the plane line of the superior border of the talus

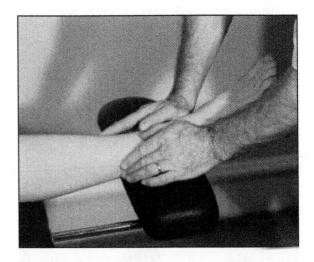

Fig. 8.10.59(b)

The thenar eminences are placed over the malleoli

Bibliography for Part Two: Joint Manipulation

Ambrosius, H. and Kondracki, M. (1992) Plantar Fasciitis. *Euro. J. Chiro.* 40(2), August.

Arnold, L.E. (1978) *Chiropractic Procedural Examination.* Florida, Seminole Printing.

Baker, W.J., Fred, W.H. and Illi, D.C. (1997) A clinical reformation in chiropractic. *ACA J. Chiro.* 34(6), June.

Bergmann, T.F, Peterson, D.H. and Lawrence, D.J. (eds) (1993) *Chiropractic Technique.* New York, Churchill Livingstone.

Blood, S.D. (1980) Treatment of the sprained ankle. *J. Am. Osteopathic Assoc.* 19(2), 680–692.

Breen, A.C., Brydges, R., Nunn, J., Kanse, J. and Allen, R. (1993) Quantative analysis of lumbar spine intersegmental motion. *Euro. J. Phys. Med. Rehab.* 3(5), 183–190.

Broome, R.T. (1984) Course Notes on Extremity Technique. Bournemouth, Anglo-European College of Chiropractic.

Broome, R.T. (1987) *Examination and Treatment of the Foot and Ankle.* Bournemouth, Anglo-European College of Chiropractic (video).

Broome, R.T. (1994) *Extremity Techniques I. The Foot and Ankle.* Self-published.

Broome, R.T. (1994) *Extremity Techniques II. The Knee and Hip.* Self-published.

Broome, R.T. (1995) *Extremity Techniques III. The Hand and Wrist.* Self-published.

Broome, R.T. (1995) *Extremity Techniques IV. The Elbow and Shoulder Girdle.* Self-published.

Broome, R.T. (1996) *The Shoulder Guide.* Self-published.

Bryner, P. (1991) *Introductory Manipulations for the Extemity Joints.* Melbourne, Australia, Phillip Institute of Technology.

Byfield, D. (1996) *Chiropractic Manipulative Skills.* Oxford, Butterworth-Heinemann.

Cailliet, R. (1964) *Neck and Arm Pain.* Philadelphia, F.A. Davis Company.

Cailliet, R. (1968) *Foot and Ankle Pain.* Philadelphia, F.A. Davis Company.

Cailliet, R. (1971) *Hand Pain and Impairment.* Philadelphia, F.A. Davis Company.

Chusid, J. G. and MacDonald, J.J. (1962) *Correlative Neuroanatomy and Functional Neurology.* Los Altos, CA, Lange Medical Publications.

Cyriax, J. (1965) *Textbook of Orthopaedic Medicine* Vol II. Treatment by Manipulation and Massage. London, Cassel.

Dohn, H. (1968) Treating the Extremities with Manipulation, British Chiropractic Association Convention lecture, October.

Droz, J.M. (1971) Indications and contraindications of vertebral manipulations. *Ann. Swiss Chiro. Assoc.* V, 81.

Dye, A.A. (1939) *The Evolution of Chiropractic.* New York, Richmond Hall.

Eisenberg, A.M. (1971) Diversified chiropractic technique. An approach to pelvic and extremity adjusting. *J. Clin. Chiro.* Archives. Edn no.1.

Faye, L.J. (1992) Manual examination of the spine. In *Principles and Practice of Chiropractic*, 2nd edn (S. Haldeman, ed.) Norwalk, CO, Appleton and Lange.

Fysh, P. (1995) Nursemaid's Elbow. *Dynamic Chiro.* 13 (16).

Gale, P. (1991) *Functional Soft Tissue and Treatment by Manual Methods.* Gaithersburg, MD, Aspen Publishers, pp.10-197.

Gillet, H. (1969) Motion Palpation and Fixation Analysis, Lecture, European Chiropractors' Union, Switzerland, May.

Gillet, H. and Liekens, M. (1964) *Belgian Chiropractic Research Notes.* Brussels, Belgian Chiropractic Association.

Gillet, H. and Liekens, M. (1981) Belgian Chiropractic Research Notes, 11th edn. Huntington Beach, CA, Motion Palpation Institute.

Gillet, H.(1972) Sternoclavicular fixations. *J. Clin. Chiro.* Archives. Edn no.2, 196.

Gillet, J. (1996) New light on the history of motion palpation. *J. Manip. Physiological Therapeutics.* 19(1), 52–58.

Gray, H. (1959). *Anatomy of the Human Body,* 27th Edn. Philadelphia, Lea and Febiger.

Grillo, F. (1969) Treatment of Adhesive Capsulitis, European Chiropractors' Union Convention Lecture, Switzerland, May.

Grove, A.B. (1979) *Chiropractic Technique – a Procedure of Adjusting.* Madison, WI, Strauss Printing and Publishing Company.

Hammer, W. (1991) *Functional Soft Tissue Examination and Treatment by Manual Means.* Gaithersburg, MD, Aspen Publishers.

Hartman, L.S. (1983) *Handbook of Osteopathic Technique.* Hadley Wood, N.M.K. Publishers.

Hearon, K.G. (1981) *What You Should Know About Extremity Adjusting*, 7th edn. Sequim, WA, Vanity Press.

Hearon, K.G. (1991) *Advanced Principles of Upper Extremity Adjusting.* Sequim, WA, Self-published.

Hertling, D. and Kessler, R. (1990) *Management of Common Musculoskeletal Disorders*, 2nd edn. Philadelphia, J.B. Lippincott.

Hollen, W.V. (1974) Examination of the Knee via McMurray's Test and the Drawer Sign. *J. Clin. Chiro.* 1(4), 35–41.

Hoppenfeld, S. (1976) *Physical Examination of the Spine and Extremities.* New York, Appleton-Century-Crofts.

Illi, F.W. (1965) Morbid predisposition of a mechanical origin inherent to the phylogenesis of man. Part 2 of 3 parts. *ACA J. Chiro.* **Sept**

Janse, J. (1976) In *Principles and Practice of Chiropactic. An Anthology* (R.W. Hildebrandt, ed.). Lombard, IL, National College of Chiropractic, pages 8, 116, 117.

Janse, J., Houser, R.H. and Wells, B.F. (1947) *Chiropractic Principles and Technique*, 2nd edn. Lombard, IL, National College of Chiropractic.

Jones, L. (1955) *The Postural Complex.* Springfield, IL, Charles C. Thomas.

Kapandji, I.A. (1983) *The Physiology of the Joints.* vol. 2. Lower Limb. Edinburgh, Churchill Livingstone.

Kendall, F.B.and Kendall, E. (1983) *Muscles. Testing and Function.* 3rd edn. Baltimore, MD, Williams and Wilkins.

Kenel, F. (1961) *Flat Foot, a cause for static insufficiency of the body.* Ann. Swiss Chiro. Assoc.V.

Kirkaldy Willis, W.H. and Burton, C.V., (1992) *Managing Low Back Pain*, 3rd edn. Edinburgh, Churchill Livingstone.

Lantz, C.A. (1988) Immobilization, degeneration and the fixation hypothesis of chiropractic subluxation. *Chiro. Res. J.* 1(1).

Lening, P.C. (1991) Foot Dysfunction and Low Back Pain – Are They Related? *ACA J. Chiro.* **May**, 71–74.

Lewit, von K., (1978) Impaired joint function and entrapment syndrome. *Manuelle Medizin.* Heft 3(48).

Logan, A.L. (1994) *The Knee. Clinical Applications.* Gaithersburg, MD, Aspen Publishers.

Logan, A.L. (1995) *The Foot and Ankle. Clinical Applications.* Gaithersburg, MD, Aspen Publishers.

MacBryde, C.M. and Blacklow, R.S. (1970) *Signs and Symptoms. Applied Pathology, Physiology and Clincial Interpretation*, 5th edn. Philadelphia, J.B. Lippincott Company.

Maitland, G.D. (1991) *Peripheral Manipulation*, 3rd edn. Oxford, Butterworth-Heinemann.

Major, R.H. and Delp, M.H. (1962). *Physical Diagnosis*, 6th edn. Philadelphia, W.B. Saunders.

McMinn, R.M.H., Hutchings, R.T. and Logan, B.M. (1982) *A Colour Atlas of Foot and Ankle Anatomy.* London, Wolf Publications.

Mennell, J.Mc.M. (1933) Joint manipulation (upper extremity). *Proc. Roy. Soc. Med.* **XXVI**(7), 881–899.

Menell, J.Mc.M. (1964) *Joint Pain Diagnosis and Treatment Using Manipulative Techniques.* London, Little Brown and Company.

Michaud, T. (1989) Aberrancy of the mid-tarsal locking mechanism as a causative factor in recurrent ankle sprains. *J. Manip. Physiological Therapeutics* 12(2), 135–141.

Mierau, D., Cassidy, J.D., Bowen, V., DuPuis, P. and Noftall, F. (1988) Manipulation and Mobilization of the Third Metacarpo-Phalangeal Joint. *Manual Medicine.*

Palmer, B.J. (1920) *A Text Book on The Palmer Technique of Chiropractic,* 1st edn. Davenport, IA, Palmer School of Chiropractic.

Palmer, B.J. (1934) *The Subluxation Specific – The Adjustment Specific.* Davenport, IA, Palmer School of Chiropractic.

Palo (1995) The short leg syndrome. *ACA J. Chiro.*

Pate, D. (1996) Acromioclavicular arthrosis. *Dynamic Chiro.* 14(24).

Peck, S.R. (1982) *Atlas of Human Anatomy for the Artist.* Oxford, Oxford University Press.

Pharoah, D. (1963) *Personal Communication.* Davenport, Iowa.

Quiring, D.P.and Warfel, J.H. (1960) *The Extremities.* Philadelphia, Lea and Febiger.

Reinert, O.C. (1972) *Chiropractic Procedure and Practice.* Florissant, MO, Marian Press.

Sandoz, R.W. (1965) About some problems pertaining to the choice of indications for chiropractic therapy. *Ann. Swiss Chiro. Assoc.* **III**.

Schafer, R.C. (1982) *Chiropractic Management of Sports and Recreational Injuries.* Baltimore, MD, Williams and Wilkins.

Schafer, R.C. and Faye, L.J. (1990) *Motion Palpation and Chiropractic Technique – Principles of Dynamic Chiropractic*, 2nd edn. Huntington Beach, CA, Motion Palpation Institute.

Schultz, A.L. (1958) *Athletic and Industrial Injuries of the Foot and Ankle.* Stickney, SD, Argos.

Schultz, A.L. (1963) *Athletic and Industrial Injuries of the Knee.* Stickney, SD, Argos.

Schultz, A.L. (1969) *The Shoulder, Arm and Hand Syndrome.* Stickney, SD, Argos.

Schultz, S. and Villnave, T.(1982) *Extremity Orthopaedic Tests.* Portland, OR, Western States Chiropractic College.

Segal, P. and Jacob, M. (1984) *The Knee.* London, Wolf Medical Publications.

Shaw, A.J. and Perth, F.R.J. (1987) An Inter- and Intra-Examiner Reliability Study of Motion Palpation of the Tarsals in the Non-Weight-Bearing Position. D.C. Dissertation. Bournemouth, Anglo-European College of Chiropractic.

Stavrou, G. (1983) *Manual of Peripheral Technique.* Sydney College of Chiropractic, Australia.

Stierwalt, D.D. (1988) *Extremity Adjusting.* Davenport, IA, The Copy Shop.

Thompson, J. Clay. (1994) Course notes, Thompson Technique Seminar. Davenport, Iowa, September.

Walther, D.S. (1974) *General Examination for the Professional Chiropractic Assistant.* Abriendo, CO, Systems DC.

Walther, D.S. (1976) *Applied Kinesiology.* Abriendo, CO, Systems DC.

Walther, D.S. (1981) *Applied Kinesiology.* Vol. 1. Basic Procedures and Muscle Testing. Abriendo, CO, Systems DC.

Wiles, P. and Sweetnam, R. (1965) *Essentials of Orthopaedics,* 4th edn. London, J. and A. Churchill.

Glossary

Much of the terminology and many of the tests encountered in this book are common to chiropractic and to other professions and no further enlargement will be needed to convey the precise meaning applied to the field of chiropractic peripheral joint technique. A few terms, however, may have a meaning peculiar to the chiropractor and it is for those terms that this short list is offered.

Adjustment — A chiropractic manipulative procedure involving a dynamic thrust utilized with varied amplitude and velocity. *See* Impulse.

Arch — The wrist is held in varying degrees of extension, hence 'high arch' (maximum extension) and 'low arch' (minimum extension). The metacarpo-phalangeal joints are flexed. This hand position facilitates the use of the pisiform as a contact.

Body drop — An adjustive thrust on a contact which can be bilateral or unilateral, with high or low velocity, utilizing a variable depth of thrust. The arm(s) held stiffly, the thrust is initiated by pressing the weight of the flexed trunk downwards directly over the contact.

Caudad — Towards the feet.

Cephalad — Towards the head.

Clasp technique — A high velocity manipulative thrust using both hands with the fingers interlocked, the contacts placed between the palms and biased by striking the thenar eminence of one hand into the palm of the other.

Compression technique — A unilateral body drop adjustive thrust applied with the support, or indifferent, hand placed under and adjacent to the contact.

Contact — That part of the anatomy chosen as a lever point on which to initiate an adjustive thrust. Apart from soft tissue techniques, it is usually as close as possible to the joint being treated.

Contralateral — On the opposite side.

Direct thrust — A commonly used chiropractic adjustive thrust employing a forward semi-flexed trunk, allowing the arms to be vertical or nearly vertical, above the contact. The thrust is made by pectoralis triceps anconius contractions utilizing high or low velocity.

Draw sign — An Orthopaedic Test performed with the patient supine, the knee flexed and the foot anchored, with no external or internal rotation. The tibia is pulled anteriorly to test for greater than normal excursion, indicating a tear of the anterior cruciate ligament, probable laxity or torn medial or lateral compartment ligaments, depending on the direction of foot rotation (Schultz and Villnave, 1982).

Drop mechanism — A mechanical device fitted to specialized chiropractic treatment equipment fitted to one or more of the sections on which the patient reclines, and which when cocked, drops down several millimetres during an adjustive thrust.

End play — The perception of elasticity to pressure, detected at the full extent of the accessory joint movement called joint play (Schafer and Faye, 1990).

Heel of hand — The anterior of the base of the third metacarpal and the capitate. Used frequently as a contact point when making an adjustive thrust.

Homolateral — On the same side as.

Hyper- — Exceeding, excessive.

Hypo- — Under, below.

Impulse — The action of the manipulative or adjustive thrust. 'An extremely skilful, balanced action demanding rapidity, co-ordination, controlled depth and prior planned direction. The culmination of the manipulative procedure following the doctor and patient positioning' (Byfield, 1996).

Ipsilateral — On the same side as.

Joint play — Small passive accessory joint movement not influenced by, and beyond the range of voluntary movement.

Kinematic — 'Motion considered abstractly without reference to force or mass' (*The Concise Oxford Dictionary*, Clarendon Press 1965).

Kinetics	'The science of the relations between the motions of bodies and the forces acting on them' (*The Concise Oxford Dictionary*, Clarendon press 1965).
Line of correction	The pre-planned direction of the impulse or adjustive force applied along the plane line of the joint being treated.
Motion palpation	The attempt to feel segmental motion and determine if it is abnormal or not (Kondracki in Byfield, 1996).
Nail point	A term coined by chiropractors when adjusting to designate a specific bone or area of the hand or elbow used as the point of contact on the lever point of the joint to be adjusted.
Patellar Apprehension Test	An orthopaedic test in which the patient reacts with fear or apprehension to lateral pressure on the medial border of the patella, indicating a probable easily dislocated patellar (Schultz and Villnave, 1983).
P.O.M.P.	Passive osteokinematic motion palpation.
Recoil technique	High velocity thrust technique with a designated depth and directed by both hands placed one upon the other. It may be used on all spinal and peripheral joints.
Scissor-type thrust	A thrust made with both hands. One which is applied equally in opposite directions.
Stabilization	The support and immobilization of the limb or joint either proximal or distal to the contact achieved by patient position, the chiropractor's trunk, arm or hand.
Support hand	The hand sometimes termed the indifferent hand, which stabilizes the joint to be adjusted.
Web of hand	The area of tissue between the base of the thumb and the second metacarpal. Used as a soft contact point.

REFERENCES

Byfield, D. (1996) *Chiropractic Manipulative Techniques.* Oxford, Butterworth-Heinemann.

Schafer, R.C. and Faye, L.J. (1990) *Motion Palpation and Chiropractic Technique Principles of Dynamic Chiropractic*, 2nd edn. Huntington Beach, CA, Motion Palpation Institute, p. 314.

Schultz, S. and Villnave, T. (1982) *Extremity Orthopaedic Tests*, 2nd edn. Portland, OR, Western States Chiropractic College.

Index

Printed and bound by CPI Group (UK) Ltd, Croydon, CR0 4YY

03/10/2024

01040345-0017